Eat

Eat Beautiful!
A LIFETIME GUIDE TO EATING RIGHT
FOR HEALTH, BEAUTY AND WELL-BEING

Patricia Long

ARROW BOOKS

This book is not intended as a substitute for medical advice of physicians. The reader should regularly consult a physician in general and particularly for any symptoms.

Arrow Books Limited
62–65 Chandos Place, London WC2N 4NW

An imprint of Century Hutchinson Limited

London Melbourne Sydney Auckland
Johannesburg and agencies throughout
the world

First published in the USA by Macmillan Publishing Company 1986
First published in Great Britain by Arrow Books 1989

© 1986 by Patricia Long

This book is sold subject to the condition that it shall not, by way of trade or otherwise, be lent, resold, hired out, or otherwise circulated without the publisher's prior consent in any form of binding or cover other than that in which it is published and without a similar condition including this condition being imposed on the subsequent purchaser

Phototypeset by Input Typesetting Ltd, London
Printed and bound in Great Britain by
Courier International Ltd, Tiptree, Essex

ISBN 0 09958150 7

*To my mothers, Perditta and Frances,
My sisters, Dayle, Doreen, Renée, Susan, Kathryn,
Elizabeth, Jane, and Bonnie,
And my grandmothers, Pauline and Edith—*

Women of sensibility and heart

ACKNOWLEDGEMENTS

I wish to thank all those who read my manuscript, offered suggestions, or located resources: Barbara Sutherland, Margo Quiriconi, Susan Walker-Kniola, Laurel Mellin, Patricia McConnell, Teri Reifer, Linda Schmidt, Barbara Mendelsohn, Judy Wenning, Susan Saperstein, Sarah Berkowitz, Kevin Carr, Bob Grossman, Frank Crawford, John Wilkes, Jennie Dusheck, and Hal Lepoff. I am also grateful for the efforts of my agent, Barbara Bova, for the editorial assistance of George Truett Bush, Alexia Dorszynski, and Jill Herbers, and for the illustrations of Iris Aguirre. Finally, I reserve my warmest thanks for my husband, Paul Kotapish.

Contents

PART 1 LIFE CYCLE

1 Adolescence: The Maiden Voyage — 13
2 Young Adulthood: Humoring the Hormones — 34
3 Pregnancy: The Blooming of the Womb — 54
4 Breastfeeding: Woman as Alchemist — 76
5 Middle Adulthood: Menopause and the Midlife Molt — 89
6 The Later Years: Never too Late — 102

PART 2 WEIGHT CONTROL, FITNESS, AND BEAUTY

7 Weight Control: The Looking-Glass War — 121
8 The Shape-up Plan: How to Make Food Behave — 157
9 Eating Disorders: When Thin is Not Enough — 170
10 The Athlete: Sharpening the Racer's Edge — 182
11 Beauty: Beneath the Makeup — 199

PART 3 DISEASE PREVENTION

12 Atherosclerosis: When the Heart Breaks — 209
13 Cancer: The Diet Connection — 223
14 Diabetes: The Sweetest Scourge — 234
15 Gastrointestinal Disorders: Gut Reactions — 242

PART 4 LIFE-STYLE

16 In the Kitchen: The Politics of the Pantry — 255
17 In the Workplace: Earning and Eating your Daily Bread — 282
18 On the Town: The Good, the Bad, and the Bubbly — 306

Appendix A
The Basics of Nutrition — 318
Table A-1 Vitamins
Table A-2 Minerals

Contents

Appendix B
Where to Find Nutrition Information — 338
Table B-1 Local Contacts for Nutrition Information
Table B-2 Nutrition Information in Popular Magazines

Appendix C
The Food Exchange — 341

Appendix D
Recipes — 346
1. Apricot-Cottage Cheese Muffins
2. Gingerbread Squares
3. Yogurt-Herb Dressing
4. Chicken Korma
5. Herb Blends to Replace Salt
6. A Precompetition Liquid Meal
7. Stir-fry Sauce
8. Lentil Soup
9. Mexican Casserole
10. Banana Bran Muffins

Appendix E
Food Sources of Nutrients — 355
E-1 Vitamin A (Carotene) in Foods
E-2 Iron in Foods
E-3 Vitamin C in Foods
E-4 Folacin in Foods
E-5 Calcium in Foods
E-6 Cholesterol in Foods
E-7 Dietary Fiber in Foods

Selected References — 363
Index — 375

Tables and Figures

Table 3-1 Sample Meal Plan for Pregnancy 69
Table 4-1 Sample Meal Plan for Breastfeeding Mothers 86
Table 5-1 Calcium Supplements 98
Table 7-1 Height–Weight Tables 125
Table 7-2 Choosing a Treatment Program for Weight Control 134
Table 7-3 Resting and Activity Calorie Needs 137
Table 10-1 What to Drink Before, During, and After Exercise 193
Table 10-2 Determining Competitive Weight 195
Table 11-1 Effects of Nutrition on Skin 205
Table 12-1 What Blood Pressure Readings Mean 214
Table 12-2 Comparison of Fat Content in Three 1,600-calorie Diets 220–21
Table 16-1 The Revised Four Food Groups 257–9
Table 16-2 Combinations of High-Quality Protein 260–1
Table 16-3 Recommended Daily Amounts of Nutrients for Girls and Women 268–9
Table 16-4 Protecting the Vitamins in Food 273–4
Table 17-1 Caffeine Content of Beverages and Foods 287
Table 17-2 Batch Cooking 302–4
Table 18-1 Energy Constituents of some Alcoholic Drinks, Average Values per 100 ml 310
Table 18-2 What Restaurant Terms Really Mean 314
Table 18-3 Tips for Ordering in Restaurants 316–17

Figure 5-1 Osteoporosis: How Older Women Lose Height 94
Figure 8-1 Food and Exercise Diaries 158
Figure 8-2 Charting Three Meals a Day 161

Tables and Figures

Figure 8-3 Charting Exercise 163
Figure 15-1 The Gastrointestinal Tract 243
Figure 16-1 The Pyramid Guide 275

PART 1
Life Cycle

"It has begun to occur to me," wrote *Boston Globe* columnist Ellen Goodman, "that life is a stage I'm going through." Life in fact is a series of stages, and at each one your nutritional needs shift slightly. Girls and boys require similar amounts of nutrients until puberty, when a girl experiences an earlier growth spurt, adds on extra body fat, and gets her first menstrual period. These changes not only affect her diet but shape her body and sense of self. In "Adolescence" and each succeeding chapter in part 1, you will discover how physical and psychological changes influence your health and eating habits. "Young Adulthood" explains how work and home pressures, menstrual periods and birth control measures increase your risk of anemia and, later in life, fragile bones. "Pregnancy" and "Breastfeeding" focus on the special dietary needs of women during and immediately after childbearing. In "Middle Adulthood" you will find out why the drop in female hormones at menopause alters nutrient requirements and can place you at risk of osteoporosis. Finally, "The Later Years" offers advice on avoiding chronic conditions, such as indigestion, arthritis, and periodontal disease, and a discussion of current theories for extending life. After you discover the major nutritional risks for your age, parts 2 to 4 will explain how to design your diet to avoid them.

1
Adolescence:
The Maiden Voyage

All those chemicals rushing around. Everything I
feel now, I felt twice as intensely then.
Bette Midler, *Seventeen*

Adolescence is that time of life when hormones grab the steering wheel, heave you into the backseat, and drive insanely over the fragments of childhood, swerving around the potholes of puberty, only to screech to a halt, flinging you headfirst into adulthood. Some people never recover.

As a popular ten-year-old, Marie was fearless. Among her friends she was a champion of movie trivia, and someday she was going to be a famous rock star—or a genetic engineer. She never stepped on the scales to check her weight, perhaps because she weighed only seventy-five pounds. By high school graduation Marie's confidence had fled, and she was left, pHisohex in hand, lying in wait for an outbreak of pimples and nervously dreading the next onslaught of cellulite.

PHYSICAL CHANGES
The fast and furious body changes

Every stage of life involves change, but rarely do the changes hit as hard and fast as they do in adolescence. In eight years Marie grew nine inches, gained forty-six pounds, and, most important, she could now have children.

Her fastest growth started when she was around eleven years old. During adolescence, most girls will shoot up about three inches, ending up taller than most boys their age. The only other age when growth is faster is the first year of life.

This rush toward growth does not happen at once. Hands and forearms enlarge before upper arms. Feet reach peak growth first, then calves and thighs, and finally hips, chest, and trunk.

Girls go through this long-limbed expansion hoping to achieve the grace of a model. But most end up feeling more like the white-gloved Minnie Mouse or the ungainly Olive Oyl, with rubbery arms and legs that always seem to be tying themselves in knots.

Soon after a girl reaches her adult height, her weight plateaus. While she is growing taller, she is also filling out, adding muscle, bone, and fat, and getting heavier. Because of their hormones, girls add a greater percentage of fat than boys. By age eighteen, one-third of a girl's pounds will weigh in as fat, and by age twenty, a girl will carry twice as much body fat as a boy.

This fat does not settle just anywhere. It gravitates toward a girl's pelvis, breasts, back, and upper arms and sculptures the contours of a woman. Girls keep most of the fat they put on during adolescence, while boys lose theirs.

A girl can be tall and slender, short and stocky, or any combination of height and build depending on her genes. At any given age, girls will be more alike in height than they are in weight because weight fluctuates with diet and exercise. Of course, it is natural for a girl to be heavier if she is tall. Though a girl inherits her rate of growth, other factors such as poor diet or stress can delay it.

Menarche: the clock strikes twelve

Growth of the arm and leg bones is stopped by the rumbling of the sex hormones, the same hormones that cause menstruation. Once a girl has had her first period, she can still grow two more inches, but rarely more. Most British girls develop breasts and pubic hair between the ages of ten and twelve and have their first period two to three years later, on average late in their thirteenth year.

Not all girls mature at the same rate. While one girl is in the locker room and all-too-loudly complaining about menstrual cramps, another is throwing on her gym suit before anyone notices that her body is dormant. For a time researchers believed a girl's ability to menstruate was related to her weight, basing their belief on work done by Rose Frisch of the Harvard Center for Population Studies. More recently, Frisch has suggested that fat levels must reach almost one-quarter of body weight before the brain can trigger menarche. Others find too many exceptions to this rule and doubt its accuracy. It is likely, they say, that a girl adds fat at the same time she is maturing sexually, both caused by rising estrogen levels. Too little fat, or overexertion, can delay menarche until an older age. If a girl is well along in physical development and does not get her first period by age fifteen, she should consult a doctor.

The arrival of a girl's first period does not necessarily mean that she is fertile. Menstrual cycles occur for a year or more without the ovaries releasing eggs. Early cycles are irregular, and all cycles are sensitive to diet and emotional stress.

PSYCHOLOGICAL CHANGES
Which way, please—the teen identity crisis

For most adolescents, events during the teen years seem to be leading to a major identity crisis. Smaller crises occur throughout life, but adolescence is when young people are programmed for the Big One—embodied in the question "Who am I?"

The identity crisis is triggered by the swirl of decisions that a girl must make. Gaining control over her life is not a small matter. Life becomes a drive down a main drag where flashing, demanding signs lure her this way and that. She flaunts her independence by conforming with her peers. Uncertain of her own abilities, she is tempted to follow fads. As she careers through her teen years, a girl tries to break her reliance on the family. She knows she has the right map for success in life and believes the only thing wrong is her parents' directions.

Society does offer a buffer period before a girl has to make all her decisions. It's called college, sometimes followed by travel or a move to another city to "find oneself." Somehow, though, when all is said and done and a girl has reached her early twenties, she is expected to have at least regained control of the steering wheel and be headed in some direction, with however rudimentary or tattered a road map.

HEALTH CONCERNS
Charting a course toward future health

Insidious diseases like heart disease, osteoporosis, and most cancers advance over many years and are not much trouble during adolescence. But poor eating and exercise habits begun at this time, if continued into adulthood, can increase a girl's risk of battling these diseases later in life.

Nutritional problems for a teenager are usually the scars of a war waged by the body's hormones against the teen's struggling sense of self. Marching regiments of fat cells attack the hips and thighs and, with taunts of "You're a fatty, you're a fatty," lay waste to the adolescent's morale. Rampaging androgens attack the face, leaving deep acne wounds. The teen retaliates with a barrage of diets that place her at risk of developing obesity, eating disorders, and anemia.

Lacking any decisive battle plan, the adolescent falls into a confused pattern of snacking, skipping meals, and relying on fast foods. There are ways for teens to get through adolescence with a minimum of damage and with a healthy attitude toward food. I offer the following strategies for winning the war.

Girth and self-worth

Compared to girls twenty years ago, today's teens are fatter. Yet thin is in style, and those whose bodies lack a certain emaciated appeal feel substandard. Of course, preoccupation with appearance is never as overwhelming as it is during the teens.

A few girls do enter adolescence with slim, boyish figures and exit the same way. They are slow at developing womanly curves and may desire rounder arms, thighs, busts, and rears. Often ignored by boys, they are left feeling inferior and backward. As they age, these girls usually have an easier time keeping their weights down, and many come to recognize their small size as a blessing.

Most girls, however, believe that they are too big. By age eighteen, as many as 80 percent of young women have tried at least one diet. Many times they are simply uncomfortable with their new womanly bodies. When shown line drawings of five body sizes and asked to choose the most desirable, a majority of girls in one study chose the figure that was 10 percent underweight.

However reluctant, a girl must adjust to her new sexuality, and that means coming to terms with her body. As she shoots up in height and blossoms physically, it is easy for a girl to be

Adolescence: The Maiden Voyage

self-conscious. At this age, she is extremely sensitive to criticism. Her sense of body space and even her center of gravity are changing radically: her feet keep getting farther away. Whether a girl learns to love or hate her body at this time sets the precedent for her future self-image. Consider the case of Carol.

A twenty-six-year-old architecture student, Carol has the fresh, rosy good looks common to women from Minnesota. She assiduously avoids caffeine and nicotine, and when she is not drawing site plans or sketching buildings, she is determinedly running her daily five miles or swimming laps at the university pool. Carol has arrived at her current state of wholesomeness only after an adolescence that she humorously describes as perpetual gluttony on doughnuts, candied apples, cereal, and Hostess cherry pies. By the time she left school she was five feet eight inches tall and weighed 167 pounds.

Her weight bothered her less than her mother's reaction to her eating. The only time Carol recalls her mother hitting her was when she refused to stop drinking a glass of milk. "If I had been thin and drunk the same amount of milk," Carol recalled, "she never would have hit me. She was reacting out of fear of seeing me blow up like a balloon." Her mother tried to convince her that she was getting too fat, but her arguments were far from persuasive: "When you eat too much, you get a bulbous nose."

When Carol entered college, she lost thirty pounds, regained it, lost fifteen pounds, and regained that, too. It took her a long time to like herself, and she now believes that dieting made it more difficult. Once she stopped worrying about her weight and started enjoying herself, the pounds began to drop.

Carol contrasts herself and her six-year struggle for self-love with the situation of her friend, Stephanie. Stephanie was a big-boned girl, but because her mother always told her she looked great, she never learned to dislike her appearance. She grew from a well-adjusted, roundish adolescent into a well-adjusted, roundish adult. Not all adolescent girls are so willing to listen to their mothers. And not all mothers are so wise. Many mothers transmit to their daughters the feelings of unhappiness about their own bodies, and it is from their mothers that girls often pick up a distorted body image.

Many girls not only have no conception of a realistic body,

Eat Beautiful!

they also try to lose weight at a time when the brain is commanding the body to grow. During adolescence, the body adds about 130,000 calories' worth of new tissue, the bulk of it between ages twelve and fifteen. The appetite awakens from its preteen slumber and growls to be fed. In *Member of the Wedding*, Carson McCullers tells the story of Frankie, a twelve-year-old girl who suddenly finds herself no longer a child. At one point, Frankie's black housekeeper complains about her insatiable appetite: "I swear, Frankie! I believe you got a tate worm. [Your father] reads over them grocery bills and he complains to me, Berenice, what in the name of holy creation did we do with six cans of condensed milk and forty-leven dozen eggs and eight boxes of marshmallows in one week. And I have to admit to him: Frankie eat them. I have to say to him: Mr. Addams, you think you feeding something human back here in your kitchen. That's what you think. I have to say to him: Yes, you imagine it is something human."

Like Frankie, most girls will experience a surge in appetite during the growth spurt. A girl's nagging appetite plus her need for calories can make her eat constantly. Her calorie needs depend mainly on her age, activity, and size. Girls who grow fast, who are active, and who prefer running to being on the debating team will often burn more calories. Lean tissues require more energy than fat ones, so physically active girls, even at rest, will need more calories than those who are less active and more plump. During the growth spurt, healthy girls take in anywhere from 1,750 to 2,600 calories daily. One way to figure out how many calories a girl needs is to use this formula to multiply a girl's weight in pounds times the number of calories given for her age group:

Age	Calories
11–14	21.8
15–22	17.3

So a seventeen-year-old girl who weighs 120 pounds would need about 2,076 (120 × 17.3) calories a day.

During the growth spurt, the body engages in all-out fat production. For some teens, especially those with obese parents or siblings, the fat remains. After the growth spurt, all girls put fat on their hips and other areas where they need it for childbearing. This fat can trigger widespread panic and prompt diets so bizarre that they can actually cause weight gain.

A girl usually becomes aware of her body by high school, and most girls, their body images mangled from self-doubt, begin to "feel fat." When I was eleven, my friend Cathy approached me at the lunch table and asked if I wanted any ice cream. When I said no, she was amazed and genuinely confused. She kept asking me how I stayed so skinny and why I didn't feel compelled to eat sweets. What was my secret?

In retrospect, the conversation was not as senseless as it seemed at the time. What had happened was this: Cathy, though my age, was years ahead of me in physical maturity. She already had the contours of a woman and was cornered by her fear of being fat. She already had begun her struggle with food. On the other hand, I still had bird legs, and my bust, waist, and hip measurements were about the same. I was a latecomer to puberty and had yet to notice that I had a body or yet to think of food as anything other than something to stuff in my mouth. (Certainly, it was nothing to be rationed.) For Cathy, whether or not to eat an ice-cream cone was a monumental moral decision. Ice cream represented a sweet, forbidden pleasure. For me, ice cream was just more food, and I simply was not hungry. It was only a few more years before I entered the same fray as Cathy and forged my own weapon against myself—a branding iron with which to stamp "guilt" on anything appetizing.

Afraid of putting on weight, some teenagers eat so little food that they slow their growth and stunt their sexual development. Dr. Fima Lifshitz, a New York pediatric endocrinologist, remembered seeing a sixteen-year-old girl who had limited her food to such small amounts that she had not gained a pound since she was ten. Once she began to eat normally, she developed breasts and other sexual characteristics. Her height remained permanently stunted, however, because once she reached menarche, her bones fused and she could grow only one or two inches more.

A number of girls, particularly those who are large-boned, mistakenly think they are fat. But others really are too fat. As a girl's growth slows and calorie needs begin to level off, she has to either cut back on food or exercise more, or she will gain unwanted fat. Losing fat is difficult for a teenager because she must forgo an immediate pleasure for some vague, future benefit. She may feel that dieting will separate her from her friends at a time when she wants to conform. Yet a teen can get in shape without risking a public display of herself.

Cutting calories in a teen's diet without cutting nutrition

A girl who wants to lose weight still needs to eat at least three meals a day. But she should limit certain foods, like fats, sweets, and alcohol, because they are high in calories and low in nutrients. Compared to lean teens, obese girls eat fewer dairy products, vegetables, and fruits, and their diets tend to be low in calcium, iron, and vitamin C. To cut calories and still get these valuable nutrients, an obese teen should substitute low-fat milk and yogurt, vegetables, and fruits for higher-calorie foods. She can order skim or low-fat milk instead of a milk shake and, for dessert, have fresh fruit instead of fudge sundaes. A girl does not have to give up any food completely, but she may need to eat smaller portions. Instead of ordering three slices of pizza, she can order one slice and have a salad on the side. She could also order pizza with green pepper, onion, or mushroom instead of pepperoni, sausage, or bacon.

Teens should avoid appetite-controlling drugs and very low calorie diets. Crash dieting or fasting can cause lethargy and depression, a loss of muscle, and slow growth in height. Even after she has stopped growing, a girl's need for nutrients remains high, and severe dieting can lead to deficiencies. It can also trigger a starving-bingeing cycle that she will find difficult to escape.

In the early teenage years, a reducing diet should provide at least 1,500 to 1,800 calories a day. If a girl's doctor prescribes a diet with fewer calories than this, she should take a multivitamin-mineral supplement and be sure to eat enough protein. A loss of muscle tissue is a *real* problem for dieting teens.

A teen will be most successful at dieting if she is not in transition between depending totally on her parents and feeling totally free of them. This interim period is a time of confusion, and motivation for dieting becomes clouded. An obese girl who is not psychologically ready to lose weight will have a difficult

Adolescence: The Maiden Voyage

time dieting, and failure will only worsen her already poor self-image.

In reaction to psychological stress, many normal-weight girls suddenly gain ten to fifteen pounds, so-called reactive obesity. Their eating results from a sense of loss—perhaps a bad sexual experience or even the death of a pet cat. When these girls are placed on a strict diet, they become even more anxious and eat more food, and consequently gain weight. The worst approach to this type of obesity is an overemphasis on weight loss and restrictive dieting. Instead, the girl should be encouraged to exercise, relax, and understand cues in her environment that trigger her eating. For most teens, these cues revolve around boredom and depression. A girl may come home from school tired and depressed only to find an empty house and a full refrigerator. Her natural reaction is to overeat. She needs to recognize how vulnerable she is during this time and to find better things to do after school, like going for a walk with a friend. For an obese teen, exercise is as important as, if not more so than, dieting.

Here is what you as a parent can do to help, whether or not your daughter is too fat:

- Help your daughter to feel good about herself and to be comfortable with herself.
- Encourage her to learn about nutrition and exercise.
- Find out why she wants to diet. If it is only because she is self-conscious about her body, work on instilling confidence.
- Give her responsibilities and teach her to be accountable for her decisions.
- Let her know that you love her regardless of her weight.

Here are ways to help an obese girl get in shape. Ask her to think about the following questions and suggestions:

- Decide how eager you are to get in shape. Are you doing it for yourself? Your parents? Your friends?
- Figure out if there are any reasons why you have *tried* to stay overweight. Do you overeat to control your life? To avoid dating? To prove that your friends like you for

yourself, not your looks? Maybe your family unknowingly gives you strokes for being fat.
- Look for times when you are most likely to overeat. Are you bored or depressed? Find enjoyable things to do during these times that do not involve eating.
- Eat three meals a day.
- Have moderate portions. Do not give up all your favourite foods, even if they are high in calories. Learn to eat them less often and in smaller amounts.
- Include fresh fruits and vegetables in your meals whenever you can.
- Start a regular exercise program and stay active. This will let you eat enough food to get essential nutrients without packing on the fat.
- Buy clothes that fit, rather than items which are too small and make you feel fat or which are too big and make you feel invisible.
- Learn to love yourself regardless of your weight. Pursue activities that interest you and make you feel you are a worthwhile person.

Parents and teens need to realize that it is normal during adolescence to be concerned about weight; but if this concern is carried to extremes, it could mean trouble. Living on one diet after another can permanently distort a girl's perception of food. Once a girl leaves adolescence and becomes a woman, she might spend her life starving and gorging and never actually enjoying what she eats. (For more on eating disorders, see chapter 9.)

The scars of acne

If you look up "acne" in the dictionary, you probably won't find "blot on the soul" as part of the definition, but it might as well be. No one really knows what causes acne, but the chief suspects are hormones, genetics, and warm, humid weather.

Some degree of acne afflicts 75 to 90 percent of all girls, and the worst years for it are between ages fourteen and seventeen. The earlier the onset, the more severe the acne. Acne could not come at a worse time, popping out when girls are emotionally insecure and anxious about appearance. Serious acne can last for ten years or more, and can take the form of blackheads, greasy skin, pimples, pustules, papules, large pores, abcesses, and cysts, usually on the face, upper chest, back, and shoulders.

One thing is known about acne: it is linked to hormones. This is why it inflicts most of its damage during puberty. During these years the adrenal glands pump out androgens, the male sex hormones, by as much as three to four times the amount in childhood. Androgens promote bone growth and sexual maturation. In some people, the oil glands are extremely sensitive to the body's androgens and respond by secreting more oil.

The oil glands lie just beneath the skin and produce sebum, a mixture of fats and waxes. The sebum flows through tiny ducts around the hair follicles to reach the skin surface, where it spreads out and lubricates both the hair and skin. Inside each duct is a skinlike lining that regularly flakes, shedding its dead cells. The sebum drags these dead cells to the skin surface.

Androgens goad the oil glands into producing a sticky sebum, gluing the dead cells together. As these sticky cells pile up, they form a plug. A plug that stays below the surface of the skin is a whitehead. If the plug enlarges, pops out of the duct, and gets stuck in the neck of the follicle, it is a blackhead. The dark color of a blackhead is not dirt: it is the skin pigments darkening from exposure to the air.

Once the dead skin cells and oil have plugged the duct and sealed up the pore, bacteria change the chemistry of the oil and stimulate the secretion of even more oil and the shedding of more cells. Bacteria do not cause acne but worsen it once it has started. If the duct cannot withstand the burden of dead cells, oil, and bacteria, it ruptures and leaks the contents through the lining into the surrounding skin. This causes the redness and swelling that results in a pimple. If the bacteria invade deep into the dermis, tissues wall off the infection to prevent it from spreading, and a hard, raised cyst appears on the skin.

Though both young women and men secrete androgens, men have higher levels of the hormone and tend to have more severe acne. The female hormone estrogen inhibits the glands from producing oil. But girls with more androgens—possibly those with square builds, irregular menstrual cycles, or facial hair—are more prone to severe acne.

Pimples habitually surface before life's most important events. That is because stress causes hormones to trigger more oil.

The only way to prevent these pimples from popping out—not surprisingly—is to avoid stress.

How nutrition affects acne

Vitamin A Though vitamin A can help acne, taking it in high doses can be dangerous. Large amounts may be safe under the supervision of a doctor, but some overzealous patients have doubled or tripled their doses or continued to take them after leaving their doctor's care. High doses can cause headaches, a dangerous loss of appetite, vomiting, increased thirst, anemia, weakness, scaling skin, scabbed lips, dry tongue, kidney pain, and hepatitis. Too much vitamin A (daily doses of 25,000 I.U. or more) can also cause rough and itchy skin, loss of hair, vertigo, insomnia, and diarrhea.

Doctors prescribe the synthetic form only for severe cases of acne because it may cause harmful side effects in persons who have liver disease or diabetes, or in those who drink too much alcohol. It should never be taken during pregnancy.

Consuming large amounts of carotene (a precursor to vitamin A in fruits and vegetables) does not produce these toxic effects. But too much carotene, say from eating a lot of carrots, can cause a temporary yellowish discoloration of the skin until you cut down on carrots. Very high levels may lead to menstrual irregularities.

Vitamin A is safer and more effective as an ingredient in facial gels or creams. Called retinoic acid, vitamin A acid, or tretinoin (Retin-A), it keeps oil ducts free from plugs by preventing sloughed-off cells from sticking together and by peeling away layers of cells that clog the pores. Your acne may seem worse at first, but after several months of treatment, your skin should be less oily and have fewer outbreaks. But beware: vitamin A is an acid, and too much can cause a burn or "blush." It also makes the skin sensitive to ultraviolet light, so avoid the sun when you are using it.

Vitamin E Some manufacturers add vitamin E to their acne products and claim it can prevent scarring. Vitamin E will not help acne because it is not absorbed through the skin—but it *can* cause severe allergic reactions.

Zinc A study of Scandinavian teenagers with acne suggests that some acne may be caused by a zinc deficiency. However, many adolescents show no improvement after taking zinc supplements. If tried, zinc supplements should be taken only under a doctor's care because too much zinc is toxic and can cause nausea, vomiting, and diarrhea.

Iodine Large amounts of iodine, such as those in some cough syrups, worsen acne. However, no evidence shows any harm from the low amounts in table salt. Sometimes fast foods are high in iodine because disinfectants used to clean the machinery contain the mineral.

Specific foods Some people say that chocolate, nuts, or fatty foods are the cause of acne because they make the face greasy and cause pimples, but scientific studies have not proven this. Some individuals may be particularly sensitive to these foods and break out after eating them. It makes sense to avoid eating any foods to which you are sensitive, but it may take two months for symptoms to disappear. It also makes sense to eat a well-balanced diet with plenty of fresh fruits and vegetables.

Acne will usually go away in time. So if all of the above remedies fail, simply try to outlive it.

The whole tooth about cavities

The hormones that race around teenagers' bodies seem to be fueled by sugar—the sweet, sticky snacks that make your teeth hurt just by thinking about them. What these sweets may also fuel is bacteria. When you eat, *Streptococcus mutans* in the mouth grab on to the carbohydrates, particularly sugars, and make a sticky goo called plaque. This plaque and the bacteria cling to the tooth's surface, where the bacteria ferment the sugars and produce a harsh acid for twenty to thirty minutes after your last bite or swallow. The acid attacks the tooth enamel and can drill a hole or cavity.

Bacteria are not partial to sweets. They also ferment apples, apricots, bananas, crackers, milk, oranges, peanut butter, potatoes, and rice. But these foods have essential vitamins and minerals and add value to your diet. While the type of snack is partly responsible for tooth decay, more important is how often you snack and how much time the teeth are in contact with food.

Some foods actually protect against cavities by being natural cleansers or by neutralizing the acid. These include fresh vegetables like cucumbers and carrots; cheeses such as Brie, Gouda, Emmental and mozzarella; fish, meats, and popcorn.

Recommendations Here are some ways teens can avoid cavities through diet:
- Eat foods that are low in sugar to reduce the risk of producing acid.
- Avoid sweets that stick to the teeth, such as caramels, soft bread, iced doughnuts, and cake—unless you can brush your teeth soon after eating these foods. Chocolate is less likely to promote cavities than, say, an acid drop, because the fat in chocolate coats the sugar and makes it less available. Be careful: even the natural sugar in dried fruits is a meal to bacteria.
- Limit snacks. The fewer times that sugar touches the teeth, the fewer chances the bacteria have to feast.
- Eat your sweets right after a meal when your saliva is flowing. Saliva rinses out the mouth and neutralizes the acid.
- Use fluoride daily in the form of fluoridated water and toothpaste. If your water is not fluoridated, use a fluoride mouthwash. Fluoride is a nutrient built into the structure of teeth that makes them more resistant to bacteria.

Losing that healthy glow—the risk of anemia

Since the 1500s, medical literature has described a disease common to adolescent girls that causes pale skin, fatigue, poor appetite, and menstrual problems. Because doctors thought the disease tinted the skin green, they called it "the green sickness," or chlorosis. In the 1800s, when it became acceptable for women to eat meat, exercise, and abandon their corsets, this disease vanished. It turned out that many of these chlorotic women had a form of iron-deficiency anemia.

Iron-deficiency anemia strikes most often in infancy and adolescence, when trillions of new red blood cells are manufactured to carry oxygen and nutrients to the ever-enlarging body. Iron is built into the hemoglobin that gives blood its bright red color. Those most at risk are girls who have heavy menstrual bleeding or who follow fad diets. The average fifteen-year-old loses about 15 mg of iron each month in menstrual blood. If her diet cannot replace the iron lost from menstruation, her body goes to work on its liver reserves. Unfortunately, because she is probably worried about weight, she might unknowingly cut out foods rich in iron and exist instead on poor sources such as yogurt, fruit, and diet soda. The result? She has too little iron to form hemoglobin, and her body produces fewer red blood cells. In short, she is anemic. A girl may not have a full-blown case of anemia, but she may be so close to it that, when stressed by increased menstrual flow, accidents, or serious illness, she slides into an anemic state.

Without a blood test a girl cannot tell if she is anemic. The symptoms of anemia—fatigue, dizziness, headaches, and irritability—are commonly displayed in other situations (for example, taking tests, being asked to do dishes, or having a date with a nerd). But unless a girl eats lean meats or legumes (dried peas and beans, such as navy or pinto beans, or split peas), and plenty of green vegetables and iron-fortified cereals, she may not be getting enough iron.

Girls who are not yet menstruating require only 12 mg dietary iron daily, but girls who menstruate heavily require more—about 18 mg. Girls who are deficient in iron will absorb more of the mineral, just like a dry sponge will suck up more water than one already soaked. An iron supplement may be recommended during the teen years and continued into adulthood, particularly if a girl is dieting or a vegetarian. (For more information on iron and supplements, see chapter 2.)

Other nutritional needs of teens

Adolescent girls win the award for having the worst diets of any age group. Worst of all are girls who are always trying to cut calories. Even with this dubious distinction, most girls are fairly well nourished.

A girl's need for nutrients reflects her physical maturity, not her actual age. Except for iron, her nutrient needs hit their peak during the growth spurt before menarche and actually surpass those of an adult woman. After menarche, they drop steadily toward adult levels.

Vitamin A Without vitamin A you could be one of those things that goes bump in the night. When you look at a bright light, a compound in your retina, called visual purple, is temporarily bleached. As the light dims, your eye must regenerate this visual purple before you can see again. Vitamin A is part of this compound, and each time your retina is exposed to bright light, a small amount of vitamin A is destroyed. If the supply of vitamin A in your blood is low, a time lag will occur before you can see again. This lapse, termed night blindness, indicates a vitamin A deficiency.

Vitamin A also wards off infection. A teen with a poor diet, particularly a diet without dairy products or vegetables, may be especially vulnerable to infections. Cells lining the stomach, intestines, urinary tract, bladder, lungs, vagina, eyes, and skin secrete mucus as a guard against microorganisms. Without enough vitamin A, these cells become hard, dry, and brittle. The tissues, like sun-baked parchment, break easily and leave the cells vulnerable to infection. Vitamin A is also needed for reproduction and bone growth.

Vitamin A refers to several compounds, all of which come from animal products, particularly dairy products and liver. Because vitamin A dissolves in fat or oil, it is called fat-soluble and is usually present in the fatty portion of food. Although whole milk, with its milkfat, is a naturally rich source of vitamin A, skim and low-fat milk are fortified with the vitamin.

Plants have no vitamin A, but they provide a precursor of the vitamin, called carotene, which the body converts into the active vitamin. Carotene is a yellow-orange pigment that colors some fruits and vegetables red, deep yellow, or orange. Others like oranges, bananas, and corn are dyed by pigments not related to vitamin A. Dark green vegetables are also usually high in carotene, though the green chlorophyll masks the yellow-orange pigment.

The liver stores vitamin A, so you need to eat rich sources only every other day. Table E-1 (see appendix E) lists food high in vitamin A. One sneaky way to make sure a teen gets enough vitamin A is to use vegetables in baked goods. Try pumpkin bread, or carrot cake. For a teen who is watching her weight, raw vegetables (carrots, green peppers, broccoli) cut up and served with a cottage-cheese dip make a tasty snack. Or fix apricot-cottage cheese muffins for a quick, nutritious breakfast (see recipe 1 in appendix D).

Calcium A teenager needs plenty of calcium because her muscles and bones are growing. Almost half of an adult skeleton develops during adolescence. The need for calcium jumps from 600 mg daily for the girl aged seven to eight to 700 for nine-to fourteen-year-olds.

Despite these high calcium needs, a teen will rarely show a deficiency because her body adjusts its calcium absorption according to its need. Girls most likely to have a deficiency are those who are growing taller much faster than they are putting on weight. A girl may not see the effects of consuming too little calcium until later in life, possibly not until menopause. But a serious bone disorder called osteoporosis has its beginnings in adolescence and may result in part from too little calcium.

The richest sources of calcium are dairy products, particularly low-fat and skim milk products. Other good calcium sources include tofu (soybean curd), sardines, canned salmon, and leafy greens. (See table E-5 in appendix E for calcium values in food.)

Zinc Teens need zinc for growth, sexual maturation, wound healing, and for the sensation of taste. It is also required for the synthesis of protein and of the genetic material DNA and RNA, and is involved in at least forty metabolic reactions.

Some teenagers, particularly pregnant teenagers, may be at risk of zinc deficiency. The richest zinc sources are oysters, herring, clams, poultry, oatmeal, corn, whole grains, meats, liver, milk, fish, eggs, nuts, legumes, and peanut butter. Usually, if you eat enough protein, you will get enough zinc, although strict vegetarians may be at risk of low levels because whole grains contain substances that bind the mineral, preventing the body from absorbing it.

Eat Beautiful!

EATING STRATEGY

Laying siege to the icebox—teen eating habits

Emotionally, a teenager often feels indestructible and immortal. She may stay up all night, drive recklessly, abuse alcohol and drugs, eat erratically, and view the future as something to contend with later. The last thing she wants to worry about is how her diet will affect her health in later years. One fifteen-year-old put it bluntly: "I don't need any nutrition information now. Maybe when I'd old and getting fat and wrinkled, I'll read a book or something on the subject." This to-hell-with-it behavior begins to change in the late teens when a girl starts to consider the long-term consequences of her decisions.

Adolescence is the first time a girl can really choose what to eat, and she makes her choices based on whether she is trying to lose weight, do what her friends do, or just be different. A girl does not want to be caught dead eating brown rice if her friends are eating french fries. On the other hand, who wants to eat french fries if everyone else is a macrobiotic?

Girls' diets show recurring patterns:

- Monotony
- Skipped meals
- Snacking
- Experimentation
- Preference for fast food

Take the example of a monotonous diet. One woman I spoke with was obsessed with cheese sandwiches when she was in junior high school. She placed a slice of processed cheese, the kind protected by its own little wrapper, between two pieces of white bread—no lettuce, mustard, mayonnaise—nothing. Just cheese and bread. She ate this every day for lunch. One day she decided to diet, but hunger pangs disrupted her sleep, and she began having wonderful dreams about cheese sandwiches. By the time she reached high school, this craving was replaced by one for ice-cream sandwiches. If her other two meals of the day were varied, or if the monotony were short-lived, she would probably not have a nutritional problem.

Teens, busy with school projects or part-time jobs, tend to eat on the run and skip meals. They may sleep all morning or get up and not have any appetite. They might be under a great deal of stress, or they might be suffering the after effects of a bag of corn chips and quart of soda from the night before.

Also common is the girl who skips meals because she is trying to lose weight. An obese teen eats fewer meals than other teens. Skipping meals, particularly breakfast, promotes her overeating later in the day, when she will tend to pile it on for one big meal. If only she would start each morning with a breakfast that includes some protein and at least 300 calories, she would have an easier time controlling her appetite the rest of the day.

Looking at what most teens eat, it is difficult to tell the meals from the snacks. Some teens choose to combine their favorite foods into one bizarre jumbo snack like M&Ms on cold pizza. "Pigging out" on snacks, an unusual form of bingeing, is popular with some teens. They consume "fun foods" like cookies and ice cream until they feel their stomachs are going to burst. Teens view the practice as a social activity. Unlike serious bingeing, it is not done alone and does not leave psychological scars. About one-fourth of a girl's calories and many essential nutrients come from snacks. Snacking is actually a good idea for teens as long as they limit fats and sweets.

Because fast-food restaurants are inexpensive, they tend to draw large numbers of teenagers. Fast foods are certainly fast, but are they food? Critics of these foods say that they are high in calories, fat, sodium, and sometimes sugar. The average fast-food meal provides anywhere from 900 to 1,800 calories. Fat often provides over half the calories, and the teen who eats often at fast-food restaurants may begin to add unwanted weight. The sodium in one meal may range from 1,000 to 2,515 mg.

Foods such as burgers, beef and fish sandwiches, tacos, and pizza provide plenty of protein, carbohydrate, and fat, with most of the calories coming from fat. They also provide some of the B vitamins and iron and, unfortunately, a lot of sodium.

French fries are high in sodium and average ninety calories per ounce. Milk shakes are high in calories. They are not always made from milk and ice cream but sometimes from milk solids, sweeteners, flavorings and thickeners.

Because most of these restaurants do not serve fresh fruits and vegetables, fast-food meals tend to be low in vitamins A,

C, pyridoxine (vitamin B_6), folacin, and biotin. They are also low in fiber and the minerals calcium and magnesium.

With a little discretion, most people can get a decent meal at these restaurants. The challenge is to get the most nutrients with the fewest calories. Restaurants with salad bars make it easier to meet that challenge.

If a teen regularly eats at fast-food restaurants, she should include in her other meals leafy greens, fresh fruit, whole grains and cereals, and low-fat or skim milk.

A question of balance

For parents, the teen years are an exercise in patience and creative coercion. Parents should encourage a young girl's independence and instill in her a sense of responsibility toward her own health. Nutrition can be sold as a way to help a teen look and feel better, especially since good eating habits are conducive to clear skin, healthy hair, and a fit body.

As a general guide, teens can follow this daily eating plan:

- Lean meat, fish, or poultry (2–3 ounces), peanut butter (3 tablespoons), or cooked dried beans or peas (1 cup)—three or more servings
- Milk or yogurt (8 fluid ounces), or cheese (1½ ounces)— four or more servings
- Bread (1 slice), cereal (1 ounce), or cooked cereal, rice, or pasta (½–¾ cups)—four or more servings
- Fruits and vegetables—four or more servings. Rich in vitamin C—one to two servings. Rich in vitamin A (dark green or deep yellow vegetables)—five times a week

No girl is going to sit still long enough to tally her day's servings. But if she has three meals a day and at each meal chooses at least one serving from each food group, as shown above, then eats nutritious snacks, she will be covering most of her needs. Once she has met these needs, an active teen who still needs extra calories can indulge in ice cream and cookies.

Eating on the run does not have to mean a poor diet if parents keep plenty of nutritious fast foods on hand, including fresh fruits and vegetables, low-fat yogurt, tortillas and beans, cold chicken, cheese, nuts, dried fruit, popcorn, whole grain crackers, and breadsticks. Bizarre but harmless eating practices should not concern a parent, either. A girl who prefers yogurt to milk is getting the same nutrients. Vegetarianism can be a healthy way to eat if done sensibly. Practices that *can* be harmful and should be avoided include strict macrobiotic diets, fasting, very low calorie diets, and smoking cigarettes as a way to lose weight.

Adolescence is a girl's last opportunity before adulthood to change bad eating habits that may become routine. The teen years are not too early to take precautions against diseases that become major threats to health and life in later years. Any girl with a family history of heart disease, obesity, diabetes, or hypertension should have regular, periodic medical screenings. The most important health goals a teen can set now are to develop a good body image, begin a regular exercise program, control her weight, moderate her intake of alcohol if she drinks, stop smoking if she has already started, find ways to release tension, and learn the kinds of eating habits that keep dieting from becoming a lifelong obsession.

RESOURCES

Francis, Dorothy. 1986. *Nutrition For Children*. Blackwell.

2
Young Adulthood: Humoring the Hormones

> The secret of eternal youth is arrested development.
> Alice Roosevelt Longworth

When adolescence catapults you into adulthood, it lands you squarely center stage, and before you can untangle your legs or smooth down your hair, the house lights dim, the curtain rises, the spotlights grow bright, and your adult performance begins. Cues come quickly. Go to college. Get a job. Get a husband. Have a family. Get a better job. (Get a better husband?) Your aspirations book you into a vaudeville one day, only to sign you up for a tragedy the next. Hormones become side-show barkers that each month may announce yet another menstrual discomfort.

There is no escape clause in your contract for adulthood. But with a little care, some thoughtful planning, and a lot of fortitude, your body can deliver a bravura performance.

PHYSICAL CHANGES
Going through your paces

Once past your teens, your body stops growing. But it continues to change, replacing cells and tissues lost to age, injury, and benign neglect. Cells do not carry lifetime warranties. They live and die. Some regenerate, others do not.

In addition, the first thirty-five years or so after puberty are your childbearing years, whether or not you choose to have a child. During these years your nutritional needs will differ greatly from a man's and from those of a younger or older woman. If you are pregnant, breastfeeding, or taking contraceptives, your needs for certain nutrients will be altered even more.

At this time, your body will begin to show the first signs of aging: laugh lines that do not vanish, the occasional gray hair.

Young Adulthood: Humoring the Hormones

But to a large degree you can slow the arrival of many such signs. When a reporter commented to Gloria Steinem years ago that she did not look forty, Steinem retorted: "This is what forty looks like!" She was right—for those women who practice body maintenance. Yet even with the best health habits, the body will change during these years—quietly, but steadily.

PSYCHOLOGICAL CHANGES
From amateur to professional

Though you cannot predict exactly when one life stage will vanish in the wake of the next, psychological and emotional changes typically occur in sequences. In the late teens and early twenties, you worry about what you are going to do with your life. The struggle begun in adolescence to define your Self and to come to terms with sexuality continues into adulthood. If you are like most young women, you spend your twenties constantly torn between making commitments and keeping your options open. You may begin to compare your progress with others only to invite feelings of inferiority. A negative self-image at this stage is common and can lead to overeating or undereating, and alcohol and drug abuse.

In your late twenties and early thirties, you reconsider your previous decisions. If you made commitments earlier, you now become aware of options. If you have been married for several years and have children in school, you may suddenly find outside work inviting. If you held on to your options you now begin to make commitments. Like many women, you may decide to marry later in life and have children when you are in your mid-thirties and early forties, choosing at the same time to remain employed outside the home. This can be a time for completing postponed goals. In short, during young adulthood, you experience some of the greatest pressures to be "successful."

HEALTH CONCERNS
The menstrual cycle: rehearsing for pregnancy

You are born with a lifetime supply of eggs. Numbering in the hundreds of thousands, the eggs huddle in your ovaries, dormant until puberty. Then each month your brain releases a hormone to the ovary, which stimulates about twenty of the immature eggs, encased in follicles, to develop. The follicles grow from the first to the fourteenth day of a cycle (a cycle begins on the first day of menstruation) and release estrogen into the blood. When the estrogen reaches a critical level, all but one of the developed follicles wither away. At ovulation, this lone follicle, a blister on the surface of the ovary, bursts and releases a mature egg that journeys down the fallopian tube to the uterus. You may experience mild pain in your abdomen when blood and fluid from the ruptured follicle irritate your abdominal wall. The pain can last from a few minutes to a couple of hours.

After ovulation (day fourteen), the ovary is left with a scar that becomes a gland—the corpus luteum. This gland pumps out estrogen and copious amounts of the hormone progesterone. Estrogen thickens the uterine lining while progesterone creates a soft, spongy, nourishing bed for the fertilized egg. These hormones work against the action of insulin, and a diabetic may find her level of blood sugar rising unexpectedly in the few days before and a few days into her period. Body temperature drops slightly at ovulation, then rises 0.5 to 1.0 degree F. To sustain this higher temperature, your body burns an extra one hundred calories a day.

If the egg remains unfertilized by the twenty-second or twenty-third day, the corpus luteum stops producing hormones, and the levels of estrogen and progesterone plummet. The blood supply to the new cells on the uterine lining is cut off, and the soft bed breaks down and is shed. This is menstruation, also known as the "poorlies" (nineteenth-century America), "the curse" (America), and "I am going to see Sophie" (France). It occurs in healthy, nonpregnant women from about age thirteen to fifty.

Most women have a predictable menstrual cycle lasting from twenty-eight to thirty-eight days, though anywhere from twenty to forty days is normal. Like a sheet catching the wind, the menstrual cycle gently billows out as estrogen and progesterone build up, then whips free, letting loose a range of menstrual symptoms that has caused more than one unsuspecting woman to doubt her sanity.

Young Adulthood: Humoring the Hormones

Premenstrual syndrome (PMS) and the histrionic womb

At least half and perhaps as many as 90 percent of all women experience some type of menstrual symptom, but only one in ten experiences symptoms they would consider severe. Along with purses and perms, menstrual discomforts may be an inevitable part of Woman's Burden.

PMS (often called premenstrual tension or PMT in Britain) can occur after ovulation and persist until the next period. Symptoms include bloating, abdominal pain, breast tenderness, migraines, depression, crabbiness, tension or anxiety, increased thirst or appetite, food cravings, and acne. This wide range of symptoms occurs regularly at the same phase of the cycle, then is followed by a symptom-free stage.

Some women are fine until a week or so before their periods, when they may experience anything from lower backache to bizarre mood swings. Some women are fatigued and need extra sleep; others get a burst of energy. Following are descriptions of some common PMS symptoms.

Increased appetite Estrogen may be a natural appetite suppressant. As estrogen levels fall before a period, women tend to eat more food. If left to their own will and freed of any guilt feelings over food, they consume about five hundred more calories a day during the ten days before their periods than during the ten days after.

Progesterone may affect appetite, too. As progesterone rises, so does your metabolic rate, and rising right along with it is your appetite. Your metabolic rate decreases at menstruation and reaches its lowest point one week before ovulation.

No matter which hormone, if either, is responsible for the change in appetite before a period, women crave more food, particularly sweet or salty items. One woman recounted that in her early twenties she would feel disturbing, suicidal urges a few days before each period. "It got to the point where I didn't bother marking my little red 'M' on the calendar," she said. "I just kept track of my cycle by noting when I felt like jumping off a bridge." Fortunately, when she reached her early thirties, the suicidal urges were replaced by overwhelming cravings for chocolate. "I'm a lot happier about the turn my body has taken, though I guess there are some purists out there would say indulging in chocolate is just another way of killing yourself. All I know is, I sure look forward to my periods now!'

This craving for certain foods is greater in overweight women, and the heavier they are, the more intense the craving. One researcher, Judith Wurtman at the Massachusetts Institute of Technology, suggests that when you are hit by a craving for carbohydrates, whether starches or sugar, you should go ahead and eat some but cut back on other foods to avoid overeating. She bases this advice on the following sequence of events: A high carbohydrate meal boosts the level of tryptophan, an amino acid needed by the body to produce serotonin, a brain chemical that controls mood. Low serotonin levels can cause depression. The only way to bring the brain serotonin levels back to normal, according to Wurtman, is to satisfy the craving.

If you eat erratically before or during your period, try to have balanced meals for the rest of the month. Researchers who calculate your daily nutrient needs assume that you are getting the essential nutrients daily. If you are eating poorly seven days out of the month, during the remaining twenty-three days your diet must not only provide the nutrients you need, but compensate for those you previously missed.

Breast tenderness At midcycle during ovulation, breasts respond to hormones by swelling with fluid and becoming heavy and tender. Some women report that eliminating caffeine from their diets relieves premenstrual breast tenderness, so they avoid coffee, tea, caffeinated colas, and chocolate.

Bloating Aristotle believed that a mirror would tarnish if a menstruating woman glanced in it. Though he was wrong, many premenstrual women look in a mirror and see their own images "tarnished" from bloating. As progesterone rises just before a period, it binds sodium, which in turn holds water in the body. You can retain sodium and the water it pulls along with it for as long as ten days before your period. Your face may get puffy, and your feet and ankles may swell. Rings become tight, shoes uncomfortable. Dentures or contacts suddenly do not fit. Bloating causes weight gain, usually about one to three pounds, but

Young Adulthood: Humoring the Hormones

in some women as much as five to six pounds. This bloating can also make you hungry and heighten your emotions.

To reduce premenstrual bloating, cut back on salt, especially in the week before menstruation. At the beginning or end of your period, you will excrete the excess water in your urine. Avoid routinely taking diuretics for mild bloating because they can aggravate deficiencies of potassium or magnesium. Low levels of these minerals may themselves cause PMS. If you must take diuretics, replace the potassium by eating apricots or bananas and the magnesium by eating leafy greens or nuts. If you want a *mild* diuretic, try caffeine. (In the US, a Food and Drug Administration advisory panel also recommends caffeine for easing premenstrual cramps, headache, and "fatigue." Of course, you may be cutting back on caffeine because of breast tenderness.)

Some women have taken pyridoxine (vitamin B_6) to get rid of excess water. In 1983, at least thirty cases of pyridoxine toxicity were reported in the US. Most patients started with 50 to 100 mg a day and steadily increased the dosage, sometimes to as high as 5,000 mg daily. A few suffered permanent neurological damage. Others had problems walking and lost their sense of touch and physical control. Smaller doses of pyridoxine may also be able to bring on these symptoms. Some researchers suspect that amounts of 200–500 mg a day can cause problems if taken over a long period of time. If you want to be sure you are getting enough of this vitamin, eat rich sources, such as meats, whole grains, leafy greens, avocado, potatoes, dried beans, fish, and dairy products.

Depression Menstrual depression is similar to that experienced by women on oral contraceptives. During menstruation, rising estrogen levels can interfere with the body's handling of pyridoxine. Without this vitamin, your body is unable to manufacture certain mood regulators, such as serotonin.

Preliminary evidence suggests that premenstrual depression might be relieved by pyridoxine in prescribed amounts of 10 mg, but the evidence is too scanty to evaluate the effectiveness, appropriate dose, and long-term consequences of pyridoxine supplements. For severe depression, a doctor may prescribe an antidepressant drug.

Nutritional therapies Because some women with PMS have low magnesium levels in their blood, a few researchers think a magnesium deficiency might be a factor in the disorder. Critics argue that there is too little evidence to link low magnesium levels and PMS, and that fluctuating levels of magnesium, like certain other minerals, may simply be part of a normal menstrual cycle. Until more data become available, you can ensure sufficient amounts of magnesium in your diet by eating dried beans, whole grains, and leafy greens.

Popular articles on PMS have recommended certain nutritional therapies, although no evidence exists as to their effectiveness. Some claim PMS results from a vitamin A deficiency. This has not been shown, and it is dangerous to take vitamin A in large doses. Others recommend vitamin C or the amino acids leucine and isoleucine, none of which has been shown to work.

Treatments for PMS are so muddled because the syndrome affects no two women in the same way. Also, research is fairly new, and the symptoms are very subjective: feeling fatigued or "out of control" are common complaints. Many things may cause PMS, and no simple treatment may ever exist. If you suffer from PMS, you can try to relieve your symptoms with the following dietary suggestions. They will not work for everyone, but there is no harm in trying them.

- Cut down on alcohol, caffeine, and sodium during your premenstrual phase.
- Eat plenty of high-fiber foods to alleviate constipation. Vary your diet with fresh fruits and vegetables, legumes, and whole grains and cereals.
- Eat small high-protein meals frequently. Low blood sugar can cause headaches, fatigue, and irritability, and eating frequent meals may provide relief.
- Restrict supplements, unless prescribed, to the one-a-day formulas that provide no more than the recommended amounts of vitamins and minerals.

Dysmenorrhea

Primary dysmenorrhea refers to the pain and cramping that strike one or two days before a menstrual period and continue

Young Adulthood: Humoring the Hormones

throughout. It is the body's response to uterine contractions triggered by hormone-like substances called prostaglandins. The more prostaglandins a woman has, the more contractions. Studies have shown that women with dysmenorrhea have two to three times more prostaglandins than women without cramps, with the highest levels on the first or second day of their periods. Prostaglandins may also trigger contractions of the stomach, intestines, and certain blood vessels and cause nausea, vomiting, diarrhea, headaches, dizziness, or fatigue. The body responds to painful cramps by releasing stress hormones, which raise the level of blood sugar. The diabetic may need more insulin at this time.

The routine therapies for dysmenorrhea vary according to the severity of the pain, ranging from soaking in a warm bath to taking powerful anti-inflammatory drugs. Preliminary research at the University of California in San Francisco indicates that nutrition may one day become part of the treatment. Carol Jessop, one of the researchers, says the daily use of pyridoxine (200 mg) and magnesium (200 mg) may dull the sensitivity of nerve cells that react to prostaglandins, lessening the intensity of cramps. The pyridoxine seems to relax the uterine muscles, while the magnesium helps the vitamin enter the uterine cells. Use of this nutritional therapy is still experimental, and final results will not be available for several years. (Because high doses of pyridoxine can cause serious side effects, do not self-medicate.)

Secondary dysmenorrhea results from disease and requires medical treatment. If you have painful periods, consult your doctor.

Amenorrhea

Primary amenorrhea describes the situation of a girl who fails to start menstruating by the time she is seventeen years old. Secondary amenorrhea is the loss of menstrual periods for at least six months once a girl has reached menarche.

In the early nineteenth century, doctors blamed the failure to menstruate on being celibate, expressing immoderate joy, lounging on the grass, or eating sherbets. Granted, the menstrual cycle is delicate, but it's not *that* delicate. It does respond to travel, change in climate, stress, illness, fatigue, weight loss, and fasting. Tumors, hormonal imbalances, disease, or certain drugs can also be at fault. The menstrual cycle is sensitive enough that most women occasionally miss a period or two, a condition called oligomenorrhea. Skipping three or more successive periods can be more distressing.

Amenorrhea is more common in women who are extremely underweight or massively overweight. For underweight women, amenorrhea may be related to low body fat, crash dieting, or eating disorders. The menstrual cycles of obese women tend to be longer (more than thirty-six days) and more irregular, and result in greater blood loss. The greater the obesity, the more striking the differences.

Menstrual irregularities are becoming more common in athletes, particularly those who run fifty miles or more a week. It is not unusual for an athlete to have fewer than two periods a year.

Writing in the *Journal of the American Medical Association*, doctors at the Rutgers Medical School in New Jersey reported a strange cause of amenorrhea. Ten women who complained of menstrual difficulties and infertility were apparently consuming too much carotene, the vitamin A precursor present in yellow, orange, and green fruits and vegetables. Some were eating as much as a pound of carrots a day. The doctors referred to an earlier study in 1971 in which six women with high intakes of carotene and irregular menses were found to have "golden ovaries." Other women have experienced menstrual problems after using European tanning preparations that contain carotene.

Infertility

A poor diet will not strongly interfere with fertility unless you are practically starving. For women, the main dietary link is to regular ovulation. Obese women or women with low levels of body fat (less than 17 percent) may have trouble ovulating on a regular basis. Menstrual periods may cease if the diet is very low in protein, calories, or cholesterol, or too high in carotene. This amenorrhea is usually temporary, and your periods will resume if you reach your desirable weight or improve your diet. Smoking cigarettes also reduces fertility.

Harnessing the Hormones Through Birth Control

Oral contraceptives Collectively nicknamed "the Pill," oral contraceptives are either combination pills with the hormones estrogen and progestogen or minipills with progestogen only. Even though you might appear healthy while taking the Pill, it affects all body cells and can prevent you from properly using certain nutrients. It is hard to understand exactly what happens and why because, throughout a cycle, shifting hormones alter many body processes.

Women taking the Pill show increased levels of iron; decreased levels of vitamins pyridoxine, B_{12}, C, and riboflavin; and, depending on which study you look at, either increases or decreases of folacin and zinc. Though vitamin A is increased in the blood, body stores in the liver are reduced, and over time a deficiency could result.

The vitamin that appears to be most affected by the Pill is pyridoxine (vitamin B_6). One study found that pregnant or nursing women were more likely to have low pyridoxine levels if they had used the Pill for more than thirty months and became pregnant within four months after stopping the Pill. Some women who become depressed as a side effect of the Pill find relief in a prescribed daily dose of 20 mg pyridoxine.

Next most affected is folacin. A few women on the Pill have developed a serious—but rare—anemia, which responds to folacin supplements. Also, an abnormal cell growth called cervical dysplasia is linked to changes in folacin metabolism possibly caused by the Pill. The condition can sometimes be improved with folacin supplements.

Your body can adapt to many of these Pill-induced changes as long as you eat a balanced diet. If you do not, you will be more prone to fatigue, depression, illness, and anemia. Women most at risk for a nutritional deficiency are adolescents, those with a malabsorption problem, and heavy users of alcohol and drugs. Supplements should only be taken if a medical test indicates a vitamin deficiency.

Some women on the Pill have higher levels of blood sugar, a problem that worsens with age, overeating, and weight gain. Because high blood sugar can be dangerous for diabetics, women

Eat Beautiful!

who are diabetic or who have a family history of diabetes should choose a different method of birth control.

Though the Pill does not cause obesity, you may gain weight from fluid retention once you start taking it. If you gain ten pounds or more, consult your doctor. During your first few menstrual cycles on the Pill, you may experience nausea or vomiting. If this happens, try to continue eating well. If it persists, again contact your doctor.

Despite its possible side effects, the Pill does have some nutritional merits. Because the Pill reduces menstrual blood loss, Pill users have higher levels of iron as well as copper. They also show less bone loss with age.

If you take the Pill and want to reduce your risk of nutritional problems, try the following:

- Limit sweet and fatty foods. They provide too few vitamins and minerals for the number of calories they contain. Saturated fats are also a risk factor for heart disease.
- Limit alcohol. Alcohol depletes the same vitamins as oral contraceptives do, so drinking while on the Pill places you in double jeopardy.
- Avoid overeating and try to reduce if you are overweight.
- If you are planning on becoming pregnant, discontinue use of the Pill for three months prior to the time you wish to conceive so your body can replenish its nutrient stores. If you become pregnant shortly after stopping the Pill, check with your doctor about taking a folacin supplement.
- Avoid taking special vitamin and mineral supplements, unless prescribed. Instead, get your nutrients from food. Here are rich sources of nutrients that the Pill depletes:

Pyridoxine (vitamin B_6) pork, organ meats, wheat germ, milk, eggs, dried beans, whole grains, peanuts, soybeans, corn

Folacin leafy greens, asparagus, broccoli, liver, lean meat, eggs, fish, dried beans, whole grains.

Vitamin A dairy products, liver, carotene (apricots, peaches, cantaloupe, spinach, kale, Chinese leaves, and greens).

Vitamin B_{12} meat, dairy products, eggs.

Young Adulthood: Humoring the Hormones

Vitamin C citrus fruits, tomatoes, cantaloupe, cabbage, potatoes, broccoli.
Riboflavin milk, meat, poultry, eggs, leafy greens, beans, yeast, enriched breads and cereals.
Zinc herring, oysters, clams, poultry, oatmeal, corn, whole grains, meats, milk, fish, eggs, nuts, dried beans, peanut butter.

Intrauterine device (IUD) The IUD does not interfere with nutrients, but it can cause excessive menstrual bleeding and lead to iron-deficiency anemia. IUD users become anemic five times more often than those who do not use IUDs. To avoid this, eat iron-rich foods (lean meats, dried beans, dried fruits, leafy greens, whole or enriched breads and cereals). Also, have your hemoglobin checked periodically and ask your doctor if you should take an iron supplement, available in multivitamin and mineral supplements. Copper-bearing IUDs do not increase the copper levels in the body because the mineral remains near the surface of the uterus.

Taking care of your parts

As women age, their health habits begin to shape their future risk of disease. At age seventeen, Rita and Anne, both active, slender high-school students, had similar low risks for chronic, degenerative diseases. By age thirty, Rita was forty pounds overweight, sedentary, a perpetual dieter, and a pack-a-day smoker who responded to stress by overeating, overdrinking, and oversmoking. Anne, by age thirty, had taken up swimming to control her weight, was a nonsmoker, and had learned how to relax under stress. As the years add up, Rita will become increasingly more likely than Anne to get lung cancer, heart disease, and diabetes.

How fast you age depends on your genes and how well you take care of yourself. Chances are that Rita, at age thirty, looked ten years older than Anne. Chances are even greater that she *felt* ten years older. Below are the major health concerns for this period of life.

Iron-deficiency anemia At age thirty-nine, Jane had finally become an officer at a large bank. Her triple degrees in math, economics, and business administration had served her well. At times, though, usually when the alarm went off at 5:30 in the morning, she found herself wondering if she was getting too old for overachieving. She enjoyed her job, but she was constantly tired and depressed, and her appetite was gone. After months of dragging herself around, Jane decided to see her doctor. The prescription, it turned out, was not to quit her job, but to start taking iron. Jane was anemic.

Each of your body's 25 trillion red blood cells lives for about 120 days. As a red blood cell dies, scavenger cells recover the iron in the cell's hemoglobin and carry it to the bone marrow, where it enriches new red blood cells, much like attorneys making sure that the family jewels are passed to the proper heirs.

As part of hemoglobin in blood and myoglobin in cells, iron carts oxygen around the body. It also helps to manufacture antibodies, remove fats from the blood, convert the pigment carotene to vitamin A, detoxify drugs, and produce energy. Once you absorb it, iron either becomes part of a cell; is stored in your liver, bone marrow, spleen, and muscles; or is incorporated into hemoglobin. Because iron is reincarnated from one red blood cell to another, very little is lost from the body. The only way you can get rid of it is through cell loss such as hair, nails, and skin; by the normal sloughing-off of intestinal cells; and by losing blood.

Even though little iron leaves the body, about 5 percent of American women have mild iron-deficiency anemia. During the childbearing years, women are most at risk of low iron levels from frequent pregnancies and the monthly loss of menstrual blood. Women lose, on average, about 40 ml of blood (20 mg iron) each menstrual cycle. One women in ten has menorrhagia, an abnormal condition in which excessive menstrual bleeding occurs. Women who lose more than 80 ml of blood with each cycle are at higher risk of anemia. If you use more than twelve pads during your period or experience damming up of blood behind tampons, you could be bleeding excessively. If you use the Pill, you will have less blood loss. If you use an intrauterine device, you may bleed more. Anemia can also result from the slow blood loss from ulcers, hemorrhoids, chronic nosebleeds,

Young Adulthood: Humoring the Hormones

or cancer. Aspirin can cause intestinal bleeding and over time can lead to a noticeable loss of iron.

When your diet is chronically low in iron, you begin to tap into your stores. Your red blood cells shrink and pale in color. Your skin looks pallid, particularly where blood comes nearest to the skin surface—the fingernail and toenail beds, around the eyes, and in the lining of your mouth and lips. With less hemoglobin your cells cannot hold or deliver as much oxygen, so you have less energy. If you become anemic, you will work less efficiently, be short of breath, be at greater risk of infection, and feel tired, sluggish, and apathetic. Even mild anemia can leave you feeling irritable and beat.

The most common test for anemia is to have your hemoglobin checked. The normal values for women are 13.8 to 14.2 g per 100 ml. Another test is the hematocrit, which determines the percentage of red blood cells in a volume of blood. The average reading for a woman is 37 to 47 percent. These values represent iron in the blood, not the bone marrow, so you can have a normal hemoglobin or hematocrit and still be depleting your reserves. To check your iron stores, your doctor would have to run a serum ferritin test.

The UK recommended daily allowance for iron during your reproductive years is 12 mg. You need only about one-tenth of this to replace iron losses, but you absorb only about one-tenth of what you ingest. The average British diet supplies this amount. But if you want to be sure you are getting enough iron, do the following:

- Include meat, poultry, and fish in your diet. Iron from these animal products is absorbed intact. Iron from vegetables and grains must first undergo a chemical conversion and so is less easily absorbed. By mixing animal products into a vegetable dish, you better absorb the iron from both. If you are going to stir-fry vegetables for dinner, throw in bits of chicken or beef. Table E-2 (see appendix E) lists iron content in foods.
- Steam vegetables in a steamer basket rather than boiling them. In large amounts of water, iron will leach out of the vegetables. The water that is left after boiling or steaming

includes iron and other nutrients and makes a good soup stock.
- Most iron is in the germ of grains, so avoid processed baked goods that contain refined, unenriched flour. Make your own desserts with iron-rich ingredients (see recipe 2 in appendix D).
- Prepare foods in cast-iron pots and pans. When you cook with cast-iron pans, especially when simmering acidic foods like tomato sauce, the iron in the pans leaches into the food. One study found that after simmering spaghetti sauce in a cast-iron pot for three hours, the amount of iron in one-half cup of sauce rose from 4 to 116 mg.
- At each meal, eat foods rich in vitamin C such as orange juice, green peppers, and tomatoes. Table E-3 (see appendix E) shows vitamin C content in foods. Because of its acidity, vitamin C boosts iron absorption. Vegetarians, in particular, need to have a diet high in vitamin C to compensate for the poorer absorption of iron from vegetables and grains. (Prescriptions for iron supplements often include vitamin C.)

Eggs, coffee, and tea can hinder iron absorption, while fiber can move food through the intestines at such a fast rate that little iron is absorbed. To offset these losses, add citrus juice to your meals or eat other high-vitamin C foods. If you cannot cut back on tea or coffee, at least try to drink them between rather than with meals.

If you are anemic or borderline anemic, let your doctor decide if you need an iron supplement. Iron can mask other underlying problems, and supplements can cause constipation, indigestion, or diarrhea. Also, supplemental iron is poorly absorbed, so it is better to get iron from food. However, if you are a vegetarian or a dieter, or if you bleed heavily during your period, check with your doctor about taking routine supplements.

If you take iron supplements, look for ferroglycine sulfate or the word "ferrous" followed by sulfate, gluconate, fumarate, lactate, glutamate, or succinate in amounts of about 18 mg. Generic varieties are as effective as brand-name ones and much less expensive. Time-release pills are not worth the added expense because you absorb iron only in the duodenum (upper

Young Adulthood: Humoring the Hormones

twelve inches of the small intestine), and any iron released after this point will be excreted.

Iron overload Your body usually controls the amount of iron it absorbs, but sometimes it is overwhelmed. Iron excesses occur from unrestricted use of therapeutic iron supplements or from drinking too much cheap wine. Iron overdose, a condition called hemochromatosis, can damage the liver, pancreas, and heart, as well as provide a feast for harmful bacteria and fungi that can cause infection.

Other anemias Any medical condition that destroys red blood cells or slows their production can lead to anemia. That is why symptoms of fatigue and irritability should be checked out by a doctor before you start routinely taking iron supplements. Deficiencies of other nutrients besides iron may even be at fault. These include folacin, vitamin B_{12}, and, to a lesser extent, zinc and copper.

Folacin or folic acid, is a vitamin needed for cells to regenerate and for the synthesis of body compounds such as the nucleic acids DNA and RNA. Your need for folacin rises whenever cells are forming or your metabolic rate speeds up—during pregnancy and breastfeeding, for instance.

With folacin deficiency, cells cannot regenerate quickly. Red blood cells lead such brief lives that they are some of the first to succumb. The result is called megaloblastic anemia because the red blood cells look bloated and are too few in number. As with iron-deficiency anemia, the red blood cells are crippled in their ability to carry oxygen to the cells, so you may feel tired and weak. Other symptoms include headaches, irregular heartbeats, sore tongue, lack of appetite, and forgetfulness. The best way to get enough folacin is to eat foods that are high in the vitamin, including leafy greens, dried beans, broccoli, orange juice, and whole grains. Table E-4 (see appendix E) shows folacin sources in food.

Folacin performs with a partner, vitamin B_{12}, and, if taken in excess, can mask a B_{12} deficiency. For this reason, the US Food and Drug Administration restricts the amount of folacin that can be added to vitamin pills to 400 mg. Though folacin can mask the abnormal red blood cells of a vitamin B_{12} deficiency, it cannot prevent the ensuing nerve damage.

Vitamin B_{12} also called cobalamin, is required for growth, nervous tissues, and the formation of red blood cells. A deficiency usually occurs when the stomach is injured or unable to absorb the vitamin. The result is pernicious anemia, a condition in which red blood cells are abnormally large, few in number, and immature. Symptoms can include weakness, indigestion, abdominal pain, constipation, diarrhea, a sore and glossy tongue, and, if untreated, permanent nerve damage. Your body can store about 2,000–3,000 µg of vitamin B_{12}, and since you need only 1–3 µg a day, deficiencies can take years to develop.

The best food sources of vitamin B_{12} are animal products, so strict vegetarians, especially women who bleed heavily during their periods, should eat B_{12}-fortified foods or take a supplement.

Zinc and copper Women who are deficient in iron tend to be deficient in zinc because both minerals are present in the same foods.

Copper is part of the enzymes needed for storing, releasing, and building iron into hemoglobin. Deficiencies are rare because most unprocessed foods contain the mineral. The richest sources are oysters, nuts, liver, kidney, legumes, shellfish, corn oil margarine, chocolate, and cocoa.

Obesity One of the most annoying changes of aging is weight gain. The gain is not always from overeating. After age thirty, your metabolic rate slows down by 2 percent for every decade of life and lowers your need for calories. Many overweight women are actually consuming insufficient calories and nutrients. Their added weight comes from too little exercise.

Toward the mid-thirties and early forties, the fat of middle-age spread begins to circumnavigate your belly. Your weight may peak in middle age, after which it slowly declines. Even if your weight stays constant, you may be adding fat and losing muscle, particularly if you avoid exercise.

Cancer and heart disease Between ages fifteen and thirty-four cancer beats out heart disease as the number-one killer of

Young Adulthood: Humoring the Hormones

women. In part this results from the natural "immunity" to heart disease that estrogen bestows on women. Only after menopause does a woman's risk approach that for men. By developing good eating habits now, you will be able to keep your risk low, even after menopause. (More on cancer and heart disease in part 3.)

Bone disease Each day your body requires a small amount of calcium to keep your blood calcium levels high enough for your nerves and muscles to function. If your diet is inadequate, your body pulls calcium from its stores in your bones, and the constant drain on your bones will make them thin and fragile. This leaves you suceptible to fractures after menopause, a condition called osteoporosis. Perhaps the best way to avoid osteoporosis is to develop sufficient bone mass when you are young. With extra bone, you can lose more before reaching the fracture point. To do this eat plenty of calcium-rich foods and start working out on a regular basis. Like having babies, this is a decision that cannot be put off forever. Once you pass age thirty-five, you are no longer adding bone mass.

You may not be getting enough calcium if you prefer coffee, tea, or sodas to milk, or if you are continually dieting. Too much protein—more than 120 g a day—can stimulate calcium loss from the bones. Other factors that can interfere with calcium are drinking too much coffee and alcohol, smoking cigarettes, and possibly eating a high phosphorus diet that is heavy in meats or soft drinks. (For ways to reduce your risk of osteoporosis, see chapter 5.)

EATING STRATEGY

Eating habits

Your eating habits depend on many things, including whether you are married, have children, go to school, or work. If you stay home caring for babies or small children, you may find yourself eating erratically, polishing off your children's leftovers, or getting a quick lift by grabbing a cup of coffee and a sweet roll while your children nap. Babies spend these early years doubling and tripling their weights. You may find your own weight heading in the same direction. And no matter how exhausting, running after children and bending down to pick up toys are not aerobic activities.

If you are a young, single woman, whether working or in college, you may not have much money and may be so busy that you are dieting half the time and eating out the other half. The more meals you eat away from home, the worse your overall diet is. By overeating from stress and haphazard schedules, coeds typically gain ten pounds in their first year. At least 12 percent of college women worry constantly about food and have serious problems with eating. Many exist solely on coffee and air or prefer to spend their food calories on alcohol.

Like many young women, you may consider cooking to be time-consuming and difficult. Gerald Nachman, writer for the *San Francisco Chronicle*, described the contents of a Single Person's refrigerator. The refrigerator, he wrote, "is full of staples like U-No bars, zipless root beer, black pears, eggs I'd rather not open, three jars of jam, each with one teaspoon of jam left—everything, that is, but actual living food." But your situation does not have to be so bleak. Cooking at home does not require more than twenty to thirty minutes, and unlike eating at restaurants, you can control the nutritional quality of your meals by cutting down on salt, sugar, and fat.

If you are a middle-management executive, perhaps married, in your thirties, with no children, you undoubtedly lead a hectic life, are constantly stressed out, and probably consume too much coffee and too many cocktails. If you are also a mother, you may have more stable meals, but your children add another dimension of stress to your life.

The eating habits of young and middle-aged women reflect the upheaval of this period of life, when there is never enough time to do what needs to be done, when home and work situations appear erratic and fickle, when your self-image rides on a wave of satisfaction only to crash onto the rocks of insecurity. To eat well during these years, you need to learn the basics of nutrition and a few simple cooking techniques. Most of all, you must decide that it is worth taking the time to do something good for yourself.

Young Adulthood: Humoring the Hormones

Recommendations

These adult years are times for storing nutrients that you will need once you reach menopause. Because women are living longer than ever, the number of postmenopausal years has risen, and the diet and eating habits you establish when you are younger become even more important.

There is no right way to eat. But if you start your day with breakfast, have a substantial lunch, and partake of a moderate dinner, you will ward off hunger and fatigue by keeping up your blood-sugar levels. Eating four or more small meals a day is another way to keep your blood sugar high, as long as you choose balanced meals and not sugary or salty snacks. But if you tend to binge, avoid eating many small meals.

The ideal diet for women is rich in iron, calcium, folacin, and zinc, without an excess of calories. To get these nutrients, eat plenty of low-fat or skim dairy products, whole grains and cereals, dried beans, lean meats, fish, fresh fruits, and leafy greens.

But diet won't take care of everything. You also need to establish a routine exercise program, have regular sleeping hours, learn to cope with stress, and stop smoking cigarettes (or at least cut back). Your body is fairly resilient and can withstand neglect—for a time. Poor habits may not show their effects until later in life, but eventually they will catch up with you. By learning sound habits, you can lessen the wear and tear on your body and possibly sidestep some diseases in your later years.

3
Pregnancy: The Blooming of the Womb

> Tonight I am halved, tonight I am doubled. Tonight I lose you forever, tonight I meet you for the first time.
>
> A woman in labor to her unborn child. From *With Child: A Diary of Motherhood*, by Phyllis Chesler

In 1953, Lucille Ball (Arnaz) and Desi Arnaz broke a long-standing television rule about no pregnancies on screen. Against the initial objections of CBS and their sponsor, they created episodes of *I Love Lucy* that dealt with Lucy's obvious forthcoming delivery. Audiences laughed through Lucy's bizarre food cravings and Ricky's sympathetic labor pains.

Today, all the hoopla over such a natural event is difficult to understand. Pregnancy is so stylish these days that you cannot watch a few weeks of soap operas without witnessing at least one character announcing the Blessed Event. Yet if all your information on pregnancy came from these popular shows, you would probably believe that the average gestational period lasts for about two months, and that during that time you might have a food craving or two, but not leg cramps and heartburn, and definitely not constipation. Here is what *really* happens.

PHYSICAL CHANGES
The watermelon look

Between conception and childbirth, your uterus mushrooms from a three-inch, one-ounce pouch into a twelve-inch, forty-ounce incubator. Entangled in it are multiplying muscles, nerves, and blood vessels that spread out like morning glories conquering a garden.

Your pelvic muscles and ligaments soften and stretch. In response to the hormone relaxin, your pelvic joints loosen. If

Pregnancy: The Blooming of the Womb

they become too loose, you will suffer backaches, and your walk will take on a distinctive waddle, a gait that Shakespeare dubbed "the proud walk of pregnancy." Backaches may plague you after delivery, since your joints take some time to tighten.

Both your uterus and embryo donate tissues to fashion the placenta. The placenta, an engineering marvel, sifts through your blood and extracts nutrients and oxygen for your fetus. It also pulls wastes from your fetus and dumps them into your blood for removal. The placenta pumps out its own hormones to keep your uterus soft and nourishing and your breasts full and tender, an exaggeration of pre-menstrual breast changes.

Your blood volume swells. To move this extra blood, your heart beats more quickly and your pulse rate speeds up. Despite your heart's heroic pumping, blood pressure usually falls slightly during pregnancy. (If your blood pressure rises, see your doctor.) Blood clots more rapidly, offsetting possible hemorrhage, and because it flows faster through your skin, your temperature may rise, causing you to perspire. A red hue may color your palms, and spidery blood vessels spread across your arms and face.

Many changes work to your advantage—and your baby's. If you eat poorly, your body will attempt to outwit you, from absorbing scarce nutrients more efficiently to lacing coffee with a bitter taste. If you invest a little energy into eating well during these nine months, you can end up in better shape after delivery than before you became pregnant.

PSYCHOLOGICAL CHANGES
As feelings come alive

Whether it is your first child or not, like all pregnant women you will experience a progression of emotions. If the pregnancy is your first, you may feel closer to your own parents, particularly your mother. If you start out nauseated and tired, expect to be disappointed and frustrated. In the first few months, fear of a miscarriage is natural. As pregnancy continues, a growing sense of responsibility toward your baby emerges, mixed with tension and irritability. One minute you may feel as if you are floating in a hot-air balloon, the next minute roped to a railroad track.

When your baby's head descends into the pelvis, you regain

Eat Beautiful!

your sense of well-being and focus more on your baby and yourself. You may lose interest in work and become less social. As delivery nears, the fears and anxieties return. Will your baby be healthy? Will the delivery have complications?

After delivery, feelings are a jumble of relief, elation, fulfillment, exhaustion, fear, frustration, depression, and weepiness. Once home, minor inconveniences, heightened by loss of sleep, can seem insurmountable.

Your feelings, during and after pregnancy, will hinge on your health and energy, and the spirit, applause, and support around you. If you can avoid the hazards and discomforts of your condition, things will be even better.

HEALTH CONCERNS

If you can answer yes to at least one of the following questions, you may be at nutritional risk during pregnancy:

1. Have you been pregnant three or more times during the past two years?
2. Have you had a problem pregnancy before?
3. Are you a strict vegetarian, or are you following any restrictive diet?
4. Do you have an existing medical condition, such as diabetes, anemia, or heart disease?
5. Are you overweight?
6. Do you smoke cigarettes, take drugs, or drink alcohol heavily?
7. Are you under fifteen years old?

If you answered yes to any question, be sure to get early prenatal and dietary counseling. Here are some of the more common health concerns of pregnancy.

Weight gain The best single indicator of your baby's future health is its weight at birth. Birth weight is determined by three things: how close to term your baby was born, your weight before conception, and your gain during pregnancy.

If you gain too few pounds, your baby might have a low birth weight (less than 5.5 pounds). Such babies are more likely to have complicated births and to contract disease and die early in

Pregnancy: The Blooming of the Womb

life. Many of these babies develop poorly in mind and body and are hyperactive as children.

If you overeat during pregnancy, you may predispose your infant to be overweight. Also, women whose infants weigh more than ten pounds at birth risk a difficult delivery. Some researchers believe that an infant overfed in the uterus may be born with extra fat cells and have a tough time losing weight as a child or adult. However, pregnancy is not the time to diet because reducing diets can lower your baby's birth weight and retard its brain development. Low-carbohydrate diets are especially dangerous. Without carbohydrates, your muscles burn fat, and keytones (by-products of fat breakdown) can harm the fetus. Delay any dieting, even for short periods, until after you have delivered.

The average gain of healthy Western women is approximately twenty-eight pounds. Only about one-third of this is your baby. What is left is amniotic fluid, placenta, water, breast and uterine tissue, and fat. The extra fat accumulating on your abdomen, back, and upper arms is an energy store for breastfeeding and for when illness or exhaustion keep you from eating well after delivery.

If you are at a normal weight, gain between twenty-four to thirty-two pounds over the next nine months. If you are underweight, gain closer to twenty-eight to thirty-six pounds. The lower your initial weight, the more critical your gain is. If you are overweight, add only twenty to twenty-four pounds, but be sure to gain at least fifteen pounds.

Gaining more than forty pounds can lead to delivery complications, including caesarean section, prematurity, fetal death, toxemia, and high blood pressure. However, if you are carrying twins or triplets, gain at least ten pounds more than recommended. The extra weight of twins may make you feel as Jean Kerr did: "I was square and looked like a refrigerator approaching."

Your weight gain should be smooth. Gain 1.5 to 3 pounds during the first trimester and .8 pound each week for the remainder of your pregnancy. If you have not gained ten pounds by the twentieth week (eight pounds if you started out overweight), you are considered at high risk. After the twentieth week, a sudden sharp increase in weight can indicate that you are retaining dangerous amounts of water, so be sure and monitor your weight.

Morning sickness Often the first sign of pregnancy is nausea, or morning sickness. This symptom has been recognized as far back as Hippocrates and in the seventeenth century was even thought by the French physician Mauriceau to be beneficial. Obviously, Mauriceau never experienced it himself.

Morning sickness is probably not beneficial, but it is normal, occurring in almost half of all pregnant women in the first trimester. It can strike at any time, and last all day, but it is most common in the morning or when your stomach is empty.

To ease the symptoms of morning sickness, try the following:

- Eat small, frequent meals.
- If your worst time is in the morning, set a few plain crackers near your bed at night time and nibble on them before rising.
- Drink liquids slowly, and drink them between meals rather than with meals. Try apple or grape juice. Skimmed milk may be easier to handle than whole.
- Eat more breads, pasta, and potatoes.
- Foods rich in the vitamin pyridoxine (meats, vegetables, whole grains) can help relieve nausea. Prescribed B-complex vitamins, taken orally or by injection, have in some cases been successful.
- Avoid any foods that bring on nausea (for many women, these include coffee and fried or very spicy foods).
- Sleep in a room that has plenty of fresh air.
- If morning sickness persists beyond three months, consult your doctor.

Morning sickness can affect your health if it changes your eating habits. Be aware of any large weight gain (from overeating) or weight loss (from avoiding foods). If you are vomiting, you may lose precious water and salts, and your weight may begin to drop. This can be disastrous if you started your pregnancy poorly nourished because your fetus is in a critical stage of development. Have your doctor check out severe vomiting.

Indigestion The hormone progesterone relaxes certain muscles,

Pregnancy: The Blooming of the Womb

one of which sits between your esophagus and stomach. When this muscle relaxes, food in your stomach leaks back into the esophagus, causing heartburn. As your uterus enlarges, it shoves your stomach upward until your stomach is perched on top. The result is indigestion, belching, and a stuffed feeling. To lessen these symptoms, eat small, frequent meals, and do not lie down after eating. When sleeping, elevate your head and shoulders. Some women find that fatty foods make matters worse. Check with your doctor before taking antacids.

Constipation Hormones also slow down the passage of food through your stomach and intestines. The good news is that you have more time to absorb nutrients. The bad news is that you may get nauseated and constipated, or as Shakespeare delicately phrased it, "She came in great with child, and longing . . . for stewed prunes."

Constipation worsens later in pregnancy as the uterus enlarges and presses against the large intestine. Hard stools and impacted bowels can cause hemorrhoids. To lessen constipation, eat fresh fruits and vegetables, prunes, figs, dried beans, and whole-grain breads and cereals. Fiber attracts water, making stools softer and bulkier. Be careful not to eat too much fiber because it binds certain minerals and can drag them from the body. You could also get diarrhea. Drink plenty of fluids and exercise regularly. Do not take laxatives or enemas without contacting your doctor.

Food cravings In centuries past, people placed such importance on a pregnant woman's special food cravings that "longing" became a euphemism for "pregnant." People said if a woman ignored her longings, she would bear a monster. In John Webster's *Duchess of Malfi*, the duchess is proved pregnant by her "most vulterous eating" of apricots. An account, published in 1725, noted that such cravings ranged from the reasonable— wheat, corn, fresh bread, out-of-season fruits and vegetables— to the odd—lizards, frogs, and scorpions. (The most bizarre longing described in this particular account was that of the woman who wished to throw eggs in her husband's face.)

Food cravings and aversions are still common. Many women find their taste for calcium foods rise, while they cannot stand the thought of alcohol, caffeine, and meat. Of course, hamburger cravings are not uncommon. Sometimes after eating a previously craved food, a woman finds that she can no longer stand the sight of it. These slight changes in food preferences are harmless. You can satisfy cravings for sweets such as chocolate by eating small amounts without sacrificing your entire diet.

Pica Some cravings, however, can be damaging to both mother and fetus. Pica is the compulsion to eat unsuitable materials, such as charcoal, ashes, stones, gravel, baking soda, cornflour, mothballs, coffee grounds, laundry starch, and even the inner tubes of tires. Eating these nonfoods is, of course, dangerous. Some women with pica have become anemic or have experienced toxemia or high blood pressure.

Many of these nonfoods contain harmful levels of toxic metals. One full-term baby was born with lead poisoning due to his mother's eating wall plaster.

Cramps One cause of leg and back cramps and muscle weakness is an imbalance of the minerals calcium and phosphorus. You can often relieve these symptoms by consuming three to four glasses of milk daily and by limiting high-phosphorus foods, such as soft drinks and processed meats. If you get a leg cramp, which happens most frequently at night, pull your toes toward you to stretch the calf muscle. Then massage the muscle and apply a warm compress.

Anemia The most common nutritional problem of pregnancy is anemia, in which there are too few red blood cells or they are mis-shapen. An anemic woman cannot get enough oxygen to her fetus, so her baby may be born prematurely or have a low birth weight or stunted growth. It can even be mentally impaired. Most anemias result from too little iron.

During pregnancy, your body needs iron, folacin, and vitamin B_{12} to form red blood cells for the more than two extra pints of blood you will manufacture. Besides the extra iron required to form this blood, your baby is storing iron in its liver for its first few months of life. Luckily, your body snatches up iron from food with twice its usual efficiency. Over the course of pregnancy, you will absorb an extra 1,000 mg of iron, half of which you lose at delivery. If your diet is deficient in iron, you will drain your body's stores and feel tired, weak, and irritable. If your iron stores are low, your baby's will be, too.

Results of hemoglobin or hematocrit tests require careful analysis because, during pregnancy, the watery part of your blood increases more than the red blood cells—making for fewer red blood cells in a given volume of blood. This can show up as a false anemia. However, since iron needs are so high, many doctors routinely recommend a daily iron supplement during the latter part of pregnancy, just for insurance.

You can also become anemic if your diet is low in folacin or vitamin B_{12}. Folacin is needed for synthesis of the gene-carrier DNA and for normal growth of red blood cells. The faster cells multiply and grow, the more folacin is required.

With too little folacin, cells cannot regenerate and growth becomes sluggish. Folacin-deficiency anemia is not uncommon in pregnancy and can cause spontaneous abortion in the early months, or hemorrhage, fetal abnormalities, toxemia, and premature delivery. You are at risk if you were on the Pill shortly before becoming pregnant, have had many closely spaced pregnancies, or are chronically anemic. The best folacin sources are leafy greens, dried beans, whole grains, fruits and vegetables, liver, and yeast (see table E-4 in appendix E). Women at low risk can obtain sufficient folacin from their diets, but others should check with their doctors about taking a supplement.

Folacin's coworker in shaping red blood cells is vitamin B_{12}. A vitamin B_{12} deficiency causes pernicious anemia, a type that is rare during pregnancy, except among strict vegetarian women who avoid all animal products and do not use any B_{12} fortified foods.

Toxemia (preeclampsia-eclampsia) and edema In the United States, the number-one cause of death in pregnant women is toxemia of pregnancy. Early symptoms (preeclampsia) include puffy face, loss of appetite, blurred vision, severe headaches, high blood pressure, loss of protein in the urine, and rapid weight gain from retained water.

In the later stages of toxemia, called eclampsia, convulsions and coma occur. Infants of toxemic mothers are often born small and later in life show mental or motor abnormalities.

Some die soon after their birth. The longer toxemia lasts, the worse it is for the infant.

No one knows what causes toxemia, but fasting, stress, or a deficiency of protein, calories, or salt can worsen it. For a long time it was thought that too much salt was at fault, but this idea has been proved false. There is no reason to restrict salt during pregnancy.

Toxemia occurs more often in women who are very young, over thirty, or in their first pregnancy. Most at risk are women who are underweight at conception and do not gain weight normally during pregnancy, or who are overweight at conception and then gain too much. The best way to prevent this disorder is to enter pregnancy well nourished and to eat a balanced diet for the next nine months.

Most pregnant women who retain water never reach the advanced stage of toxemia. They simply get swollen ankles and legs (edema), which sometimes lead to varicose veins and lightheadedness.

If this happens, avoid standing or sitting for long periods of time. Put your feet up and lie on your side to rest or sleep. Exercise can help rid your body of water. Do not restrict sodium or salt, and do not use diuretics or other medications unless your doctor advises them. Do not worry about swollen legs or ankles unless the swelling is sudden. But if your face or hands swell up or you have any of the early symptoms of toxemia, see your doctor immediately.

Gestational diabetes Gestational diabetes is the form of diabetes that develops during pregnancy. No one knows whether pregnancy causes the diabetes or whether the stress of pregnancy unveils an existing but hidden condition. As your fetus grows, it demands more and more glucose (blood sugar). As you eat more food, your pancreas secretes more insulin, the hormone that allows cells to pick up glucose. The glucose of a woman who produces only marginal amounts of insulin may remain in her bloodstream and spill into her urine. Pregnancy may be the first time that she shows signs of diabetes, and that is one reason your doctor will check your urine.

You have a greater chance of becoming diabetic during pregnancy if you have a family history of the disease, have high

Pregnancy: The Blooming of the Womb

blood pressure, obesity, high levels of blood sugar, or have previously given birth to a large baby or one that was congenitally malformed. If you previously experienced gestational diabetes, see your doctor as soon as you suspect you are pregnant. By monitoring and controlling her blood sugar, a diabetic woman can deliver a healthy, full-term baby.

Here are some ways to control diabetes:

- Eat properly spaced meals to keep your blood sugar constant. This usually means three meals plus snacks at midmorning, late afternoon, and before bedtime.
- If you require insulin shots, take them on time and plan your meals accordingly. Keep a record of daily urine or blood tests.
- Keep your diet low in fat and sugar. Eat plenty of starches like dried beans, rice, and pasta.
- Eat enough calories so your baby can grow normally. Check with a dietitian about an appropriate meal plan.
- Exercise regularly.

If you become diabetic during pregnancy, you have a higher risk of becoming diabetic again later in life, so maintain a desirable weight, exercise regularly, and eat well.

Substances to avoid

Alcohol Alcohol damages babies—that much has been known for centuries. But only recently has one of the most devastating effects of alcohol (suspected for years) come to light.

Fetal alcohol syndrome, estimated to affect one out of every two thousand children born in the United States, causes growth and mental retardation, defective heart and organs, misshapen faces, central nervous system damage, and malformed arms, legs, and genitals. These children are often hyperactive and nervous, with a short attention span.

Because alcohol easily passes through membranes, it flows from a woman's blood through the placenta to the fetus. The fetus's liver is not fully developed and cannot detoxify the alcohol. If the mother is drunk, so is the baby.

The more you drink, the greater the risk. Even drinking one to three ounces of alcohol a day (to to six drinks) can lead to still-births and babies with low birth weights or with sleeping difficulties. Binge drinking, even if the total amount of alcohol is low, can cause these same effects. Cigarette smoking and drinking together create a nightmare for the fetus.

If you are pregnant, try to avoid alcohol completely. Short of that, have no more than one drink a day. Luckily, many women lose their taste for alcohol when they become pregnant. If you are trying to become pregnant, cut down on alcohol now because you can hurt your fetus during the time you are not yet aware that you are pregnant.

Caffeine Based on animal studies, some researchers suspected caffeine of causing birth defects, but the best and most recent study on humans refutes this (more on this in chapter 17). Though caffeine may not cause birth defects, heavy coffee drinking (four to six cups a day) can lead to babies who have a lower weight, are less active, and have poorer muscle tone. They may or may not exhibit abnormal behavior soon after birth. The risk of miscarriage, still-birth, and breach birth (a baby born buttocks first) increases.

When pregnant, you take more than half as long again to eliminate caffeine from your system as when you are not pregnant. Your fetus is even slower to get rid of it. Fetuses and newborns lack a certain enzyme, so it takes them three to four days to eliminate a dose of caffeine that an adult could metabolize in five to six hours. While pregnant, switch to decaffeinated coffee, weak tea, grain beverages (Postum or Benger's), or warm milk.

Saccharin Saccharin is a weak carcinogen for bladder cancer. That does not mean it causes a weak form of cancer, only that it affects fewer people. Saccharin can enhance the activity of other cancer-causing agents, like cigarettes. Certain individuals may be at higher risk of bladder cancer—among these are cigarette smokers and pregnant women. (Pregnant women who smoke are at even greater risk.) Many foods and beverages are no longer sweetened with saccharin but with aspartame, a product that some researchers believe has been inadequately tested. If possible, skip the diet soft drinks altogether and drink fruit juices and milk.

Pregnancy: The Blooming of the Womb

Prescribed and over-the-counter medications Most women take at least one medication during pregnancy. These include vitamin supplements, aspirin, antacids, diuretics, antibiotics, antihistamines, and barbiturates. Do not assume that if a drug is safe for you, it is safe for your baby, especially since your baby will receive a much higher dose for his weight.

When pregnant, never megadose with vitamin-mineral supplements, particularly vitamins A, D, C, and pyridoxine, and the minerals iodine and zinc. Vitamin A in daily amounts of 35,000–150,000 I.U. causes abnormalities in the kidney, urinary tract, and nerves of infants. Excess vitamin D can lead to abnormal calcium deposits and birth defects, so limit daily amounts to 10 mg. Megadoses of vitamin C can make babies so dependent on large doses that they exhibit deficiency signs after birth when the massive doses are discontinued. Cases of infantile seizures have been reported in infants whose mothers took megadoses of pyridoxine. Excess iodine can cause congenital goiter (an enlarged thyroid gland), but overdoses of iodine are rare unless you take kelp tablets (ten to twenty tablets a day) or supplements that contain iodine.

Nicotine Women who smoke tend to weigh less before pregnancy and gain fewer pounds during pregnancy. Nicotine can reduce the size of the placenta and indirectly lessen the amounts of nutrients your fetus receives. Smoking is so strongly associated with low birth weight in babies that some researchers at the Center for Disease Control in the United States suggest the problem be formally termed "fetal tobacco syndrome."

If you continue to smoke during pregnancy, at least stop as soon as labor pains begin. Your baby will get more oxygen during delivery.

EATING STRATEGY
Nutrient needs and the growing fetus

A good diet can reduce the risk of complications, improve your chances of delivering a healthy baby, put you in better health after pregnancy, and help ensure success with breastfeeding. That probably comes as no surprise. But did you know that your diet before pregnancy is just as critical? You could conceive

Eat Beautiful!

and be six weeks along in your pregnancy before you realize it (you may have missed one period). And during this time, much is happening.

For the first two weeks, the dividing cells are nourished directly from nutrients in your blood. Early in the fourth week, the placenta will take command of extracting nutrients from your blood and passing them on to your fetus. A poor diet, by stunting the size of your placenta, undermines these efforts and raises the chances of your fetus dying in the uterus.

In the early weeks of pregnancy, the rapidly dividing cells demand large amounts of vitamin B_{12} and folacin. From the fourth to the twelfth week, organs develop, and by eight weeks the central nervous system constitutes one-fourth of fetal weight. A poor diet at this time (including too much alcohol) can cause defective organs, yet you may still be unaware of your pregnancy.

As pregnancy progresses, you require more protein to build new tissue for the fetus, uterus, breasts, and blood. Too little can stunt your fetus's body and mind. Most British women consume enough protein unless they are dieting or eating only one or two meals a day.

At seven weeks, your fetus's skeleton begins to harden from cartilage into bone, and in the twentieth week its teeth calcify. Both events demand large amounts of calcium. If your diet is inadequate in calcium or vitamin D (which is needed to absorb calcium), the mineral will be pulled from your bones, a loss that can weaken you later in life.

Each day, consume three to four glasses of milk, whether whole, low-fat, skim, or buttermilk. Or substitute cheeses, yogurt, cottage cheese, or ice cream. You can add powdered milk to almost anything: casseroles, baked goods, meatloaf, soups, and desserts. If you cannot digest milk properly because of lactose intolerance, try low-lactose products such as natural cheeses, yogurt, buttermilk, or acidophilus milk, or add lactase enzyme (sold as Lact-Aid) to your regular milk. Other calcium sources include broccoli, spinach, kale, figs, nuts, or blackstrap molasses, though the calcium in these foods is less well absorbed. Table E-5 in appendix E shows calcium sources. If you cannot consume about 1,200 mg of calcium daily while pregnant, check with your doctor about taking a supplement.

Pregnancy: The Blooming of the Womb

To form strong bones and teeth you also need fluoride. If the water in your area is not fluoridated, check with your doctor about a supplement.

In the last months of pregnancy, your fetus grows longer and heavier. Organs, muscles, and bones have been constructed, but very little fat has been added. A baby born too early will have skin clinging to bone, with few fat underpinnings. During this time, be sure to eat enough calories and gain a sufficient amount of weight.

In the last trimester, your baby must also store nutrients for the future. If you are neglecting your diet, your baby may be born small or have immature systems. Such babies have a harder time surviving and, as infants and children, have more infections and illnesses.

Other critical nutrients Your need for other nutrients jumps during pregnancy, though not as much as for those already mentioned. To use the extra calories you are consuming, you need more thiamin, riboflavin, and niacin. Pyridoxine is required for you to use protein, vitamin A to form healthy epithelial tissues, and vitamin C to construct connective tissue. With too little vitamin C, fetal membranes may rupture. To obtain these vitamins, eat a balanced and varied diet.

Planning your meals

The three worst dietary habits you can adopt while pregnant are not eating enough food, not spacing meals throughout the day, and eating lots of junk food. As mentioned earlier, you can avoid the first and second by eating enough food to achieve a smooth, continuous weight gain and by eating small, frequent meals to keep up your blood sugar. Don't skip meals.

The third bad habit, eating the wrong foods, is just as easy to avoid. Over the nine months of gestation, you require about 80,000 extra calories, or 300 extra calories a day. Do not waste these extra calories on sugary and fatty foods. Instead select milk, cottage cheese, lean meats, eggs, dried beans, whole grains, fruit, and leafy greens. In your last two trimesters, eat the following each day:

- Milk or dairy products—1½ pints (2 pints for teenagers)

- Meat, fish, poultry, cheese, eggs, vegetable protein combinations—three to four servings
- Fruits and vegetables:
  Rich in vitamin C—one to two servings
  Rich in vitamin A—five servings a week
- Cereals and grains—four servings
- Vegetable oil—one to two tablespoons
- Fluids—six to eight glasses, plus milk

Table 3-1 shows a sample meal plan.

Improving your diet at any point in pregnancy will raise your infant's chances of surviving in the womb and having a healthy life after birth. It will also give you more energy after delivery to handle child care and breastfeeding.

Supplements

Take supplements only under your doctor's supervision. Some doctors will prescribe iron supplements, sometimes folacin and calcium and, for the strict vegetarian, vitamin B_{12}. Iron comes in different forms. Ferrous sulfate is the most easily absorbed. Any iron supplement may cause constipation (and black stools), so eat plenty of high-fiber foods, such as iron-fortified cereals, dried beans, and dried fruits such as prunes, figs, raisins, and apricots. If one iron supplement upsets your stomach, try another. Take iron in frequent small doses over the course of a day, preferably with a glass of orange or grapefruit juice. Vitamin C in the juice boosts iron absorption.

Exercise

In the 1952 summer Olympics, Juno Irwin won a bronze medal in platform diving—she was three and one-half months pregnant. Trina Hosmer, a United States Olympic cross-country skier in 1972, gave birth to her first child just two hours after running four miles.

Trina, like Juno, is unusual. Many women have trouble running four miles even before pregnancy. Though exceptional in her level of fitness, Trina knew what many women are just beginning to discover: Exercise during pregnancy can increase flexibility, decrease fatigue, lessen constipation and leg swelling, build up stamina and endurance, promote an easier delivery

Table 3-1 Sample meal for pregnancy

BREAKFAST

Start with one of these:

Egg (1)
Cheese (1 ounce)
Meat (2 ounces) or cooked legumes (½ cup)
Cooked cereal (½ cup) or dry cereal (1 cup), with 4–6 ounces of milk

Add:

Whole-grain bread (1 slice)
Butter or margarine (1 teaspoon)
Milk (6–8 fluid ounces)
Fruit: juice (4 fluid ounces) or grapefruit (½) or orange

LUNCH

Start with one of these:

Any choice from breakfast or serving of Soup or stew
Casserole

Add:

Vegetable, cooked
Vegetable, raw
Whole-grain bread (1 slice)
Butter or margarine (1 teaspoon)
Milk (6–8 fluid ounces)
Dessert (optional): some combination of milk, eggs, or fruit, such as puddings, custard, or fruit salad with yogurt

DINNER

Start with one of these:

Meat (2 ounces) or cooked legumes (½ cup)
Cheese (1 ounce)
Egg

Add:

Vegetables, cooked (1 or 2)
Vegetables, raw
Whole-grain bread (1 slice)
Butter or margarine (1 teaspoon)
Milk (6–8 fluid ounces)
Dessert: See lunch

SNACKS

Fruit juices with a cracker or slice of whole-grain bread
Small pieces of fruit or raw vegetables
Small pieces of cheese with cracker or bread
Yogurt with fruit

Eat Beautiful!

with fewer complications, and speed recovery. And you can have all of this without being an athlete. What is important is overall conditioning.

Before starting a workout program, check with your obstetrician. There may be special precautions if you have diabetes, hypertension, or cervical defects, or have previously experienced pregnancy loss.

The key to a successful exercise program is to get fit *before* pregnancy. If you are out of shape when you get pregnant and have no history of pregnancy-related problems, go ahead and exercise twenty to forty minutes at least three times a week. Try walking, swimming, or calisthenics, but be sure your heart rate returns to normal fairly quickly and is less than one hundred beats per minute five minutes after stopping. To avoid overheating, make certain that your temperature after exercising is no more than 101 degrees F. If it is higher, then the next time you exercise, work out for a shorter time. Avoid exercising in hot weather, wear light clothing, drink more fluids, and rest more frequently. If you need a nap after exercising, you are probably overdoing it.

For the first three months, your fetus should be safe, secure in the womb. But do not go beyond 65 percent of your maximum heart rate and do not exercise to exhaustion. (To determine heart rate, see chapter 7.) In the second trimester, the uterus rises up out of the bony pelvis that protects it. A healthy fetus will not shake loose, but avoid sports like skiing or climbing where you might fall or have a blow to your abdomen. As you put on weight, certain sports may stress your back and breasts. Swimming and stationary bicycling are good exercises to try at this time.

The level of exercise during the final three months depends on what you have been doing and how you feel. Avoid vigorous exercise unless it is part of your normal routine. If you have been extremely sedentary, stick to light exercises. For many women, the final three or four weeks are best spent stretching and going for short walks. Because of your heavier body and increased blood volume, you may tire more easily. Loose ligaments put strain on your lower spine, hip joints, knees, ankles, and feet. To avoid sprains and dislocations, warm up for at

Pregnancy: The Blooming of the Womb

least ten minutes before exercise. Also, do not exercise on an empty stomach.

Postpartum

Right after delivery you will lose weight equal to the weight of your baby, plus 1½ pounds for the placenta and 2 pounds for fluid. In the next two weeks, seven more pounds will drop from body fluids and decreased blood volume. In six weeks, you will have lost about twenty-one pounds if you are bottlefeeding and twenty-five pounds if you are breastfeeding. Since your body does not know if you intend to breastfeed, it packs about eight to nine pounds of fat on your abdomen, back, and thighs during pregnancy. If you do not breastfeed, you will have to eat less and exercise more to lose this fat.

After delivery, get your hemoglobin checked. Blood loss during delivery can be heavy, and iron losses may drain you of energy. Many women become so tired that for the first few months they give up eating, preferring to catch a few extra hours of sleep. If you find yourself in this situation, plan simple meals like sandwiches and soups and have on hand fresh fruits and vegetables, crackers, cheese, yogurt, canned beans, milk, and peanut butter. Even spaghetti sauce, made in batches and frozen, is easy to prepare.

After you give birth, eat adequate protein and vitamin C to help heal tissues torn during delivery. Women at greatest risk of nutritional deficiency are those with many closely spaced children. Delaying a second pregnancy for two to three years allows you to replenish any lost nutrients. This will favor your next child's health as well as your own. Get rid of any extra weight added during pregnancy before you get pregnant again.

Getting back in shape Exercising after pregnancy can not only firm up your body but help vanquish 'baby blues.' To tone stretched abdominal muscles, do simple isometric exercises. Start your first day postpartum. Progress slowly to more strenuous exercises, not so quickly that you find you are constantly fatigued. Try walking forty-five to sixty minutes a day. To avoid inflamation in your cervix, wait at least three weeks after delivery before you swim. Five to six weeks postpartum, try swimming or bicycling for forty-five minutes a day. At this time, competitive athletes can resume serious training.

Terminated pregnancies

If you have had a miscarriage, or a spontaneous or induced abortion, you may have lost enough blood to require extra iron. You should be screened for iron-deficiency anemia and be prescribed supplements if your iron reserves are low. Despite some claims, no evidence supports the notion that vitamin E supplements can prevent miscarriages.

A checklist for pregnancy

To help you make sense of all the information in this chapter, here are the basic rules you should follow when pregnant:

- Limit your overnight fast to twelve hours.
- Eat three meals a day, plus healthful snacks.
- Eat a variety of foods, including fresh fruits, vegetables, whole grains and cereals, dried beans, dairy products, eggs, lean meats, and fish. Avoid foods that offer little besides calories.
- Take supplements only if prescribed. These may include elemental iron daily and for two to three months postpartum, and folacin daily (not to exceed 1 mg).
- Drink at least six to eight glasses of fluid a day, not counting your milk intake.
- Use iodized salt. Do not restrict salt or use diuretics unless your doctor directs you to do so.
- Exercise—in particular, walk, swim, or attend prenatal exercise classes.

SPECIAL CONSIDERATIONS

The older mother

If you are one of the increasing number of women who become pregnant after age thirty-five, you have special needs. Generally, if you are healthy and at normal weight before pregnancy, your chances of a problem pregnancy are not much different from those of a younger woman. Though you are at a slightly greater risk for high blood pressure, other complications increase only if you are obese, or have diabetes, cardiovascular disease, or kidney disease. Because weight tends to increase with age, if you are overweight, try to reduce before getting pregnant. Even if you are normal weight, your metabolism has slowed down somewhat, so you need fewer calories. However, your need for protein, vitamins, and minerals does not drop, so it is essential that you eat high-quality foods.

The young mother

A girl can bear children even before she can perceive of herself as a mother—and often before she can understand the full impact of pregnancy. Yet a girl who becomes pregnant suddenly has to face two separate developing beings—her baby and herself. The younger a girl is, the greater her risk of toxemia, iron-deficiency anemia, and of delivering a premature baby or a baby with a low birth weight.

The diet must provide calories and nutrients not only for the growing teenager but for her developing baby. If a girl is not fully grown, she must gain beyond the recommended twenty-five to thirty pounds. One-forth of teenage pregnancies are complicated by to much weight gain, while many girls gain too little. Some teens worry so much about their figures that they begin a feast-and-fast routine.

The American College of Obstetrics and Gynecologists has formulated a general guide to daily energy needs for pregnant girls:

For ages 11–14   2,700 calories
For ages 15–18   2,400 calories

A pregnant teen can eat well and still enjoy such favourite foods as hamburgers, milkshakes (made with milk), pizza, and chili. Snacking can work to a pregnant teen's advantage if she avoids soft drinks, sweets, and other high-calorie but low-nutrient snacks. Nutrient needs are so high during pregnancy that a doctor may recommend daily supplements of iron, calcium and folacin. Of particular danger to pregnant teens are fads like macrobiotics, megavitamins, and severe weight-loss diets.

The vegetarian mother

In 1978, a six-month-old boy was admitted to the hospital in a coma. At birth, he had weighed 6.6 pounds and had appeared healthy. He developed normally on breast milk for four months. But then something happened. He began to eat poorly and became cranky. He could not control his head, his eyes wandered randomly, and when examined, he did not respond. Doctors diagnosed him as being severely anemic, but not from lack of iron. It was a vitamin B_{12} deficiency.

For eight years his mother had been a strict vegetarian, shunning all animal products and taking no vitamin supplements. Though she herself showed no deficiency symptoms, her infant was unable to store enough vitamin B_{12} while in the womb, and after birth he received little of the vitamin from his mother's milk. Once vitamin B_{12} therapy was begun, he became alert and responsive—and smiled.

This case does not suggest that if you are a vegetarian, you should not become pregnant, or that if you become pregnant, you should start eating meat. It suggests that if you are a vegetarian, you cannot afford to be careless. There are different degrees of vegetarianism, and the more you restrict animal products, the more you need to plan. The one diet to avoid is the highest level of the Zen macrobiotic diet, which limits you to grains and water.

Because vegetarian diets are high in fiber and tend to fill you up quickly, many vegetarian women eat too few calories. These women may begin pregnancy at low weights or they may gain too few pounds during pregnancy. If you are not gaining weight at the appropriate rate, eat more high-calorie foods.

If your calories are too low, your protein probably is, too. To use protein, your body needs all the eight essential amino acids in the right proportions. This means combining grains, beans, and vegetables (see chapter 16). Vegans, those who eat no animal products, including eggs, milk, and cheese, will have the hardest time getting all the essential nutrients, but with some care it can be done.

Pregnancy: The Blooming of the Womb

Complications in pregnancy

Certain situations require special nutritional needs. Women who know beforehand that they will deliver by caesarean section should plan for it by eating extra servings of leafy greens, two more servings of whole-grain cereals and breads, an extra serving of protein, and an extra daily serving of a vitamin C-rich fruit or vegetable in the week prior to surgery. These foods are rich in nutrients that help speed recovery and reduce the chances of abnormal bleeding and infection.

If you have ever delivered a premature or stillborn baby or one with a low birth weight, you have a special reason to eat well during pregnancy. If you are late in delivering your baby, continue to eat a balanced diet because your baby is still growing and relying on you for nourishment.

4
Breastfeeding: Woman as Alchemist

> She had the distinct impression that his lips were
> pulling from her a thread of light. It was as if she
> were a cauldron issuing spinning gold.
>
> Toni Morrison, *Song of Solomon*

Searching for a universal cure for human maladies, medieval alchemists concocted various potions, always hoping to find *aurum potable*—liquid, drinkable gold. They believed that gold, being perfect, could bestow its perfection on the human frame. This golden nostrum eluded them and their successors, yet it was as close as the nearest wetnurse. The liquid is breast milk.

The perfect baby food

Benefits to your baby Like the alchemist's mythical elixir, breast milk is perfect—at least for your baby. High in two proteins, lactalbumin and lactoglobulin, it stays soft when drenched with stomach acid and forms a curd that is easy to digest. The amino acids in breast milk are arranged in the right proportion for a baby's growth, whereas cow's milk is high in the amino acid phenylalanine, which babies may have difficulty metabolizing.

Breast milk has less saturated fat than cow's milk and is high in the essential fat called linoleic acid. It also contains an enzyme that digests fat even before it has reached a baby's intestines. Breast milk is rich in cholesterol, which babies need to form cell membranes and nerve tissue. The carbohydrate lactose is plentiful in breast milk and is easily handled by a baby's immature system.

Breast milk resembles the alchemists' remedy in another way. It contains factors that help babies resist infection. Bifidus factor, for instance, is fertilizer to intestinal organisms that fight harmful bacteria. Breast milk can even pass on antibodies. What all this means is that breastfed babies have fewer infections of the ear and lower respiratory tract, less vomiting and diarrhea, and fewer allergies. Your baby will benefit from any amount of breastfeeding, even if you stop after six weeks instead of persevering for the recommended four to six months.

Breastfed infants are less apt to become obese. Your milk is half-fat at the end of a nursing period, so it fills up your baby and cues it to stop feeding. A woman who bottlefeeds will be less certain when her baby is full and may urge him to polish off the last few ounces in the bottle, unintentionally stuffing him. Sucking at the breast exercises muscles and develops well-formed jaws and straight teeth.

Benefits to Mom   Oxytocin, a hormone that releases milk from the breast, contracts the uterus and shrinks it more quickly to normal size, lessening the chance of hemorrhage. These contractions, plus the calories you lose through breast milk, can help whittle down your figure. Breastfeeding can delay ovulation but is not a failsafe method of birth control.

PHYSICAL CHANGES

Anatomy of a breast

Fat and glandular tissue give your breasts their size and shape. As you age or have children, you add on more fat, and your breasts may get bigger. But big breasts do not guarantee more milk. Breast milk comes from the glandular tissue, and even if your breasts appear small to you, you should have enough of this tissue to nurse.

Within each breast are twenty or so lobes bunched together like grapes with ducts leading to collecting pools. In a mature woman, each lobe is further divided into lobules, and each lobule into several small sacs. Lining the sacs are cells that produce and expel milk. Surrounding the sacs are cells that squeeze the milk through the ducts, into the pools, and out the nipple.

As soon as your infant suckles, this apparatus kicks into gear. Nerves from your breast relay the message "Kid is nursing" to your brain. The pituitary gland in the brain releases the hormone prolactin, which wends its way through your blood to milk-producing cells and starts them working. The more your infant suckles, the livelier this process.

Your baby's suckling also triggers the let-down reflex—that is, the release and ejection of milk through your nipple pores into your infant's mouth. When first put to the breast, your infant might suck for a minute or two before your milk is let down. Once let-down starts, your breast will tingle, a sensation that ranges from sexually exciting to quite painful, at least at first. Other things can stimulate this reflex: the cry of your infant (or any infant!) or even thoughts of your baby. The reflex is inhibited by fear, anxiety, depression, embarrassment, or pain.

For the first few days after delivery, your breasts secrete colostrum, a thin, watery fluid that resembles diluted orange juice. This early milk provides fewer calories than later mature milk but is loaded with several factors that fight infection. It is also a laxative and cleans out the dark feces (meconium) from a newborn's intestines. Between the third and tenth day, colostrum changes to a thin fluid, bluish like skim milk.

The more often your infant nurses during the first few weeks of life, the more milk you produce—a basic supply-and-demand situation. When your infant sucks your breast dry, you release more milk at the next feeding. When he does not empty the breast, you produce less milk in the next round. If your baby stops sucking or if you give formula during the first two weeks, your milk supply may start to dwindle—or stop altogether—and any milk waiting in the collecting pools will be reabsorbed.

After two weeks of breastfeeding, an occasional bottle should not decrease milk supply, especially if you express the milk from a skipped feeding into a sterile container and save it for the next bottle feeding. By the end of the second month, give your baby a bottle or two so that when you're away during a normal feeding, sucking from a bottle will be more routine and less traumatic. For the first four to six months, breast milk alone can provide complete nutrition for your baby's needs.

PSYCHOLOGICAL CHANGES

During the first few months of nursing, common feelings range from ecstasy to depression to inadequacy—even resentment. First-time mothers often fret over whether they are producing enough milk, especially since they cannot actually see what their babies are consuming. Others worry about their figures or feeling chained down.

If you are anxious or frustrated, you could set up an endless cycle of problems. Anxiety reduces your milk secretion; your baby is frustrated, bawls, and shakes her little fists at you; you become more anxious and insecure; you secrete less milk. Women with too little milk usually have no physical problem but are anxious or overtired. Learn relaxation techniques and breastfeed when you are relatively unstressed (if such a time exists for the new mother).

Breastfeeding bonds mother and child. The hormone prolactin fosters "nurturing" feelings. You can experience similar feelings if you bottlefeed, but if rushed, you may "prop" the bottle—effectively cutting off bonding. Ultimately, however, how you feed your infant is less important to bonding than a relaxed, comfortable environment.

HEALTH CONCERNS

You may start out enthusiastic about breastfeeding, but a few days or weeks into it, you may hit a snag: your breasts hurt, your milk supply appears to have dried up, your infant is howling and always seems hungry. The problems you may encounter with breastfeeding will affect your infant's nutrition more than yours, but that, of course, is just as important at this point. Usually the problems can be overcome with a few changes and a little patience. By knowing beforehand what situations may develop, you can deal with them calmly and without immediately calling your womanhood into question.

Fatigue Breastfed babies feed more often than bottlefed babies—at first every two to three hours, then slowing down by the end of the first month. An inexperienced mother may allow her baby to nurse for an hour on each breast, only to find that after two hours it is (sigh) time to start over. A baby gets most of your milk in the first five minutes of nursing, and though a baby needs to suckle even when full, nursing for fifteen to twenty minutes on each breast is sufficient.

Night feedings are another immense joy for new mothers. A

newborn's digestive system cannot hold large amounts of milk, yet he grows faster in this first year of life than at any other time. As a result, he get hungry during the six to eight hours when you want to sleep. To avoid chronic fatigue, rest during the day while your baby naps.

Poor let-down The first sign of poor let-down is a baby who sucks for a while and soon becomes frustrated, squirmy, and decidedly annoyed. Your breasts will not tingle or feel full and tender. To bring on the let-down reflex, relax. Before nursing, have something warm to drink. Take a hot shower or bath, or apply a warm towel or heating pad to your breast. Gently massage your breasts. Feeding on a fairly regular schedule can make the reflex more automatic. If your milk refuses to budge, contact your doctor.

Sore nipples To toughen your nipples and prevent soreness, alternate your breasts at each feeding and limit the nursing period on each breast to five minutes until your milk supply is established. (It helps to start toughening your nipples two to three months before delivery by rubbing them with a rough washcloth, exposing them to air each day, or rolling the nipples between thumb and forefinger once or twice a day.) If your baby has not grasped the entire areola (the brownish area around the nipple), only the end of the nipple, her efforts to squeeze out milk will be futile. She will be frustrated and hungry, and you will have one *sore* nipple.

Before removing your baby from your breast, break the suction by inserting your little finger between your breast and your baby's mouth. Do not use soap or alcohol on the nipples; this can dry and crack them. Keep your nipples supple with baby oil or cold cream. Allow air to circulate around the nipple area.

Nipple soreness is temporary, but if you stop nursing, your milk ducts may become clogged, engorging your breasts and possibly causing infection. Follow your doctor's advice on alleviating the condition.

Clogged ducts If your milk ducts fail to drain completely, the remaining milk can clog them. Your glands continue pumping milk into the duct, where it builds up, causing breast swelling

Breastfeeding: Woman as Alchemist

and tenderness. Unremedied, the situation can cause infected glands—an extremely painful experience. To avoid this:

- Nurse more often and for a longer period of time
- Let your baby empty the affected breast first
- Change position for each feeding so your baby will exert pressure on different ducts
- Express milk from the sore breast, removing as much as possible.

Breast infection Breast infections result from a clogged duct or staphylococcal infection carried from your baby. You may feel hot and have aches, a headache, and fever. If your breast becomes infected, contact your doctor. Go to bed and apply heat to your breast. Continue to nurse, but offer your baby the sore breast first so it is more likely to be emptied of milk. This clears up the infection more quickly. (Your baby will not become ill from an infected breast—she probably has got the same germs you do.)

Swollen breasts In the first few days after delivery, your breasts may swell from the pressure of newly produced milk. When engorged, breasts become hard and tender. If they swell, your baby may only be able to fit the end of your nipple into her mouth. Again, her fruitless sucking on the nipple tip will cause soreness.

Breast engorgement is a serious—but common—problem. Ice bags or cold cloths on the breasts can reduce swelling and dull the pain. Switch to heat on the breasts right before feeding to trigger the let-down reflex. Massage your milk down to the pool, and hand-express it to reduce some of the fullness so your baby can get a solid grasp of the breast. Call your doctor for further advice.

Too little milk If your baby loses weight, she may not be getting enough milk. To establish a good milk supply:

- Place your baby on a frequent and flexible schedule.
- Nurse often in the first few weeks after delivery.
- Leave your baby at each breast for at least five minutes to establish the let-down reflex.

Drink plenty of fluids and eat foods high in calcium and protein. If your baby's weight continues to drop, contact your doctor. You may have to switch to bottlefeeding.

Substances to avoid

Alcohol Alcohol passes through breast milk, and large amounts affect not only your baby but your ability to breastfeed. But a couple of glasses of beer or wine will not harm your baby and may relax you enough to aid the let-down reflex.

Caffeine and nicotine Caffeine in breast milk can make an infant jittery. Newborns may require three to four days to eliminate a dose of caffeine that takes an adult only five to six hours to metabolize.

Smoking can decrease your milk supply, but so can the stress of giving up cigarettes. Much of the nicotine from cigarettes that gets into breast milk is detoxified in a baby's liver and kidneys. Yet infants may still become nauseated, vomit, have diarrhea, or have a rapid heart rate. So try to stop smoking or cut back.

Drugs Breast milk can transport over one hundred different drugs and chemicals, particularly fat-soluble ones. Because the toxicity of a drug depends on the body weight of the user, an infant can receive a full dose even if your breast milk contains only small amounts. Also, your baby's enzyme system is immature and its kidneys poorly developed, so it has a tough time detoxifying drugs. Older infants can better tolerate them.

Drugs to avoid include aspirin, antibiotics (penicillin, ampicillin, chloramphenicol, Flagyl, and others), psychoactive drugs (Valium, Lithium, Thorazine, chloral hydrate), thyroid drugs, and anticancer drugs. Check with your doctor before taking any drug. If you are on prescribed drugs and your doctor says to continue breastfeeding, take the drug shortly after nursing so you can detoxify as much as possible before the next feeding.

Marijuana The active component of marijuana is fat-soluble and passes into breast milk. Though the long-range effects are unknown, reports have indicated that its active ingredient gets concentrated in breast milk and absorbed by the baby. Breastfed infants have been known to become drowsy after their mothers smoked marijuana.

Oral contraceptives and IUD Infants of nursing mothers who use the Pill grow at a slower rate. Little is known about the effects of these hormones on a baby's developing endocrine system, but taking the combination Pill before six weeks postpartum can diminish milk production. Women who have an IUD inserted any time during the breastfeeding period stand a greater risk of a perforated uterus.

Pesticides Pesticides such as DDT, DDE, hexachlorobenzene and industrial chemicals such as PCBs and PBBs have been found in human milk. Most nutritionists and pediatricians believe the advantages of breastfeeding far outweigh the risks, but to minimize your infant's exposure:

- Avoid excessive weight loss while nursing because this quickly turns over fat cells and any fat-soluble chemicals they contain, pushing them into the bloodstream and into your milk
- Choose low-fat foods because most pesticide residues are fat-soluble
- Avoid using aerosol sprays containing pesticides
- If you live in an area where there has been an industrial accident, have your breast milk checked for these chemicals and discuss the issue with your doctor.

Nutrient needs

Assuming that you ate well during pregnancy, the only changes to make now are getting more calories and fluids. While breastfeeding, you need about 600 extra calories a day. (You are spending closer to 1,000 calories a day, but remember that fat you added during pregnancy? Now is the time to burn it up. It will last you for about three months, then you need to eat more food.) You might require even more than 600 extra calories a day if you gained fewer than twenty-six pounds during pregnancy, nurse more than one infant, or continue nursing after three months if your infant is getting only breast milk.

Breastfeeding takes so much energy that many nursing

mothers, after weaning their babies, end up weighing less than they did before pregnancy. If you are overweight, this is a good time to get in shape.

If you want to diet while nursing, wait until after the first month. For the first couple of weeks, establish your nursing pattern and follow the dictates of your appetite. Then begin cutting back on sugary or fatty foods. Eat plenty of dried beans, low-fat dairy products, lean meats, whole grains, and fresh fruits and vegetables. Find creative low-fat recipes (see recipes in appendix D). If you find weaning stressful, put your diet on hold. Continue to cut back on calories as long as your infant is growing well and shows no signs of unrelieved hunger and as long as your breasts remain full. If your weight falls below that desirable for your height, you may be restricting calories too severely.

If you do not drink about three quarts of fluids a day, you may become dehydrated. This extra need for fluids usually leads to greater thirst, but if not, make a conscious effort to drink a glass of water, juice, or milk right before or during nursing. (You do not have to drink milk to produce milk.) Try homemade soups. They can be frozen and easily reheated. Avoid drinking a lot of coffee or tea because these are diuretics and can pull water from your body.

A poor diet may reduce your milk supply, but what you produce will still be high quality. How this happens is simple: your body drains its nutrient stores. The flip side is that during your breastfeeding months, your body's efficiency at absorbing nutrients—like iron and calcium—jumps. So by eating well, you can end up healthier after nursing than before you were pregnant.

Recommendations

You can get all the nutrients you need for nursing by following this daily guide:

- Milk (or the equivalent in dairy products)—four servings (nursing teenagers should make this five servings)
- Meat or other protein sources—at least two servings
- Fruits and vegetables—at least four servings
  Vitamin C source—one

Vitamin A source—four to five times a week
- Bread and cereals (enriched, fortified, or whole grain)—four servings

In theory, you need extra protein, but chances are you probably already get enough. Instead of eating more meat, drink extra milk so you get your extra protein, calcium, fluid, and calories all at once. Table 4-1 shows a sample meal plan.

For the extra servings of food, indulge in a midmorning and midafternoon snack. No foods, including spices, need to be avoided unless they upset your infant. In some babies, cabbage, cauliflower, broccoli, brussels sprouts, onions, garlic, and rhubarb can cause gas within hours. Too many sweets or fruits can give some babies diarrhea.

Supplements Your doctor will probably recommend that you continue any multivitamin-mineral supplements from pregnancy. Because your menstrual flow is scanty while you breastfeed, you can use this time to build up your iron reserves. (You lose this advantage if you are bottlefeeding, so you may be given a supplement for a few months.) If you cannot consume milk or dairy products, you will need a calcium supplement. If you were a long-term user of the Pill before pregnancy, you may need a pyridoxine supplement. Vegetarian mothers who do not eat any animal products should have a reliable source of vitamin B_{12}, even if it is a supplement. (More on vegetarianism in chapter 16.)

Megadosing with vitamins or minerals can be risky. Toxic levels of vitamin A in particular can enter breast milk.

SPECIAL CONSIDERATIONS

The working woman

When my husband and I first decided to get married, we were referred to a woman minister. We arrived at her office and knocked, but the only response was a strange, rhythmic, mechanical noise. My husband said it sounded like a broken Xerox machine. "No, Paul," I replied, "*that* is a breast pump." Looking back, I can think of no more appropriate introduction to modern marriage than a woman at her office desk struggling to pump her milk.

Table 4-1 Sample meal plan for breastfeeding mothers

BREAKFAST

Start with one of these:

Egg
Meat (2 ounces) or cooked legumes (½ cup)
Cheese (¾–1 ounce)
Cooked cereal (½ cup) or dry cereal (1 cup), with 4–6 ounces of milk

Add:

Whole-grain bread (1 slice)
Butter or margarine (1 teaspoon)
Milk (8–10 fluid ounces)
Fruit: juice (4 fluid ounces) or grapefruit (½) or orange

LUNCH

Start with one of these:

Any choice from breakfast or serving of soup or stew
Casserole

Add:

Vegetables, cooked (1)
Vegetables, raw (1)
Fruit juice (4 ounces) or piece of fruit
Whole-grain bread (2 slices)
Butter or margarine (1 teaspoon)
Milk (8–10 fluid ounces)
Dessert: some combination of milk, eggs, or fruit, such as puddings, custard, or fruit salad with yogurt

DINNER

Start with one of these:

Meat (2 ounces) or cooked legumes (½ cup)
Cheese (1 ounce)
Egg

Add:

Vegetables, cooked (1 or 2)
Vegetables, raw (1)
Whole-grain bread (1 slice)
Butter or margarine (1 teaspoon)
Milk (6–8 fluid ounces)
Dessert: See lunch

SNACKS

Fruit juices with a cracker or piece of bread
Small pieces of fruit or raw vegetables
Small piece of cheese with cracker or bread
Yogurt with fruit
Drink plenty of fluids, such as water, juices, decaffeinated beverages

Breastfeeding: Woman as Alchemist

Nursing on the job is not easy, but then again it is not impossible. And it can be well worth the extra time and frustration. Here are suggestions to make it easier:

- Take two to six months' maternity leave to get your milk supply established.
- Go back to work part-time and keep flexible hours. If your baby is good for a four-hour stretch, you should be able to make all but one feeding.
- If you work full-time, feed your baby in the morning, say at eight, then try to get home for the evening feeding, at four or five.
- If you work close to home or your baby's day care center, nurse at lunchtime. If not, see if your sitter, mother, or friend can bring him to work for his midday feeding. (Find a comfortable place to nurse, even if it's your car.)
- If you cannot nurse at lunchtime, express your milk into a sterile container by hand or with a hand pump (admittedly, both can be difficult to do) or rent the more efficient electric pump. Breast milk will keep forty-eight hours in a refrigerator, two weeks in a refrigerator freezer (several months if the freezer is kept at 0 degrees), or two years in a deep-freeze. Thaw the milk by leaving it in the refrigerator for a few hours and then running it under warm tap water. This milk can be given to your baby when you are away. Expressing your milk helps to maintain your milk supply, but if this is too troublesome, buy a formula for these times.

Work and home pressures may begin to intrude into your nursing time. But make an effort to relax. Take a warm bath, put on some music, drink a warm beverage. Have a quiet, leisurely nursing period with your baby. Enlist the help of your partner. Let him take care of the house and run household errands. Forget about making any major career moves for a while, particularly if they will add more pressure on you.

If your milk supply falls off, take a day off from work, rest, drink a lot of fluids, and nurse almost continuously. Your milk supply—and you—will be rejuvenated.

For many women, the hardest part about returning to a job after giving birth is that their thoughts keep straying to their infant. Continuing to breastfeed after resuming your job may soften the separation. "With the onset of the first pangs of birth pains, one begins to say farewell to one's baby," Princess Grace of Monaco once remarked. "With the child at one's breast, one keeps the warmth of possession a little longer."

RESOURCES

La Leche League of Great Britain, PO Box BM 3424, London WC1V 6XX.

FURTHER READING

Messenger, Máire. 1982. *The Breastfeeding Book*. Century.

Stanway, Drs Andrew and Penny. 1978. *Breast is Best*. Pan.

5
Middle Adulthood: Menopause and the Midlife Molt

> Middle age is the time when life really begins. The kids have finished college and got jobs and the dog has died.
>
> Carol Saline, *Philadelphia Magazine*

If "life" is over at menopause, *somebody* forgot to tell Annabel Marsh. At age sixty-one, Annabel and her friend Caroline Merrill, forty-two, became the first women to run across the United States—from Boston to San Francisco. At a rate of fifteen miles every morning and fifteen miles every afternoon, they wore out twenty-four pairs of running shoes and devoured uncountable mounds of hot fudge sundaes. Interviewed afterward, Annabel said that she planned to return to golfing; Caroline hoped to pursue tap dancing.

Not only is one in every five people in Britain between ages forty-five and sixty-five, but, after menopause, close to a third of a woman's years are left.

PHYSICAL CHANGES
Menopause: when estrogen packs its bags

The climacterium is the stage of life when your reproductive years bid farewell. Menopause is but a small part of this leave-taking.

From puberty until your forties and fifties, hundreds of follicles in your ovaries have matured into eggs while thousands more have degenerated and disappeared. Only the least responsive ones remain. Exhausted, your ovaries allow their estrogen and progesterone production to dwindle.

With menopause, your estrogen levels drop. Your adrenal glands continue to pump out a less powerful form of estrogen called estrone, converted from weak male hormones in your fat cells. Obese women with their extra fat cells produce more estrone and may bleed for a longer time after they have stopped ovulating.

Shorter menstrual cycles may last for two to seven years, but menopause is "official" when your periods have stopped for one year. This usually happens between ages forty and sixty. At the turn of the century, the average menopausal woman in the United States was forty-five. Now American and British women are reaching menopause closer to fifty or fifty-one, though cigarette smoking hastens it.

Surgical menopause refers to a young woman who has both of her ovaries or uterus surgically removed. Removing the ovaries leads to more severe symptoms than removing only the uterus, for with the ovaries goes the estrogen. Surgical menopause seems to bring on more severe symptoms than natural menopause, especially after age thirty.

The good news is that if you have suffered for years with premenstrual syndrome, menopause will bring relief. The not-so-good news is that menopause presents its own discomforts, the most common complaints being sweating, vaginal dryness, and hot flashes.

As many as three out of every four menopausal women experience hot flashes. In general, thin Caucasian and Asian women seem to be affected the most. Heavier women, who have more fat cells to produce estrone, have the mildest symptoms. However, some obese women have severe hot flashes while some thin women have none.

As annoying as hot flashes can be, they will not affect your health unless they interfere with your eating a balanced diet. They usually subside within two years.

What little information is available on how nutrition can lessen the discomforts of menopause is based on doctors' reports of successful treatments. These reports point the way for future research, but they cannot serve as a common recommendation for every woman.

Some doctors recommend vitamin E (30–300 mg) to minimize hot flashes. They say it may take two to six weeks for the symptoms to lessen. Other researchers have found that vitamin E has no effect on these symptoms. Only take these massive doses under your doctor's supervision.

Middle Adulthood: Menopause and the Midlife Molt

PSYCHOLOGICAL CHANGES

How you react to menopause depends a lot on how you feel about yourself and about aging. If you are in good health and spend time doing things that make you feel productive and give you a sense of worth, you are less likely to experience severe symptoms. If you had an easy time of menarche or pregnancy, you will probably have no trouble with menopause. If you found these earlier stages of life threatening, you will probably feel the same now.

Besides menopause, other midlife challenges materialize. Some women begin to assess their lives up to this time and find their self-questioning not unlike that of adolescence: Who am I? Where am I going? How on earth did I get here? Ursula DeVane, forty-four, one of the main characters in Gail Godwin's *The Finishing School*, proclaims to her fourteen-year-old protégée: "We are both at crucial turning points in our lives. In a strange way, the adolescent and the middle-aged person are neither one thing nor the other: they are both in the process of molting, of turning into something else."

After reviewing her life, one woman may retreat, depressed at what she sees. Her sense of worth, if tied to her children, may vanish as the children leave home. She may feel unappreciated and possibly burdened if she is caring for her elderly parents. Misunderstandings may develop with her spouse. Time presses in, and she realizes she is not going to live forever.

Another woman may look at herself and decide to expand her horizons. She may join an aerobics dance class, revamp her diet, restyle her hair, and be delighted to find that she actually looks and feels better in her fifties than when she was younger. Many women consider it the best time of life.

HEALTH CONCERNS

Until you reach forty, you assume your body will respond to your commands. Sometime in middle age you begin to hear the faint rumblings of trouble. After that tour of Bavarian cafes, an extra five pounds of fat hugs your waist, resisting all efforts to pry them loose. Suddenly, rich foods, long a staple of your diet, trigger heartburn. You decide to take up an exercise program but the walk from your car to the gym leaves you breathless.

At the turn of the century, a menopausal woman could count on about five more years of life. Today she can look forward to twenty-five to thirty more years. As a result, conditions that develop over time—arthritis, heart disease, cancer, hypertension, and diabetes—begin to threaten. Some of these disorders are associated with your lifelong eating habits. How you lived your life as a young woman and what you choose to do in your later years can determine whether or not you are better off than your great-grandmother.

Osteoporosis

Margaret had always been small for her age. Her slim figure and short, curly blond hair gave her an ageless look. She was always a pack-a-day smoker and relied on coffee to keep her going at the office when she had no time for lunch. She rarely exercised, except to bend down to get the morning paper.

At age forty-six, Margaret had a natural menopause. Nothing was too uncomfortable, just sporadic hot flashes and occasional headaches for a year. She was in good health up until her sixty-seventh birthday, when she fractured a wrist prying open a stuck window. Not long after, her lower back began to ache, and within a few years she suffered crushed vertebrae in her spine, shrinking three inches in height. In a few years' time, Margaret had lost her youthful appearance and spent her later years hunched over, her shoulders drooped as if in defeat.

Margaret has osteoporosis, a condition compared to an overbent wire in which the bones become so weak and porous they easily break. Osteoporosis affects one out of every four women over sixty. It causes 190,000 broken hips a year. Of those women who fracture a hip, one in five will die from complications such as pneumonia or blood clots caused by prolonged bed rest. Of those ninety or older, one in six will die within three months.

The beginnings of osteoporosis After age thirty-five, both men and women lose bone mass as a natural part of aging. In the first five to six years after menopause, the rate accelerates, then drops off. If your bones lose too much mass, they become so

Middle Adulthood: Menopause and the Midlife Molt

fragile that a blow, a fall, or stress from lifting a light weight—things that pose no problem for the average woman—may fracture them.

The early signs of osteoporosis are easy to miss. But there are clues. Periodontal disease, for instance, can be a sign that your lower jawbone, like other osteoporotic bones, has become weak and porous. Another clue is low back pain. Most women simply dismiss this pain.

A woman can fracture a hipbone by falling, or the fracture can occur first, causing the fall. Wrist and arm fractures are also common. In fact, once you reach age sixty, the risk of your fracturing a forearm jumps ten times over that of a man. Osteoporosis progresses so slowly that small fractures may heal before a complete break occurs. Other times the break is not clean but "shattered bone," which does not heal easily. Standing up quickly or raising a window can cause a vertebra in the spine to collapse, so that four or five vertebrae may fit in a space previously occupied by only three. In serious cases, this compression tilts the rib cage downward and settles it on the top of the hipbone, the ribs pushing out the internal organs. A woman will develop an outward curve or "dowager's hump" of her upper spine, an inward curve of her lower spine, a protruding abdomen, and lose one to eight inches or more in height (see figure 5-1). Because of this shift, she may feel pressure on the nerves, pulled muscles, and joint pain that can lead to arthritis.

Added to the physical pain is the emotional trauma of suddenly being disabled and disfigured. For many women, whether they are thirty-five or seventy, fracturing a bone is the first time they feel old.

Risk factors Whether your bones become excessively porous depends on two things: how much bone you had at age thirty-five or so, and how fast you lose that bone. These things depend on your genes, diet, and health habits. Here are the risk factors for osteoporosis:

- Heredity: Having a grandmother, mother, aunt, or sister who has osteoporosis
- Being female: Women have smaller bones and more time for bone loss because they live longer

Eat Beautiful!

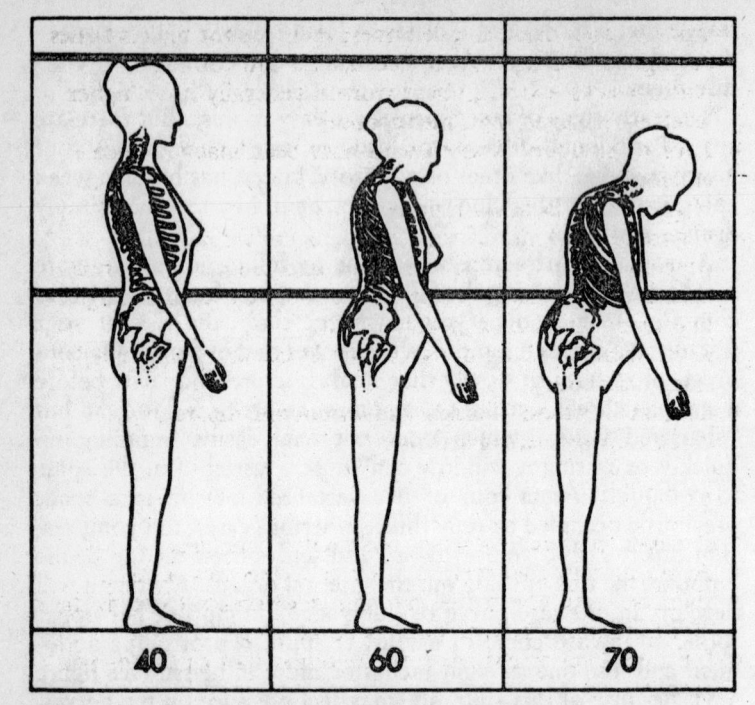

Figure 5-1 Osteoporosis: how older women lose height Spinal vertebrae weakened by osteoporosis collapse causing loss of height (from the upper part of the body), inward curvature of the lower spine, outward curvature of the upper spine, and protruding of the abdomen.

Highest risk: Women who become pregnant or breastfeed *and* whose diets are low in calcium
- Menopause: The earlier the menopause, the higher the risk
Highest risk: Women who have had a surgical menopause
- Ethnic Background: British, Northern European, Chinese, or Japanese; Jewish women are at moderate risk
- Stature and Build: Short, medium-height, and slender women
Highest risk: The anorexic because she is extremely thin, consumes very little food (or calcium), and may stop menstruating, a condition that accelerates bone loss (obese

women rarely have fragile bones; their weight makes bones stronger and denser. Also, because fat can convert androgens to estrone, obese women generally have higher levels of estrogen after menopause)
- Lack of Exercise: Women who have been inactive since childhood
  Highest risk: Bedridden patients
- Cigarette Smoking: Three-fourths of the women who develop osteoporosis are smokers, and most smoke more than a pack a day (smokers reach menopause an average of five years earlier than nonsmokers)
- Diet: Women whose diets are low in calcium, particularly since childhood
- Certain Diseases: Women with endocrine disorders, diabetes, rheumatoid arthritis

To reduce your risk:

- Eat well, particularly when pregnant or nursing.
- Avoid forcing your weight down to a very low level.
- Exercise regularly, especially from adolescence through the mid-thirties when bone mass is developing.
- Stop smoking or cut back on the number of cigarettes you smoke.
- Eat calcium-rich foods such as skim or low-fat dairy products, leafy greens, and soybeans.
- Take a supplement if you cannot get adequate calcium in your diet.

Treating osteoporosis

Hormone-replacement therapy (HRT) Replacing estrogen prevents bone loss, even six years after menopause, but it does not make bone more dense, nor does it strengthen already weakened bones. Some studies show a 60 percent decrease in hip, wrist, and spine fractures in women whose HRT began within a few years of menopause. (If the estrogen is discontinued, bone loss once again accelerates.)

HRT is not without its side effects, the main hazard being increased risk of endometrial cancer. Because all the data are not in, many doctors reserve HRT for women at high risk of osteoporosis—those with a premature menopause from surgery or disease or those chronically disabled or bedridden.

Nutritional therapies Calcium is not as effective as estrogen in preventing bone loss, but an adequate diet can slow the process. The currently recommended calcium allowance for British women is 500 mg a day, though the US National Institute of Health has recommended higher levels:

1,000 mg for premenopausal women
1,000 mg for postmenopausal women on estrogen therapy
1,500 mg for postmenopausal women without estrogen therapy

The average calcium intake of British women is 960 mg. The best sources of calcium are dairy products because they contain vitamin D and lactose, two substances that aid calcium absorption. But if you are lactose intolerant or a strict vegetarian, other sources are available. Table E-5 (see appendix E) lists food sources of calcium.

Here are easy ways to increase the calcium in your meals:*

- Make your own soups. Add a small amount of vinegar when preparing the stock from bones. Vinegar dissolves the calcium in the bones, so a pint of homemade soup will have the same calcium content as a quart of milk. The vinegar taste disappears.
- Before cooking, add vinegar to tenderize meat. Use the juice for gravy; it contains dissolved calcium. The vinegar taste again disappears.
- Instead of buttering your vegetables, add a touch of grated cheese.
- Garnish salads and soups with bits of cheese or tofu.
- Make salads from dark green lettuce leaves. They are rich in calcium, vitamins A, D, E, B vitamins, and many minerals.
- If you pickle fruits or vegetables, use calcium chloride instead of salt (sodium chloride).
- Add nonfat, dry, powdered milk to cream soups, casseroles,

---

* Adapted from the book *Stand Tall! The Informed Woman's Guide to Preventing Osteoporosis*, by M. Notelovitz and M. Ware (Triad, 1982).

meatloaf, desserts, anything. Each teaspoon of dry milk contains 5 mg of calcium—and no fat.
- When baking, add about one-quarter cup nonfat dry milk to recipes.
- Find creative ways to use yogurt (see recipes 3 and 4 in appendix D).

Even if your diet is loaded with calcium, any of these factors can reduce the amount available to your body:

High-fat diet
High-protein diet
Possibly a high-phosphorus diet (heavy intake of meat, processed foods, soft drinks)
Too much sodium
Oxalates (in spinach, chard, beet greens, rhubarb)*
Phytates (in the bran of whole grains)*
Alcohol
Coffee (four or more cups a day)
Fasting or crash dieting
Megadosing with vitamin A
Drugs, such as tetracycline, corticosteroids, anticonvulsants, antacids containing aluminum, diuretics, thyroid supplements

If you cannot get enough calcium from your diet, take a supplement. Some supplements contain only small amounts of calcium, so you need six to eight tablets of these daily to reach the desired amount. Also, calcium in supplements is not as well absorbed as that from food, so try to improve your diet at the same time. Table 5-1 compares available calcium supplements.

Take your calcium supplements throughout the day, preferably with small amounts of milk or yogurt. During sleep your immobility and overnight fast signal the body to extract calcium from your bones, so save your final dose for bedtime. Establish a routine and take the supplement at the same time each day.

If you have a history of kidney stones, take calcium supplements only under your doctor's supervision. Dosing yourself

---

* These should not pose a problem if you have rich sources of calcium in your diet.

Table 5-1 Calcium supplements

Calcium carbonate (tablet, elixir, or "Tums") 40% calcium	Most calcium per tablet. Cheapest. Not well absorbed by those with low stomach acid (elderly)
Calcium lactate 13% calcium	Less concentrated than calcium carbonate—must be taken in larger quantities. Avoid if you are lactose intolerant
Calcium gluconate 9% calcium	Small amount of calcium per tablet; must be taken several times during the day; may be too sweet for some people

with supplements of 1,000–2,500 mg calcium a day should cause no side effects for healthy women. Those individuals with certain existing health problems, such as sarcoidosis or tuberculosis, may suffer problems at this level.

To absorb calcium, you need vitamin D. Your body can manufacture vitamin D if you expose your skin to sunshine. However, if you rarely go outside or you wear heavy clothing, be sure to eat vitamin D-rich foods. The only naturally rich sources are fatty fish (mackerel, swordfish), eggs, and chicken liver, so drink vitamin D-fortified milk. Ignore advertisements that promote large doses of vitamin D to protect bones. Doses of 600–800 I.U. and over are toxic; too much vitamin D does nothing to strengthen your bones and can even speed their loss.

Fluoride Just as fluoride strengthens teeth, bones with fluoride built into them are less likely to lose mass. In experiments, fluoride plus calcium stimulates bone formation, but this new bone is brittle and more vulnerable to breakage. Patients may experience stomach upset and joint pain from the fluoride, and many do not respond at all. Because of these effects and the fact that fluoride is toxic in large doses, it has not yet been approved in Britain or the United States for treating osteoporosis.

Exercise Exercising may not prevent osteoporosis, but *not* exercising certainly hastens it. Bones enjoy being physically stressed. Weight-bearing exercises stimulate new bone formation and reduce the amount of bone lost after menopause. The best exercise includes walking, jogging, cycling, dancing, gymnastics, skipping, basketball, and tennis. Swimming and calisthenics do little to strengthen the bones.

Check your daily routine for these simple ways to stress bones:

- Take the stairs, instead of an elevator, when possible.
- Stand instead of sit.
- Walk instead of drive.

If you are bedridden, move around as much as possible. Ask your doctor for special exercises.

While it's all very well to say "Get out there and exercise," this advice has its hazards. Women who become exercise fanatics may become amenorrheic and begin to show bone loss. The long-term consequences are unknown. Another hazard concerns women who already have severe osteoporosis. These women should avoid any exercise that puts too much stress on already weakened bones. Walking is always a good bet, and even swimming can help at this stage. Check with your doctor for other activities you can enjoy.

Weight control

As you get older, you will feel social pressure to remain, if not youthful, at least fit. Yet once in your forties, you may find yourself overweight for the first time. If you have always had a weight problem, it may worsen. After menopause, it is easy to gain weight because your metabolism slows, you lose energy-consuming muscle, and you typically become inert. You may eat less food than when you were younger and trimmer, and still the pounds pile on. You not only gain weight, but your body becomes proportionately fattier.

Over a quarter of all middle-aged women in Britain are overweight. Weighing over 130 percent of your desirable weight places you at risk of diabetes and cardiovascular disease, so see your doctor about a diet. If you are less than twenty pounds overweight, it is important to watch what you eat, but you are better off staying somewhat overweight than attempting a severe weight-loss diet. Instead, get your body moving. Exercise pares down body fat and strengthens the muscles that support body organs, improving both figure and posture.

Cancer and heart disease

For British women aged thirty-five to fifty-four, cancer is the number-one cause of death (followed by heart disease, stroke, accidents, and suicide). The highest rate of cancer of the cervix is between ages fifty-five to sixty; for the lung, sixty-five to seventy-four; and for both breast and ovary, sometime over age fifty. (Details on cancer in chapter 13.)

A man is ten times more likely to die from a heart attack than a woman—that is, before the woman reaches menopause. After menopause, when the protective effect of estrogen is lost, a woman's risk catches up.

High blood pressure (hypertension) can promote heart disease by injuring the lining of the arteries. If you are healthy, get your blood pressure checked once a year. If you have hypertension, you should have it checked more often. Control your high blood pressure by taking your drugs (if prescribed), eating right, exercising, and giving up smoking. (More on heart disease in chapter 12.)

EATING STRATEGY

Eating habits

In your middle years you tend to follow the eating habits of your previous decades. If you are financially secure at this age, you may decide to eat out more often. Your children may also have left home, so it is easier to escape the kitchen. Some women become tired after years of cooking and find easy-to-prepare processed foods more appealing. Relying heavily on such foods can make for a diet high in sodium and low in some vitamins and minerals, so be sure to add fresh fruits and vegetables whenever possible. Or try the batch-cooking ideas in chapter 17.

Recommendations

If you have neglected your diet for most of your life, now is the time to pay attention. Suddenly faced with the realization that cancer and heart disease are real threats, you may find that for

Middle Adulthood: Menopause and the Midlife Molt

the first time in your life you have the motivation to change. It is not too late.

Chapter 16 offers practical guidelines for improving any diet. Cutting fat, sodium, and cholesterol from your meals should be a priority, as well as getting sufficient vitamins and minerals (particularly calcium). One advantage of passing menopause is that your need for iron drops. Yet you can still have low iron levels if you eat poorly, have a chronic disease, or take certain medications, so be *sure* to eat right. Your diet should provide only enough calories to maintain desirable weight. Besides eating well, exercise remains just as important as when you were younger.

FURTHER READING

Mayes, Kathleen. 1987. *Brittle Bones and the Calcium Loss*. Thorsons.

6
The Later Years: Never Too Late

Keep breathing.
Sophie Tucker

At age sixty-seven, Eula Weaver had angina; at seventy-five, a heart attack; and at eighty-one, congestive heart failure. She could walk about three blocks from home but sometimes had to be carried back. Her poor circulation forced her to wear gloves in the summertime. At five feet three inches and one hundred pounds, Eula was in bad shape.

Faced with the specter of permanent disability, Eula changed her diet dramatically and began a structured exercise program. In a few years, she could walk three miles, ride ten on a stationary bicycle, and jog a quarter mile. Five years after she first started exercising, she entered the American National Senior Olympics and over a period of another five years won ten gold medals.

To have made it into your seventies or beyond, you are either doing something right or your genes are fairly rugged. If you have managed to reach these later years with poor health habits and are now suffering the consequences, it is not too late to change. Remember Eula.

PHYSICAL AND PSYCHOLOGICAL CHANGES

Certain cells can no longer reproduce, and your tissues progressively degenerate as you age. Different parts of your body vary in how fast they age, but to some degree you can delay the onset of aging signs.

As you age, muscle ligaments weaken and become less elastic. Small fibers grow between muscles and their surrounding sheaths, and this cross-linking prevents muscles from sliding past one another. Inflexible muscles can make bending over to tie a shoe or reaching into the hall closet for blankets a painful task. Staying active can slow this process and keep muscles looser, particularly in your legs, lower back, shoulders, and neck.

Connective tissues in the arteries become less elastic and the artery walls thicken with age. Your heart has a tougher time moving blood and is less efficient at carrying oxygen to your lungs. Blood pressure rises. The sacs in your lungs, less flexible from age, no longer expand as easily. But regular exercise can improve circulation, reduce blood pressure, and even raise levels of "good" cholesterol.

With age, your carbohydrate tolerance decreases, raising your risk of diabetes. But regular exercise can make cells more responsive to insulin and offset this rise.

If you are physically and emotionally healthy, your life can continue to expand past your eighties and nineties. This can be a creative time. Grandma Moses began her painting career at age seventy-six. It can be a time of wisdom. You develop "crystallized intelligence"—that is, the ability to tap into an accumulated store of knowledge to make judgments and solve problems. It can be a time to take a stand. Malcolm Cowley, the critic and historian (age eighty-seven), writes: "Then there is the matter ... of finding a purpose in continued living that is beyond simple instinct for survival. Always, there is something to be done or something to be said that nobody else seems willing to do or say." This can be a time of intensity. "Age puzzles me," wrote Florida Scott-Maxwell (age eighty-two) in *Measure of My Days*. "I thought it was a quiet time. My seventies were interesting, and fairly serene, but my eighties are passionate." Though you have no guarantee that this time of life will be your most glorious, there is no reason for it to be your worst.

HEALTH CONCERNS
Negotiating for time

Though most degenerative changes eventually come with time, to a large degree you can speed up or slow their onset. And you can definitely control how much you let them interfere with your life. "I am enjoying myself," wrote Agatha Christie at age seventy-five. "Though with every year that passes, something has to be crossed off the list of pleasures ... fillet steaks and apples and raw blackberries (teeth difficulties) and reading fine print. But there is a great deal left. Operas and concerts, and reading, and the enormous pleasure of dropping into bed and going to sleep. ... Almost best of all, sitting in the sun ... remembering."

Your calendar does not indicate when your body will display the telltale signs of lost youth. Your calendar age has nothing to do with your "real" age—the one that marks your physical vigor, your intellect, and your willingness to endure.

Weight control Over time, body fat, like a migration of flesh, begins to shift. Fat from your arms, neck, and breasts seems to slide to the rib cage, abdomen, and back. Your breasts and upper arms sag. Your waist thickens. A great proportion of body fat moves from under the skin inward to pad organs.

Yet even with these changes, proper diet and exercise can keep you in shape and looking fit. Diet gives you the energy to be active, and exercise keeps your weight down, your muscles toned, your posture erect, and your bones strong.

Despite the notion that your best weight is the one you had at age twenty-five, recent evidence shows that your healthiest weight may change over your lifetime, rising somewhat with age. One reason is that you need more nutrient reserves to fall back on in case of illness. Also, added weight strengthens your bones. This does not justify being obese. Too much weight puts pressure on joints and can aggravate arthritis.

Being underweight at this age can be a problem, too. Loneliness and isolation can reduce the desire to eat and lead to the tea-and-toast syndrome, sometimes swallowed with large amounts of expensive vitamins and minerals. Too little body fat can leave a woman vulnerable to hypothermia, an abnormally low body temperature (usually 95 degrees F or lower) that can damage vital organs and lead to death.

Gastrointestinal problems As you age, your intestinal muscles weaken, your stomach secretes less acid, and you lose certain digestive enzymes, the result being constipation, heartburn, and indigestion.

Because of less stomach acid, you may have difficulty digesting

The Later Years: Never Too Late

red meats and certain vegetables, and you may absorb less iron. The stomach also makes less of a protein called intrinsic factor, needed for the absorption of vitamin B_{12} supplements.

If you have chronic indigestion:

- Avoid alcohol, coffee, tea, colas, and pepper.
- Eat three small meals a day plus snacks at midmorning and midafternoon.
- Eat slowly
- Include a small amount of fat in each meal.

Occasional use of antacids can provide relief from heartburn or indigestion, but long-term use for chronic conditions like ulcers can inhibit the absorption of iron, magnesium, and phosphorus. Antacids containing aluminum and calcium carbonate can be constipating, while magnesium-containing ones can cause diarrhea. Those with both aluminum and magnesium have fewer side effects, but they are usually high in sodium. Also, anyone who frequently takes antacids (which reduce stomach acid) may be at risk of iron-deficiency anemia because stomach acid actually helps to absorb iron.

Fiber can relieve constipation because it absorbs water and makes stools softer and bulkier. If you add bran to foods, do so gradually and drink more fluids. (Fiber does not do much if there is no water to absorb.) Take laxatives or cathartics only on your doctor's advice.

If you suffer from constipation, try these simple dietary changes before you resort to medications:

- Eat at regular times.
- Drink a hot beverage first thing in the morning.
- Eat breakfast.
- Drink six to eight glasses of fluids a day.
- Get plenty of fiber.
- Exercise daily.

(More on gastrointestinal disorders and fiber in chapter 15.)

Heart disease and cancer The leading causes of death in women aged fifty-five to seventy-four are (in order) heart disease, cancer, stroke, and diabetes. Once women reach seventy-five, the order of diseases shifts to heart disease, stroke, cancer, and pneumonia or influenza. The highest death rates for many cancers occur before the seventies, so survivors reach their later years having to face the threat of heart disease. For ways to delay or avoid these diseases—or at least lessen their damage—see part 3 of this book.

Arthritis Osteoarthritis results from wear and tear on the weight-bearing joints, mostly from overuse, stress, or injury. The strain of massive obesity can worsen it. Cartilage that normally cushions the joints erodes from weak tendons, ligaments, and muscles. The two end bones thicken, causing bony, knobby lumps. Bone ends up rubbing against bone. This type of arthritis affects one joint at a time, mainly in the lower back, hips, knees, ankles, and feet. The last joints on the hands are especially prone to misshaping, a condition called Heberden's nodes.

Osteoarthritis worsens with age, and if you live long enough, you will get it. If you are obese, try to lose weight to relieve the stress on your joints. If you are athletic, you may have to cut back on certain sports, though you should stay active. By strengthening ligaments and cartilage, non-weight-bearing exercises like swimming can even help prevent this disorder.

Rheumatoid arthritis is potentially the most crippling form of arthritis. It primarily inflames the small joints of the hands and feet, elbows, wrists, and ankles but can also affect other body tissues, causing weakness, fatigue, loss of appetite, and weight loss.

Treatment depends on how severe your symptoms are and which joints are affected. Common prescriptions include rest, moderate exercise such as swimming or walking (when the inflammation has subsided), physical therapy, sometimes surgical replacement of the joints, and aspirin or aspirin substitutes. In high doses, aspirin acts as an anti-inflammatory agent. However, long-term use and repeated high doses can cause tiny vessels in the gastrointestinal tract to hemorrhage. This tiny but chronic loss of blood can increase requirements of iron, vitamin D, and folacin. To reduce stomach upset, take your aspirin with or just after meals, even if the aspirin is buffered. Eat plenty of iron-rich foods, such as meat, whole and enriched grains, dried beans, and dried fruits, and have your iron levels checked frequently.

Rheumatoid arthritis patients may develop osteopenia, a loss of bone, from inactivity and possibly the use of cortisone-related drugs. To avoid this, exercise whenever possible, even if you just go for leisurely walks.

Sometimes severe rheumatoid arthritis is treated with penicillamine. This drug interferes with the absorption of pyridoxine, so check with your doctor about a vitamin supplement. If untreated, rheumatoid arthritis can cause permanent deformities in the joints.

Neither type of arthritis is caused or cured by diet, but both can affect nutrition. Acute pain can prevent you from preparing food, while chronic pain can cause loss of appetite. Morning stiffness can turn the making of breakfast into torture. If this happens, eat a midmorning snack instead.

As yet there is no cure for arthritis. The famous cod liver oil treatment, claimed to lubricate joints, does not work because the body digests the oil long before it reaches the joints. (Cod liver oil also is high in certain fat-soluble vitamins like A and D, which can be toxic.) Vinegar, another sham remedy, is said to dissolve calcium salts on the joints. But again, vinegar is digested before it could ever do its work. For some unknown reason, rheumatoid arthritis patients have higher blood levels of copper and lower blood levels of zinc, but supplements are not the answer. They do not improve the condition, and in large quantities, copper and zinc can cause kidney damage.

Folklore holds that certain "nightshades"—potatoes, tomatoes, green peppers, aubergines—and dairy products worsen arthritis. No scientific evidence exists to back up such tales, nor is there such a thing as a legitimate "arthritis diet" or "arthritis cookbook," despite the claims.

Periodontal disease Three-quarters of Britons aged fifty-five to sixty-four have lost all their teeth, and eighty-seven percent of those over seventy-five. When the teeth go, eating becomes a bit tricky.

The number-one reason for tooth loss after age thirty-five is periodontal disease. It gets worse with age, and since women live longer than men, they are more at risk. Once started, periodontal disease spreads rapidly in individuals with poor dental and eating habits.

Your first line of defense is to be meticulous about your teeth, removing plaque and getting regular check-ups. Next, look at your eating habits. If your diet is low in calcium, your body may be extracting calcium from your bones—jawbone included. Also, the tissues between your teeth and gums, which block the passage of harmful substances, grow rapidly and require continual supplies of nutrients, particularly vitamin C, folacin, and zinc. Without them, your resistance to infection drops.

To keep your gums healthy:

- Eat a well-balanced diet that provides all the essential nutrients in recommended amounts.
- Eat calcium-rich foods; if possible, eat plenty of dairy products.
- Avoid high-protein diets; eat only moderate amounts of red meat.
- Avoid short-term diets that promise to cure or reverse periodontal disease (particularly if they do not mention the need for regular dental care).

If you have trouble chewing, experiment with cooking, soft, nutritious foods:

applesauce	juices
rice pudding	yogurt
lentil soup	oatmeal
omelets	soufflés
pureed vegetables, meats	puddings

Drug use Drug use is not limited to the older adult, but as you age, you tend to accumulate multiple prescriptions. Drugs, especially those taken over a long time, can interfere with nutrients. They can affect how well you eat by changing your appetite or making food taste terrible. Once you eat, drugs can destroy nutrients, prevent your body from absorbing or using them, or make you excrete them in large amounts. If a drug causes fatigue, nausea, vomiting, diarrhea, constipation, and dizziness, you may lose weight. Be sure to monitor your weight and report any substantial loss to your doctor.

A drug's effectiveness often depends on whether or not you take it with meals. Some drugs, such as ampicillin, penicillin, and tetracycline, are destroyed by acid and should therefore be taken before meals. Others, such as aspirin and tolbutamides, irritate your stomach and should be taken with food. Sometimes food affects how well you absorb the drug. One of the most dangerous interactions is that of tyramine-containing foods (hard cheeses, aged soft cheeses, liver, pickled herring, salami) and drugs called monoamine oxidase inhibitors. The combination can cause severe hypertension, and sometimes stroke or death.

To lessen the chances of a harmful interaction between drugs and foods, take only the drugs you need and ask your doctor if those you will be taking for a long time interfere with any nutrients.

Senility Senility is a generic term covering over a hundred different conditions. It is often a side effect of disease (arteriosclerosis, anemia, walking pneumonia, malnutrition), drugs, or depression. Claims to the contrary, neither supplements of lecithin nor the nucleic acid RNA prevent senility.

SPECIAL CONSIDERATIONS

The woman alone

Eating is a social experience, so find companionship for meals. By preparing and eating meals alone, you may soon decide it is not worth the effort and stop eating altogether. Or you may just grab whatever is handy. If you tire easily by the end of the day and cannot face your kitchen, eat your main meal for lunch. If you live alone, take turns with friends to cook meals. Or start a lunch club that meets at a nice restaurant a couple of times a month. If you live at home but cannot prepare meals, Meals on Wheels provides a hot noontime meal. (For information, check with a doctor, social worker, or visiting nurse, or look in your phone book under Women's Royal Voluntary Service.)

The woman on a tight budget

Impulse buying is the worst enemy of budgets, and stores are designed to promote just that. To win the battle of the budget:

Eat Beautiful!

- Plan your menus in advance so you can limit your trips to the store to once a week.
- Keep a notepad in the kitchen to write down needed supplies, and shop with your list.
- Check advertised specials and "money-off" coupons for products that you need. Plan to shop on the days the specials are offered.
- Do not shop on an empty stomach.

When you get to the store, be prepared to make last minute substitutions if a lower-price product is on sale. Read labels for products low in sugar and fat. Compare costs according to:

- Different brands of the same food when unit prices are available
- Large quantities instead of small (if you can use extra before the food goes bad)
- Different forms of the same food: frozen, canned, fresh
- Store brands or generic products (store brands may be identical to brand-name products but have a different label; generic foods are nutritionally equivalent to brand names, but their appearance may alter somewhat from can to can, or box to box)
- Interchangeable products (peaches for pears)

Buy lower grades of meat: they often contain less fat. Also, try cheaper protein sources: fish, eggs, dried beans, peas, lentils, and tofu. In the dairy section, choose bulk cheeses over grated or individually wrapped ones, and mild over aged. Low-fat powdered milk is an inexpensive alternative to fresh milk, especially for baking. Buy only fresh fruits and vegetables that are in season. Frozen foods can be as nutritious—or more so—but canned foods have fewer nutrients and are often high in sodium. For snacks, forget costly cookies and cakes and try fresh fruits and vegetables, whole grain crackers, low-sugar cereals, and yogurt. Avoid frozen convenience foods; instead, prepare and freeze your own. Leave dented cans or crushed packages on the shelf, even if they are on sale. Make your own salad dressings, gravies, and sauces.

Extending life

Fannie Thomas of San Gabriel, California, died in 1981 at age 113 years, 273 days. Alice Stevenson of the United Kingdom lived for 112 years, 39 days. Considering the scientists estimate the human life span at 115 years, Fannie and Alice did well.

Life span, the greatest possible age humans can attain, is the age when the body free of disease and any other interferences simply poops out, like an electric light bulb that one minute glows brightly and then, with a brittle flash, expires. But life span is calculated for a species and does not have much to do with real people who contract illnesses, overeat, overdrink, smoke cigarettes, and live in a polluted, stressful world. For populations, we discuss life expectancy, or average age at death, and for individuals like Fannie Thomas, we talk about longevity.

Since before the turn of the century, women in the United Kingdom have shown a greater survival rate than men. Currently, women live on average to age seventy-seven, men to age seventy-one. In fact, half of all people on earth who ever lived past age sixty-five are alive today.

Antiaging theories and nutrition Pushing longevity beyond its usual limits is big business these days. Several years ago, authors Durk Pearson and Sandy Shaw wrote a popular tome called *Life Extension: A Practical Scientific Approach* (Warner, 1982), in which they explained how we can live to a vibrant 150 years or so by taking a somewhat expensive array of vitamins, minerals, amino acids, food additives, and drugs. No need to worry about butter, cream, and eggs. And exercise? Don't bother. Of course, no scientific evidence exists that this regimen works. But if it doesn't, what have you lost? William Bennett, contributing editor to *American Health* magazine, estimated it would cost him $39,000 (£22,000) of supplements for each extra year presumably plunked onto his lifeline—and that's quite a gamble.

A later book, *Maximum Life Span* (W. W. Norton, 1983) by Roy Walford, a researcher at the University of California at Los Angeles, offered its readers hope of a longer life through a rigorous adherence to a Spartan diet, boosted with vitamin and mineral supplements. Bits of data from laboratory studies sup-

Eat Beautiful!

port Walford's approach, but again, there's no solid evidence to guarantee you a return on your money.

But what are the data backing antiaging regimens? One line of research involves free radicals, highly reactive molecules with only one electron in their outer shells. Free radicals form naturally as the body uses oxygen. The danger of free radicals is that they can wrest electrons from other molecules, which then become free radicals themselves, causing chaos for the cell membranes and DNA. The buildup of free radicals, some say, causes aging.

To prevent free radicals from forming, some scientists have been studying chemicals known as antioxidants. Antioxidants such as vitamin E react with free radicals and tie up their delinquent electron to render it harmless. In theory, vitamin E supplements should retard aging, but research with cell cultures, lab mice, and humans has not be convincing. The body itself manufactures two antioxidants: glutathione peroxidase and superoxide dismutase. (Don't bother with oral supplements of superoxide dismutase, or SOD, because the enzyme is digested and does not reach your cells intact.)

The antioxidants selenium, vitamin C, and carotene should also react with free radicals and slow aging, but so far no strong evidence points to their value either. Dosing yourself with massive amounts of these nutrients may even interfere with getting enough oxygen to your cells. However, there is no reason not to get plenty of these nutrients in your diet. Here are some good food sources:

- Vitamin E: whole grains, wheat germ, nuts, legumes, avocado
- Vitamin C: citrus fruits, leafy greens, broccoli, melons, strawberries, papayas, tomatoes
- Carotene: leafy greens, broccoli, carrots, pumpkin, squash
- Selenium: fish, meats, while grains

Also, avoid taking special antiaging supplements, such as Gerovital H-3, a solution of an anesthetic, a preservative, and an antioxidant. This product does not retard aging or prevent any disorder associated with the elderly.

Besides antioxidants, another way to thwart free radicals is by limiting food intake, according to some scientists. Undernutrition can extend life in laboratory animals and theoretically could do the same in humans. However, no one is recommending that we start starving our children so that they will live longer. Underfeeding can stunt growth, impair mental development, and cause later reproductive problems. Also, few scientists believe that data from current research on aging will increase the species' life span of about 115 years. At most—and it is a big most—it will stretch some of the vigorousness of youth and vitality of middle age into the last third of life.

What you can do The idea that changing your diet can extend your life expectancy may lead you to assume that you can battle heredity and environment—and win. This is slightly optimistic. Yet nutrition can prolong your survival within the time your genes allow. Because cardiovascular disease and cancer account for 70 percent of all deaths, taking measures to reduce your risk of these killers can help you live longer. Lifelong exercise and proper diet can delay osteoporosis, another crippler and killer of women. There is no guarantee that improving your health habits will extend your life, but it can make your years much more pleasant. Here are some steps to take:

- If you drink alcohol, do so in moderation.
- Know your family history of disease, and take the necessary steps to reduce your own risks.
- Follow a regular exercise routine that includes stretching, aerobics, and strength building.
- Maintain normal weight through diet and exercise.
- Eat a balanced diet, with regular meals.
- Do not smoke cigarettes.
- Have regular sleep hours.
- Find ways to handle stress and take time to relax.

EATING STRATEGY

Nutrient needs

The nutrition paradox for this age is that you need fewer calories than when you were younger, but you must obtain as many, if not more, nutrients. Why? Because you absorb nutrients less efficiently, your risk of chronic disorders rises, and you are probably taking one, if not more, drugs.

Little research exists on specific nutritional needs for older women, though some doctors emphasize vitamins A, C, and E, and the mineral calcium. Vitamins A and C maintain tissues and bones, vitamin E keeps cells intact, and calcium delays bone thinning. Because you are less efficient at metabolizing glucose, you may need extra chromium. (Chromium is part of the "glucose tolerance factor," which helps insulin do its job.) The richest sources of chromium are

> brewer's yeast   liver
> beef   whole grains
> potatoes   oranges
> wheat germ

If you neglect your diet, you may experience general malaise, loss of appetite and weight, fatigue, headache, insomnia, confusion, and depression. Many older people cannot think straight, not because their mental acuity is gone, but because they are depressed, and depression can lead to malnutrition. A vicious cycle may begin.

Eating habits

"Some elderly people do enjoy their food. Others couldn't care less," observed Norman, one of the four central characters in Barbara Pym's *Quartet in Autumn*. His comment underscored one of the main differences between the two women characters: Letty, a woman given to serious reading, who decided upon retiring to learn about "social studies," and Marcia, who was "ageing, slightly mad" before retirement, only to become more so afterward. After leaving her job, Letty becomes more careful of her appearance, arriving for a luncheon with her former office mates dressed in "her best tweed suit and carrying a new pair of gloves." Marcia shows up "thinner than ever," wearing on her head "an unsuitably jaunty straw hat from which her strangely piebald hair straggled in elflocks." For Letty, eating becomes one of life's main enjoyments, and she is absolutely thrilled over a meal of chicken "*forestière*," white wine, apple pie, and ice cream. Marcia would typically skip lunch and then have bits of bread and a cup of tea for dinner. Letty and Marcia, both alone, represent two reactions to aging: one attempts to make it a time of growth and adventure, while the other succumbs to her isolation and rapidly slides toward death.

With age, many older women choose certain foods because they evoke pleasant memories from earlier years. Including such old favorites is fine, even if they are not nutritious, as long as they do not overwhelm the rest of the day's meals.

Physical impairment causes other older women to avoid certain foods. Bone loss from the jaw can make old dentures uncomfortable and new ones hard to fit. Hard or sticky foods may have to be banished. Because of tooth loss or a diminished sense of taste, many older women eat soft, sweet foods, which only promote further tooth decay.

Your senses of smell and taste may become less acute, particularly if you are a heavy smoker. Avoid sprinkling on extra salt to flavor "tasteless" food. Instead, perk up your foods with spices and herbs (see recipe 5 in appendix D).

Some older women rely on fast foods or inexpensive restaurant food, which is often loaded with salt, sugar, and fat. Others exist on frozen dinners. For those with little money, the hot plate is always a challenge.

Food habits will hinge on your previous eating patterns, your state of health, and your financial status—all of which reflect a lifetime of choices. Even now, though, you can change your habits, improve your diet, and learn how to plan meals around a tight budget.

Recommendations

If it were possible to define a good daily diet for all older women, included would be:

Vegetables (raw or cooked) and fruit—two to three servings of each
  Vitamin C source—one
  Vitamin A source—four to five a week
Whole-grain breads and cereals—three to four servings
Dairy products—two servings
Poultry, lean beef and pork, fish, and dried beans and peas—one to two servings

Such a diet would limit sweets, alcohol, and soft drinks and provide only enough calories to maintain desirable weight. Unless you are overweight, do not avoid naturally fatty foods like whole milk or meat, but do remove unnecessary fat by trimming meats and baking, broiling, or boiling foods instead of frying them. Unless you are on a special diet, do not avoid eating eggs. They are a cheap source of high-quality protein.

Eat plenty of fresh fruits and vegetables, or frozen vegetables if fresh are unavailable. If you take supplements, find one that provides recommended daily intakes of vitamins and minerals. Take larger doses only on your doctor's orders. Check with your doctor about taking a calcium supplement.

With age, you become less sensitive to thirst, so to be sure you get enough liquid, drink six to eight glasses of fluid daily, particularly plain water and fruit juices. Moderate amounts of alcohol, coffee, and tea are okay but do not count as part of your daily fluids because they are diuretics.

With age you have more aches and pains, and getting to the store may sometimes be difficult. Set up an emergency food shelf in your cupboard for times when bad weather or sickness prevents you from shopping. Items to stock include:

Cans	*Packets*	*Jars*
tuna	pastas	peanut butter
chicken	noodles	applesauce
baked beans	dried fruits	nuts
spaghetti	instant soup	Ovaltine
soups	nonfat dried milk	vegetable oil
vegetables	instant cocoa	coffee
fruits	rice	
juices	hot and cold cereals	
bean salad		
macaroni cheese		

Besides eating well, you should exercise daily, keep regular sleep hours, take time every day to relax, let others help you when necessary, and find enjoyable ways to spend your days. T. S. Eliot once wrote that old men should be explorers. So, Mr. Eliot, should old women.

RESOURCES

Laver, Mary, and Smith, Margaret. 1981. *Diet for Life: Cook Book for Arthritics*. Pan.

Arthritis Care, 6 Grosvenor Crescent, London SW1X 7ER. Free diet fact sheet and other pamphlets.

PART 2
Weight Control, Fitness, and Beauty

"Give me a dozen such heart breaks," wrote Colette, "if that would help me lose a couple of pounds." To lose a few pounds many women would suffer heartaches and worse, gladly handing over their Visa cards for the latest gizmo that promises quick relief from prodigious fat cells. In "Weight Control" I describe how your body image affects your sense of self-worth and how different factors mingle to cause obesity. This chapter suggests realistic ways to get fit and stay that way, while "The Shape-Up Plan" offers a structured weight control program aimed at changing your eating and exercise habits. "Eating Disorders" describes what happens when a woman's distorted perception of her size leads her to self-destructive practices, such as starving, bingeing, and purging. For the woman whose level of fitness is a professional concern, "The Athlete" provides special advice on improving performance during training and competition. Last, in "Beauty" you will discover how diet affects the sheen of your hair, the smoothness of your skin, and the strength of your nails. Taken together, these five chapters illustrate the beauty of being fit and healthy—that is, the beauty beneath your makeup.

7
Weight Control: The Looking-Glass War

> When we see a woman made as a woman ought to be, she strikes us as a monster.
>
> Harriet Beecher Stowe, 1830s

If mirrors could speak, they would make nasty remarks like "My, we're looking pudgy today," or "Isn't it about the time we took up weight lifting?" Though some mirrors are kinder than others, they are all rascals. Gazing into them, thin girls are horrified to see blobs of fat clutching their thighs while fat women strangely disappear below the neck.

That image you see every morning in the bathroom mirror might look better or worse than the real you. Chances are it looks worse. So for the moment, ignore your mirror's morning antics. Forget about whether it scowled, glared, howled with laughter, or quietly wept. You are about to discover that you have been duped.

Body image—in the mirror of your mind

The image you hold of your body is formed by two things: how you see yourself and how you think others see you. This image has nothing to do with your actual body dimensions. It is the reflection of your body in the mirror of your mind—a mirror strangely cut and framed in the shape and size that your mind calls "ideal." Your body image rarely matches the contours of this mirror—usually overlapping the frame—because you believe, like most women, that you are too fat.

The truth for many of you is that you are not overweight. That ripply, funhouse mirror of your mind uses your insecurities to distort your sense of personal size. A clumsy, slender girl might see herself as fat simply because she is always bumping into things. A middle-aged woman whose marriage has entered a slump may suddenly decide her thighs are too big.

Try this experiment. Stand in front of a full-length mirror and take a long look at yourself. Look at your feet, then your legs. Move up to the trunk, arms, and face. Give your most confident assessment. Now read an article on some successful career woman who "has it all"—loving husband and children, respectful colleagues, devoted dog—and who wears a size 10. Look in the mirror again. Don't you look fatter than you did a few minutes ago? So much for real mirrors.

Being fat: prohibition of the 1980s

Today's ideal is slowly but steadily shifting toward a thin, boyish form. A survey of Miss America Pageant entrants from 1959 through 1978 showed that winners weigh less than other contestants. In the 1984 pageant, the California entrant, Donna Grace Cherry, told a reporter for *Newsweek* that, to prepare for the contest, she existed for months on 600 calories a day.

Over the last twenty years, the average weight of *Playboy* Playmates of the Month, when adjusted for age and height, has decreased. Measurements of Playmates have also changed: busts and hips have become smaller, while waists have become larger.

So much for beauty contestants and *Playboy* Playmates. Where does this leave most women? While the ideal body has slimmed down over the past twenty years, the average woman has not. Today women in their early twenties weigh three to six pounds more than young women twenty years ago; those in their mid- to late twenties weigh one to four pounds more. The disparity between the ideal and real weights of young women is growing so much that we find ourselves in the middle of a cultural obsession with weight that affects women of all ages and shapes. Consider that Elizabeth Taylor, long a survivor of Hollywood gossip, created her biggest scandal simply by getting fat.

Women who already weigh less than their desirable weights feel pressure to attain even lower weights. Though government statistics claim that 25 percent of women between the ages of twenty and seventy-four are overweight, almost 50 percent of all women consider themselves so. Why do even normal-weight women think that they are overweight? (And why do many men agree with them?) One reason is that ads portray an image that is almost impossible to attain.

Models are paid to stay slim and look even slimmer. One young model described a photo session in which she wore designer jeans so tight that, during the shooting, she had to hold her breath because the jeans' snug fit prevented her from breathing. She was helping to fashion the unattainable standard by which millions of young women judge their bodies, a standard that also does not fit.

Another problem is that magazines and television have instilled the belief that bony thinness is a symbol of self-control and success. Control means dieting and consciously refusing to indulge in large amounts of food even though you are surrounded by it.

No matter who you are, this thin ideal has its price. Whether you are working in or out of the home, you will probably find that following a very low calorie diet and trying to keep up your everyday pace will leave you tired and grumpy and start your weight yo-yoing up and down erratically.

If a woman wants to be fit, she must first realistically appraise her body. She may not need a diet at all. She may simply need to look at herself in the mirror, smile, and learn to be happy with what she has got.

Risks to happiness and health

Being fat is socially uncomfortable. We are actually offended at the sight of fat people. Eating, according to *Boston Globe* columnist Ellen Goodman, is the "last bonafide sin left in America." In a column entitled "The Perils of Pounds," she wrote: "I have heard the same people who talk about alcoholism as a 'disease' and crime as a 'social disorder' ... speak of fat as unforgivable. They may express all kinds of sympathy for an amphetamine junkie, but someone who has gained 10 pounds is accused of 'letting herself go.' Someone who has a new tube around the middle is guilty of having 'no will power.' "

It is not surprising that psychological problems emerge from the social stigma of being obese. Many obese women are passive and isolated, behaving like victims of ethnic or racial discrimination. And the discrimination is very real. Even those who are internationally recognized in their fields suffer from such prejudice. A letter to the editor published in *Time* magazine about a cover story of Boston opera conductor Sarah Caldwell stated: "I am proud to see women take their place in music. However, one cannot regard Sarah Caldwell as anything but a big blob of blubber."

Besides creating psychological problems, obesity can pose risks to health. It can contribute to cardiovascular disease, gallbladder disease, and can worsen, though not necessarily cause, such a serious disorder as osteoarthritis of the knees, hips, or spine. The pressure and obstruction from excess fat can lead to abdominal hernias and varicose veins. Higher rates of cancer of the breast, pancreas, uterus, and gallbladder are linked to moderate obesity, and people who have an inherited tendency toward diabetes may trigger the condition if they put on excess fat.

Obese women suffer more menstrual disorders than lean women, and may have difficulty conceiving. The obese are also at greater risk from complications of surgery, anesthesia, and pregnancy. Finally, fat below the skin of an obese person can cause skin irritation and chafing.

Not every obese person will experience these disorders. In general, the more obese you are, the worse your problems. You need to exceed your desirable weight by 30 percent or more before your risk of heart disease or cancer increases. If you are less than 30 percent overweight but smoke cigarettes or have diabetes or high blood pressure, the risk remains high.

Recent research indicates that risk of disease depends on where your fat is deposited. Fat above your waist (arms, chest, abdomen) increases your risk of diabetes and heart disease while fat below the waist (thighs, buttocks) does not.

Your age is also a factor. Risk of heart disease is higher for those who become obese between the ages of twenty and forty than for those who add their fat after age forty. Women who get slightly heavier as they age may be healthier than those who force their weights to stay low—even as they push into their fifties and sixties.

The debate continues over whether mild obesity (28 to 40 percent over your recommended weight) without other health complications shortens life expectancy. But no matter how this controversy is resolved, most researchers agree on a few things. Anyone over forty who is overweight should be regularly screened for high blood pressure, high levels of blood sugar (a sign

Weight Control: The Looking-Glass War

of diabetes), and elevated levels of cholesterol. Also, two of the greatest hazards to the obese are the adoption of dangerous diets and yo-yoing cycles of weight loss and gain.

Body weight versus body fat

To be overweight is not the same thing as to be obese. A height–weight table will tell you if you are *overweight*. But height–weight tables themselves are inconsistent with each other. At a 1973 conference, for instance, obesity specialists devised a set of weight recommendations. Then in 1983 the Metropolitan Life Insurance Company revised their own table and set levels for desirable weights higher than their 1959 table. Both of these tables for women appear in table 7-1.

Another quick way to estimate your desirable weight is to use

Table 7-1 Height–weight tables

Height	Obesity Conference, 1973 Weight (lbs)	Metropolitan Life, 1983 Weight (lbs)
4'10"	92–119	100–131
4'11"	94–122	101–134
5'0"	96–125	103–137
5'1"	99–128	105–140
5'2"	102–131	108–144
5'3"	105–134	111–148
5'4"	108–138	114–152
5'5"	111–142	117–156
5'6"	114–146	120–160
5'7"	118–150	123–164
5'8"	122–154	126–167
5'9"	126–158	129–170
5'10"	130–163	132–173
5'11"	134–168	135–176
6'0"	138–173	

The weight ranges are for a woman not wearing shoes or other clothing. The Metropolitan Life table is for women, aged 25 to 59 years; the table from the 1973 Obesity Conference did not include ages.

Sources: 1973 recommendations of the Fogarty Center Conference on Obesity; Metropolitan Life Insurance Company.

this formula: Allow 100 pounds for the first five feet of height. Then add 5 pounds for each additional inch. If you are 5 feet 5 inches tall, you start with 100 pounds for your first 5 feet, then add 25 pounds (5 pounds times 5 inches) to get 125 pounds of desirable. If you are short, subtract 5 pounds for each inch under 5 foot. This is only a ballpark figure, of course.

A drawback to both height–weight tables and this formula is that they do not take into account your individual physique. For instance, if your current weight is greater by 10 percent of your recommended weight, you are considered overweight. But body weight includes bones, muscles, and water as well as fat. And muscle is heavier than fat, so you may actually gain weight when you start an exercise program. If you retain water, as many women do right before their menstrual periods, your weight will go up. Because weight measures many things besides fat, it makes a bad indicator of fitness.

While being overweight refers to *body weight* and how you rank on a height–weight table, obesity refers to *body fat*. Some amount of body fat is natural, and women throughout the world accumulate fat from their teens through their fifties. Both men and women need about 3 percent of their total weight as body fat, called "essential fat," to live. This fat is present in cell membranes, bone marrow, and tissues of the nerves, spinal cord, and brain. It pads the heart, lungs, liver, spleen, intestines, and kidneys.

Besides this essential fat, women have "sex-specific fat" that accounts for an additional 9–12 percent of their weight. This fat is necessary for childbearing and settles around the breasts and hips. What other fat you have is "storage fat," for times when food may be scarce. For women, the desirable range of total body fat is 20–25 percent of their weight. The range for men is lower (15–20 percent). Women athletes might have as little as 18 percent body fat, but once a woman drops below 17 percent, she is likely to stop menstruating. Women are usually defined as obese if they have greater than 28 percent (some say 30 percent) body fat.

Some people may be overweight but not obese. Athletes are often overweight by height-weight tables as a result of their well-developed muscles—but they are far from obese. Some women may even be *underweight* and obese. Elderly women who weigh less than their recommended weight are often so sedentary that they have a large percentage of body fat and few well-developed muscles. Having too much fat is more likely to affect your health than simply being overweight from heavy bones, well-developed muscles, or water retention.

However, obesity *is* often more conveniently defined in terms of weight. A given body has only so much bone and muscle, so if a woman weighs over 20 percent of her recommended weight, it is assumed that the excess is fat and she is therefore considered obese.

You can measure your body fat by being weighed underwater. You sit on a seat suspended from a scale. Fat floats, so it does not register on the scale. Muscle sinks, so it will register. From this underwater weight you can derive your percentage of fat. (To get your fat levels measured, check with your local private health clinics.)

Another method is to use skinfold calipers, an instrument that measures the thickness of skin folds pinched at various places on the body. These calipers are sold by numerous firms that market weight-loss gadgets. Be advised that it takes much training to get accurate readings.

To determine whether you are too fat, a few other, less precise methods exist:

1. The Ruler Test: Lie on your back and place a ruler along the midline of your body, touching your ribs and pelvis. If the ruler does not lay flat, it could indicate too much fat around your waist.
2. The Belt Test: Adjust a belt snugly around the lower rib cage and try to slip it down over your waist. If the belt does not fit over your waist (and you are not pregnant), you are too fat.
3. The Pinch Test: If you can pinch more than one inch of fat (not muscle) from one of the following places—above the hip, along the navel, or midway on the upper arm—there is a good chance you are plump.

Eat Beautiful!

WHY PEOPLE GET FAT

Americans as a group are fatter than ever, but instead of eating more food, they are eating less than they did in the early 1970s. So it seems clear that gluttony is not the reason for obesity. No one really knows what causes obesity, but chances are that many types of obesities exist and result from any number of factors: genetics, hormonal imbalances, external cues, emotions, and poor food choices.

Genetics

"I come from a long line of fat people."

The fat-cell theory At the moment of conception, you are handed a legacy of genes that you cannot alter, trade, or toss away. Studies of obese and lean families show that genetic heritage may influence your chances of obesity. Statistically, if neither of your parents is obese, you have only a 7 percent chance of becoming obese yourself. If one of your parents is obese, your chances rise to 40 percent. And if both your parents are obese, your chances jump to 80 percent. This escalating risk can be attributed partly to overweight parents who pass bad eating habits on to their children. But a biological reason also seems likely.

Researchers have proposed several theories to explain how genetics might influence the risk of obesity. According to the fat-cell theory, you lay down fat cells only during certain periods of life: the last three months of fetal development, between ages one and three, and in adolescence. Gaining weight as an adult usually does not involve adding new fat cells but overstuffing existing ones.

Regardless of how you got your fat cells, they tend to regulate your appetite. If you have many fat cells, you will find yourself hungrier than someone with fewer fat cells. This is one reason why people who become obese during childhood have a harder time losing weight than those who become obese as adults. Such a person, when dieting, will experience persistent hunger that keeps her preoccupied with food.

The setpoint theory According to the setpoint theory, your body is programmed to reach and stay at an ideal biological weight and to have a certain amount of fat. Your setpoint is supposedly determined by the number of fat cells in your body. Like a thermostat that clicks a furnace on or off to keep a room at a desirable temperature, your fat cells send out chemicals to signal the body to stop or start eating if your level of body fat rises above or falls below this setpoint. It may be possible to lower your setpoint over time, so you could lose fat and maintain the loss with less effort and much less agony. Though you have no way to measure your setpoint, theoretically it is the weight to which your body returns when you are eating normally—not trying to lose or gain weight.

According to the setpoint theory, if you gorge, say, at Thanksgiving or Christmas, you will feel bloated until you have worked off your holiday gain. For dieters, it means that if you lose too much fat, your body will automatically try to put it back on. And if your setpoint is high because you have so many fat cells, you are doomed either to be fat or to fight a near impossible battle to say thin.

Both the fat cell and setpoint theories suggest that the obese may have to contend with internal antagonists far stronger than mere eating habits: fat cells clamoring to be satiated. Both theories are still controversial.

The brown fat theory The brown fat theory holds that the body gets rid of extra calories through strange cells known as brown fat cells. The brown color is due to their iron content. Brown fat is a special type of fat that reacts to cold by generating heat, which burns off calories. It is possible that some obese persons may have fewer brown fat cells, or perhaps the ones they do have are defective. Either way, their bodies are unable to burn off calories as efficiently as a lean body. This theory might also explain why some people can eat twice as much as others, yet never have a weight problem. These people are simply more efficient fat burners.

Hormonal imbalances

"I have a problem with my glands."

A small number of people are obese because their bodies release insufficient amounts of the thyroid hormone. Too little of the hormone can cause your energy needs to be so low that you do not have to eat much before you have overshot your limit.

External cues

"I have to pass by this doughnut shop on the way to work, and, well, the smell of those honeybuns draws me in."

Eating is an emotional experience. Everywhere you go there are external cues urging you to eat: the clock on the wall, the smell of a bakery, or an advertisement for Chicago-style pizza. Everyone responds, in some degree, to these signals.

A few years ago researchers thought that the obese responded to these external cues more than they did to the internal ones of strong stomach contractions. Data seemed to support this view until researchers took another look. The differences in response to external cues were not a function of how fat a person was, but of how much she tried to restrict her eating. A chronic dieter who severely limits her food cannot rely on her internal cues of hunger because she is *always* hungry. Instead, her diet forces her to ignore hunger and look for other signs of when to eat.

These restrictive eaters, whether they are fat or thin, are more likely to gorge on food once they have dented their armor of restraint. Fat people who complain that they often eat "because it is there" are probably strict dieters, and the presence of food has temporarily defeated their self-control and their latest diet. Once a container of food is opened, they feel compelled to eat the entire contents.

Alcohol, possibly marijuana, and the slightest infraction of a diet can trigger bouts of bingeing. Binge eating is sudden, compulsive eating of very large amounts of food in a short period of time, followed by a wave of guilt. Some restrictive eaters, after indulging in one sweet, feel their control snap and start gorging on mountains of sugary foods. Once they break their diet or eat a forbidden food, their rationale becomes "Well, I might as well pig out now and get a fresh start in the morning."

Restrictive eaters often become compulsive eaters who think about food all the time. People who quit smoking frequently turn into compulsive eaters when they grab for food in response to a cigarette craving.

Emotions

"I don't know why I ate it. I was just so depressed."

Obese women as a group are not more neurotic, depressed, or anxious than lean women and are not more likely to eat to soothe inner conflict. Yet some women, whether fat or thin, eat for emotional security. Children who are rewarded with food for good behavior often grow up into adults who seek solace in food. Many women, when depressed, insecure, lonely, ill, or homesick, gorge on "comfort foods." After moving to a unfamiliar city to start a new job, one depressed eater wrote in her journal: "Depression takes many forms. Tonight it took the form of 15 distinctive Milano cookies and three glasses of Grenache rosé."

Stress can trigger binge eating. In night-eating syndrome, a person has no appetite in the morning but eats enormous amounts of food in the evening and then is unable to sleep. Night eating is preceded by stress, often the stress of hunger caused by chronic dieting. The stress builds through the day until eating at night relieves it.

Women, especially chronic dieters, tend to gain weight when their emotions overwhelm their resolve to stay on a diet. During times of stress, the pounds accumulate, and middle-age obesity slowly creeps up on a woman as she loses and gains, loses and gains, always with a net gain in weight. The increase might be only two to ten pounds at a time. Paule Marshall, in *Praisesong for the Widow*, described the plight of fifty-eight-year-old Clarice: "With each crisis her weight had increased, the fat metastasizing with each new sorrow."

Poor food choices

"Look, when you get right down to it, I would much rather eat a piece of chocolate cake than a plate of cottage cheese."

Some people may have a hard time keeping their weights down because their genes and cells are working against them, but others make matters worse by choosing to eat too many fatty and sugary foods. When psychologists Anthony Sclafani and Deleri Springer at Brooklyn College studied the effects of a rich diet on laboratory animals, they got some fascinating results. When animals were fed standard lab chow, even in unlimited amounts, they did not overeat, and they maintained a normal weight, just as animals do in the wild. But when these laboratory animals were given the choice between lab chow and a "supermarket diet" of chocolate chip cookies, milk chocolate, salami, marshmallows, peanut butter, and condensed milk, the animals ignored their standard chow and gobbled up the supermarket goodies. Some animals actually tripled their weights.

Humans also share this desire to eat fatty and sugary foods. In a society where there is an abundance of such delicacies, individuals, both fat and thin, may have to fight strong impulses to avoid these foods. No evidence, though, indicates that fat people are more likely to have a sweet tooth than lean people.

In short, obesity results as much from biology as behavior. With so many different causes of obesity, it is no wonder that dieters have trouble losing weight and keeping it off. And though some body fat is natural, beyond a critical point, doctors say, it starts to kill us. The difficulty is knowing where naturalness ends and the threat to health begins.

THE DECISION TO LOSE WEIGHT

It takes over forty pounds of excess fat to get most men to consider dieting, but for women a mere ten pounds of flabby veneer will cause them to begin starving themselves to peel the pounds. But successful dieting does not require starving—only a little planning and patience.

Before you diet, consider why you want to lose weight:

- Are you unhappy with your body? Are you unhappy with things that you can change (being physically out of shape), or with things that are fixed (your height)?
- Are you overweight according to height–weight charts but generally in good shape?
- If you are overfat, are you content with your body but feel pressure from others to lose weight? Are you miserable with your body? Does your extra fat prevent you from participating in activities and relating to others?
- Has your doctor suggested you lose weight because of a medical problem?

Weight Control: The Looking-Glass War

Once you know your motive(s) for wanting to lose weight, you can get a better idea of your chances of success. Some people actually function better with their extra weight. Those who keep losing and gaining may do more harm to themselves than if they remained slightly overweight. They will be losing muscle tissue but gaining fat. Also, cholesterol levels rise with weight gain and increase the chances of cholesterol deposits in the arteries. These levels do not always drop with weight loss, so a woman whose weight is yo-yoing may inflict irreversible damage on her body.

Once you have assessed your current weight and degree of body fat, check table 7-2 for the treatment program best for you.

Planning a diet

What is a calorie? Calories are not nasty little creatures running around your bloodstream packing fat cells onto your body. A calories is not a thing at all. Like a gallon or inch, it is simply a unit of measurement, and what it measures is energy.

Everyone needs energy. Without it, you could not play tennis, read a book, or breathe, and frankly, you wouldn't be much fun at parties. The energy in food is technically measured in kilocalories, but for practical purposes we call them calories. If you substitute the word "energy" every time you read "calorie," you will get a new perspective on food.

You get energy from only three essential nutrients: carbohydrates, fats, and proteins. Each gram of carbohydrate or protein gives four calories; each gram of fat provides more than twice that amount—nine calories. Though not an essential nutrient, alcohol can also be broken down for energy—seven calories per gram—again more than either carbohydrate or protein.

Nutrient	*Calories/Gram*
Carbohydrate	4
Protein	4
Fat	9
(Alcohol)	(7)

All calories count, and too many add unwanted pounds. Consuming too much carbohydrate, fat, protein, or alcohol can

Table 7-2 Choosing a treatment program for weight control

If you are   *Program*

Overweight and overfat

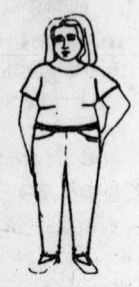

Your weight is above that desirable for your height and you have too much body fat. Begin a moderate reducing diet. Work on improving eating habits and getting more exercise. (This is the only condition that calls for a reducing diet.)

Overweight and normal fat

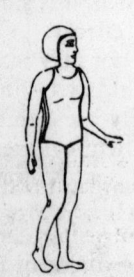

You are probably heavy-boned or muscular, possibly an athlete. If you are unhappy with your body, you may need to learn self-acceptance. Heavy bones or muscular builds are not factors you can change.

Normal weight and overfat

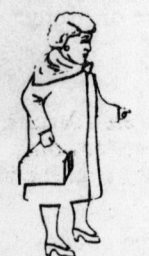

Your weight falls within the desirable range for your height, but you have too much fat relative to your lean tissues. You are out of shape. Establish good eating habits, but more important, start exercising.

Weight Control: The Looking-Glass War

If you are	*Program*
Normal weight and normal fat	Congratulations! You are doing fine. However, if you think you weigh too much, you could have a distorted body image. Try to learn self-acceptance.
Underweight and overfat	Your weight may be slightly under the desirable for your height, but you have few muscles and have proportionately too much fat. Exercise.
Underweight and normal fat	You have no problem if you are naturally slender, perhaps tall and slim. However, if you are maintaining this low weight only by chronic dieting, try to eat regular meals and get more exercise, even if you end up gaining a few pounds.
Underfat (regardless of weight)	Low fat levels are common in athletes, dancers, and models. If you have stopped menstruating, you might be losing bone. The long-term effects of such bone loss are unknown.

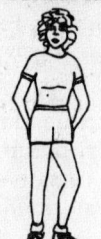

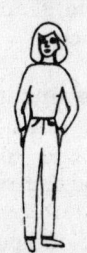

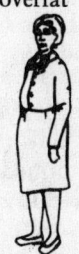

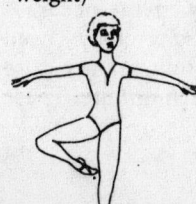

Eat Beautiful!

make you plump, but the calories add up fastest from fat and alcohol. (Vitamins and minerals are needed to release energy from fat, carbohydrate, and protein but they do not provide energy themselves. See appendix A.)

Perhaps the greatest myth in dieting circles is that carbohydrates make you fat. Wrong. Carbohydrates are a blessing to dieters. Remember, they provide only four calories compared to fat's nine. Potatoes are okay, but fat-laden sour cream glopped on top adds a mountain of calories. Bread is okay, but nix the butter. Pasta is okay, but the fatty sausage in the tomato sauce is the calorie heavyweight. Also, rich carbohydrate foods are high in fiber, and fiber curbs the appetite.

Though protein provides only four calories, it is not a better choice than carbohydrate because rich protein foods (meats, dairy products) are often high in fat. Also, your body has to remove and excrete the nitrogen from protein, and too much can tax the kidneys.

Most cells can operate on energy from either carbohydrate, fat, or protein. But nerves, muscles, and red blood cells need a constant supply of glucose, and glucose can be formed only from carbohydrate and protein—not fat. (Fats can release energy in other ways.) If you consume too little carbohydrate, your body, desperate to maintain its blood glucose level, may be forced to tap into such protein stores as hair, skin, and muscles. You will be left with loose, sagging skin and a dreadful appearance, another reason to avoid low-carbohydrate diets.

How many calories do you need? You burn off calories in two ways: by keeping your body's life-support systems functioning and by moving the body, as in exercise. The energy for the internal work of your body is measured when you are resting and is called your basal metabolic rate (BMR). You need this amount of energy just to stay alive—to keep your blood pulsing through your veins, your lungs drawing in oxygen and pushing out carbon dioxide, your glands secreting hormones, and your body temperature hovering around 98.6 degrees.

The BMR accounts for a large part of daily energy needs. A woman who requires 2,000 calories a day may need 1,200–1,400 calories just for her BMR. Certain factors raise your BMR and help you burn more calories each minute. These

Weight Control: The Looking-Glass War

include large body size (being male), rapid growth (infancy, pregnancy), muscular body, exercise, and cold weather. Other factors, such as small body size (being female), old age, a fat body, dieting, and low levels of thyroid hormone, lower your BMR so you burn fewer calories and consequently find it harder to lose weight.

Most of us do more than lie around all day like sofas, so we need energy above our BMR. Any type of movement, whether it is jogging ten miles or simply opening one eye to see if it is worth opening the other, adds to your energy needs. Exercise is one way to really control the number of calories your body burns. Use table 7-3 to figure out your resting and activity levels. This will give you an overall picture of how many calories you need each day.

How many calories should a reducing diet provide? One pound of body fat stores about 3,500 calories. Generally speaking, any time you consume 3,500 calories more than you burn off, you gain one pound. And any time you burn off 3,500 calories more than you consume, you lose a pound. (Of course, some bodies can burn off calories better than others.) It is difficult to burn off 3,500 extra calories rapidly, so if you have

---

Table 7-3 Resting and activity calorie needs

1. Determine resting level:
   (weight in pounds) × 11 = _____ calories

2. Determine activity level:

Your rate of activity	Adjustment factor
Very light	1.2
Light	1.3
Moderate	1.5
Strenuous	1.75
Very Strenuous	2.0

   Adjustment factor × resting level (from above) = _____ calories

Example: A moderately active woman who weighs 135 pounds
Resting level = 135 × 11 = 1485 calories
Activity level = 1.5 × 1485 = 2227.5 calories for total energy needs

lost one or more pounds in a day, it was probably from loss of fluids, not fat.

You should consume at least 1,000 calories on any reducing diet. Below this level you may not obtain enough vitamins and minerals, and you will probably surrender to hunger and regain the weight.

The dos and don'ts of dieting

The concept of dieting is negative. You hear dieters groan, "I am going to deny myself certain foods," or, "I am not going to allow myself more than one thousand calories." Dieting is deprivation. This negativity is a bit ludicrous because you need food to live, be healthy, and look good.

Psychiatrist Hilde Bruch, an authority on obesity and eating disorders, recounted a conversation with a friend of hers that gave another perspective on dieting: "What I resent about dieting," said her friend, "is that it makes one so terribly self-centered, so much aware of oneself and one's body, so preoccupied with things that apply to oneself only, that there is scarcely any energy left to be really spontaneous, relaxed, and outgoing . . . it makes one less of a human being."

Some women have found that after years of watching their weight wax and wane in cycles that seemed as inevitable as the seasons, they gained control over their eating and their weights by making a single decision: they simply stopped dieting.

Dieting is often a burden and taxes how you look, feel, and relate to others. Instead of thinking of your diet as denial, think of it as giving your body what it needs. Instead of thinking about what you are *not* going to eat, think about what you *will* eat to stay healthy and look good.

First, your body needs a *regular* supply of energy. Stomach growls, light-headedness, and fatigue are signals that your immediate energy reserves are low. A woman who has spent most of her life dieting may be oblivious to these cues and never know when she is hungry. Hunger is an unpleasant sensation that, if ignored, builds toward an explosion. A woman who denies herself food is stretching her limits to contain her hunger. Suddenly, it will blow up into a binge. The best way to avoid hunger is to eat food at regular intervals in reasonable amounts.

Second, to be healthy your body must get the energy it needs.

Weight Control: The Looking-Glass War

If you eat too little food, your body will lose lean tissue as well as fat, and you will begin to look like a homemade Halloween costume. Instead, you can lose weight without harming yourself by temporarily consuming a diet that has slightly less—about five hundred calories less—than your daily needs. Your body will draw slowly from the stored energy in fat cells.

Third, your body needs protein, carbohydrates, fats, vitamins, minerals, water, and fiber. Without adequate amounts of any of these, your diet will begin to take its toll on your health and looks.

Last, and just as important, your body needs exercise to stay in shape. Dieters often neglect exercise in their weight-loss programs, but it can determine the success or failure of your long-term weight control.

Diet products—are they worth it?

Artificial sweeteners Surprisingly, artificial sweeteners have never been shown to aid weight loss, and some researchers speculate that they may even frustrate efforts at reducing because they perpetuate a dependency on sweet foods. Here are descriptions of the two most common sweeteners:

Saccharin is three hundred times sweeter than sugar but has a major weakness—it leaves a bitter aftertaste. In late 1976, the US Food and Drug Administration released the results of a study that found an increased risk of bladder cancer in humans from the use of saccharin. Subsequent studies failed to confirm this, and it is now generally agreed that saccharin is at most a relatively weak carcinogen, though it seems to enhance the ability of cigarettes to promote cancer. Children who are not diabetic and pregnant women should avoid saccharin completely. Premenopausal women should avoid heavy use, and everyone should avoid excessive use. Though attempts to ban saccharin have been made, the ban may never come. One reason is that it is rapidly being replaced by aspartame.

Aspartame (sold as "Canderal" to consumers and "NutraSweet" to manufacturers) is not a sugar, but a hybrid of two amino acids: phenylalanine and aspartic acid, which are digested as protein. Technically, aspartame provides the same number of calories as protein (four calories per gram) but because it is about two hundred times sweeter than sugar, it can be used in tiny amounts. Aspartame that is equal in sweetness to one teaspoon of sugar provides less than one calorie.

Aspartame holds certain advantages over saccharin. It tastes like sugar, has no metallic aftertaste, and when combined with saccharin can even mask the bitter aftertaste of that sweetener. Like saccharin, it is safe for diabetics. Among its drawbacks are the fact that it breaks down under prolonged and high heat (such as in baking) and gradually breaks down in liquids (do not store soft drinks sweetened with aspartame beyond one year).

Not all researchers give aspartame a clean bill of health. Large amounts, say some researchers, could affect behavior. But spokespersons for Searle, aspartame's manufacturer, insist that the levels of phenylalanine in soft drinks are so low as to be negligible. Some people have reported side effects from using aspartame, including headaches, dizziness, stomach upset, allergy-type reactions, and menstrual changes, but such reports are common when a new product appears on the market. Also, a certain percentage of the population is always sensitive to any product and should avoid its use. Anyone with the genetic disease phenylketonuria should avoid using aspartame-sweetened products. Unfortunately, though labels indicate whether a product contains aspartame, restaurant food may not.

Diuretics and diet pills Diuretics, by pulling water out of the body, can cause a temporary weight loss, but they do nothing to shrink fat stores. Once you stop taking the pills, the weight returns. Never take diuretics without a doctor's prescription. Misusing diuretics can cause dehydration, an imbalance in body minerals, and heart problems. If you tend to hold water, cut back on salt instead.

Appetite suppressants supposedly work by curbing the appetite so the dieter is not tempted to overeat. These suppressants are usually amphetamines and amphetaminelike substances. Most of these drugs have undesirable side effects, such as insomnia, nervousness, increased pulse rate, heart palpitations, dry mouth, diarrhea, and a temporary rise in blood pressure. To offset these effects, some diet pills also contain barbiturates and other tranquilizers. Phenylpropanolamine (PPA), an ingredient in over-the-counter diet pills, not only reduces the appetite but also dulls the sense of taste and produces anxiety, agitation, dizziness, and high blood pressure. If you are nervous or suffer from heart or kidney disease, diabetes, or high blood pressure, avoid taking appetite suppressants. If you experience dizziness or headaches, stop taking the drug immediately.

Another type of diet pill is the starch blocker. This product comes from kidney beans and is supposed to contain a natural inhibitor of the intestinal enzyme needed to digest starch. A dieter on these pills presumably could eat as much carbohydrate as she wanted and not gain weight. However, no study has shown that this product works. If the starch blocker itself manages to survive digestion, any carbohydrate that it blocks will be a feast for intestinal bacteria, causing cramps, gas, and diarrhea. Though the US Food and Drug Administration has taken starch blockers off the market until their safety and effectiveness are proven, retailers continue to sell them.

The case against fad dieting

The humorist Art Buchwald once suggested that the word "diet" has its root in the verb "to die." Most dieters would agree. But then most chronic dieters follow fad diets that promise quick results and ignore moderation, variety, and, oddly enough, exercise. These diets rely on starvation, protein supplements, drugs, hormones, and other unpleasant remedies and lead to such common side effects as fatigue, irritability, anxiety, and depression. Fad diets have one thing in common: they are bad for your health. Beyond that, they are usually monotonous and difficult to follow for long periods of time. Here are descriptions of a few short-cut methods to weight control, most of them best avoided.

Low-carbohydrate diets Low-carbohydrate diets have surfaced under different names: the Mayo Clinic diet and the Air Force diet (disowned by both the Mayo Clinic and the air force), the Stillman diet and the new Stillman diet (apparently the first one didn't work), the Atkins diet, the liquid-protein diet, the Scarsdale diet, and the fructose diet. Each allows you to eat only small amounts of carbohydrate—60 grams or less. Some diets even replace the carbohydrate with fat.

The problem with these diets is that your body *needs* carbohydrate. When it is drastically reduced, you enter ketosis, an unhealthy state in which your body cannibalizes itself for energy. By the fourth or fifth day of ketosis, you may experience fatigue, nausea, and dehydration. The body, unable to get carbohydrate for energy, burns fats instead. But it needs carbohydrates to break down fats completely, so some of the fats are incompletely metabolized and form products called ketone bodies, or just plain ketones, which you can actually smell on your breath or measure in your urine with special colored strips of paper.

The easiest way to reverse ketosis is to eat some carbohydrate. If you don't, other problems can follow. First, protein from muscle is broken down to provide some of the energy that normally would have come from carbohydrates. The waste products from protein breakdown, together with the ketones, can stress the kidneys and lead to serious losses of water, sodium, and other minerals. The rapid loss of water explains the sudden initial weight loss on these diets, a loss that is only temporary. Abnormally low blood pressure, nausea, fatigue, and dehydration are other possible side effects.

Another reason to avoid these diets is that, for some people, a craving for starchy or sweet snacks is related to a drop in a brain chemical called serotonin. If such a person restricts carbohydrate for a few weeks, serotonin levels drop, and she begins to desire starches or sweets. She may even feel irritable or have trouble concentrating. A subsequent snack of these carbohydrates can trigger an eating binge. To avoid the binge, she should eat enough starches and sweets to satisfy her craving before it rages out of control.

One category of low-carbohydrate diets includes supplemented fasts, such as liquid or powder protein supplements. The most popular ones in recent years were the "last chance diet" promoted by Dr. Robert Linn and the Cambridge diet of Dr. Allen Howard. Reported side effects of such diets include vomiting, nausea, diarrhea, constipation, fainting, muscle cramps, fatigue, hair loss, dry skin, and intolerance to cold. Even deaths have occurred.

Weight Control: The Looking-Glass War

Fasting Total fasting causes side effects similar to those of supplemented fasts. There is a drop in blood pressure and loss of body water and minerals. Fainting spells are common. During fasting, close to two-thirds of the weight loss is from muscle, not fat. So in terms of percent body fat, fasting can actually make you fatter. These diets do not help you learn new eating habits, and any weight lost is usually regained—plus more.

Single-food diets Diets that stress one food or food group pop up every year or so. Take, for instance, the rice diet, the prune diet, the banana diet, the hard-boiled egg diet, the grapefruit diet, and the all-meat diet. Any weight loss on these novelty diets is from eating less food, usually as a result of boredom, and the loss is short-lived. These diets can lead to serious deficiencies because no single food is nutritionally complete. They also encourage bingeing.

Anticellulite therapy Cellulite, those dimply lumps that overtake thighs and hips, is claimed to be a special kind of fat that includes water and toxic wastes. Strangely enough, scientists can find no difference between cellulite and regular fat. A cellulite program combines "elimination" of toxins, breathing exercises, massage, physical exercise, and relaxation, with a one-thousand calorie diet that prohibits sugar, salt, alcohol, and artificial sweeteners. The total treatment is quite expensive and will only take the bulge out of your wallet.

The only successful way to lose these fat lumps is to reduce the amount of fat in fat cells, preferably before age thirty-five to forty while the skin is still elastic enough to shrink.

Surgical removal of fat A new method for getting rid of large fat deposits in the buttocks, thighs, and abdomen is called suction lipectomy. It actually vacuums fat cells from under the skin and leaves little tunnels that eventually collapse, reducing the area of fat. If the skin is not elastic, it will simply hang. Such treatment can leave permanent distortions in your shape and can cause serious dehydration if done by inexperienced doctors. It is no substitute for dieting and exercise because it works only on local fat deposits, not overall obesity.

Eat Beautiful!

Side effects of fad diets Besides the fad diets discussed here, you can find thousands more to keep you hungry. Although I believe that women should not follow these diets, I realize that many will. So for those of you committed to a life of food denial, I am giving you a list of symptoms, any one of which could mean that you are too severely restricting calories and nutrients and are heading for trouble. Listen to your body, and watch for the following:

- Fainting when you stand up (could be a sign of low blood pressure)
- Headaches or light-headedness
- Decreased concentration
- Heart palpitations
- Skin pallor
- Loss of hair
- Weakness or fatigue
- Insomnia
- Irritability
- Food preoccupation or dreams
- Diarrhea or constipation
- Mood swings
- Depression or anxiety
- Loss of menstrual periods

Sound appealing? Now for those of you who do not mind suffering these side effects, consider this: Dieting can make you fat! You have probably heard the complaint, "I don't know why I'm fat. I've been dieting for fourteen years." There is a good reason for this. After you lose weight, your metabolic rate slows, and you burn fewer calories each minute just to stay alive. To keep weight off, you might have to eat less than a person of the same weight. Your body also becomes more efficient at storing fat, so you have a hard time losing weight and an easy time gaining it back.

By disrupting your appetite regulator, dieting can make it difficult for you to judge feelings of fullness and hunger. After losing weight, many people are continually hungry. This constant gnawing in the stomach and obsession with food all too often leads to bingeing. For many, relief comes only with weight gain.

Weight Control: The Looking-Glass War

Dieters, by limiting what they eat, inadvertently set themselves up for defeat. If they indulge in a "forbidden food," they lose all restraint, eating anything and everything, vowing in between mouthfuls to "start over tomorrow." Close to 90 percent of dieters regain the weight they have lost, plus a few pounds more.

Many women who manage to lose weight and keep it off are forced into a lifetime of semistarvation, hunger, and obsession with weight. If a woman continually ignores feelings of hunger, she may develop a full-fledged eating disorder, such as anorexia nervosa or bulimia, risking not only her health but her life.

You can choose the sage way to look and feel your best. The key here is "your best." You may not end up looking like your ideal, but you will be able to enjoy eating, free from obsession with food, and know your body is in its best possible shape.

Exercise: rolling with the paunches

Controlling weight Exercise as a way to control your weight is far from a new idea. At the turn of the century, weight-conscious women were instructed to do the turkey trot for an hour each morning and night and to "pirouette while you peel potatoes." When you exercise, you burn calories. The more intensely you exercise, the more calories you burn. But exercise does far more than this.

A certain amount of activity keeps you attuned to your body's cues for being hungry and, after eating, being satisfied. If your activity falls below this level, you will miss these cues and overeat. If you try some intense aerobic activity, like cycling, you drive up your body temperature and shunt blood away from your stomach. This temporarily decreases hunger. But if you exercise and find yourself ravenous, it may be because you are exercising in short bursts.

Vigorous activity raises your metabolic rate and keeps it high for several hours after you have stopped exercising. Up to fifteen hours later, you may be burning extra calories. By exercising one to three hours after eating, you will burn calories faster than if you wait until your stomach is empty. So try to make breakfast and lunch your heaviest meals, and take a twenty-minute walk after eating.

Besides speeding up your metabolism, exercise burns calories by toning your muscles. Muscle is metabolically more active than fat, so the more muscle you have, the more calories you use each minute just to exist. Because muscle is denser than fat, you can gain muscle weight and lose inches. It is not uncommon for a sedentary woman to start a workout program and drop two dress sizes but gain two pounds. Horrified with the weight gain, she decides to stop exercising.

Dieters who exercise can afford to eat more food than those who do not, so they are less likely to feel the stabbing hunger pangs of a low-calorie diet. And while the deprivation of dieting can leave you depressed, exercise bestows a sense of well-being. Dieters who exercise are less likely to look in the mirror and feel fat.

The best way to lose fat is to combine exercise with a good diet. If you only diet, you tend to reduce your metabolism and lose muscle as well as fat. You can actually lose one pound of muscle for every three pounds of fat. But if you also exercise, you increase your metabolism and build up your muscle.

The exercise bonanza You will find no end to the benefits of exercise. Besides helping to control weight, exercise lowers risk of heart disease, high blood pressure, and diabetes. Modest exercise, by stressing the bones and joints, keeps bones dense and may even reverse the loss of bone. As an added benefit, the more you exercise, the more food you can afford to eat, including rich sources of calcium.

By stimulating the gastrointestinal tract, exercise reduces your chances of constipation and kidney stones—problems that worsen over the years. It can also help keep you free from colds and infections by raising body temperature, which in turn kills bacteria.

As you exercise and become better conditioned, your stamina will improve. You will perform the same amount of work with less energy. Even after an exhausting work week, you will have energy to enjoy your weekends. If you are feeling tired in the afternoon, a short walk outside can give you a greater energy boost than you would get from snacking on a candy bar. Being in shape also improves your power, agility, flexibility, speed, and strength.

Exercise is not an activity for young women only. It slows the degenerative changes of aging. A sixty-five-year-old woman, by maintaining her level of fitness, can have the stamina, suppleness, and strength of an inactive thirty-year-old.

Not all the benefits are physical. Exercise lifts a depression through a natural tranquilizing effect. After you exercise, you have an elevated level of endorphins, naturally occurring painkillers released by the brain. Many women find that they can work out their frustrations with exercise and become calmer, more alert, and better able to cope with the stresses in their lives. By coping with stress through exercise instead of overeating, they also gain a better self-image.

Which exercise should you choose? Before you begin a workout program, decide which types of exercise you are most likely to enjoy and which have the most benefits to offer. Your first goal should be physical fitness—and this involves much more than keeping your weight down. Depending on your age and your fitness goals, you will need to work on the following:

- Endurance—the ability of the heart and lungs to handle vigorous exercise. This usually involves rhythmic movement of the large muscles, forcing a continuous flow of blood through the muscles.
  How to get it: Start slowly with walking, gradually increasing your distance and speed. Work up to a one-hour brisk walk. Once you can do this, feel free to substitute other aerobic activities (skipping rope, running, bicycling).
- Flexibility—a wide range of movement in the joints.
  How to get it: Do ten to fifteen minutes of stretching exercises each day. Hold stretched positions for several seconds, working up to from thirty to sixty seconds.
- Strength—the maximum amount of force that a muscle can exert through a specific range of motion.
  How to get it: Each day do several calisthenic exercises, such as sit-ups (with knees bent) and push-ups. Breathe normally and do not strain.
- Body Composition—maintaining fat levels within the desirable range for your sex.
  How to get it: Do aerobic exercises regularly.

Aerobic exercise For overall fitness, aerobic exercises are the

Eat Beautiful!

best. These exercises require a sustained effort that makes your cardiovascular system work very hard for at least twenty minutes. They force a continuous flow of blood through the muscles and burn a large number of calories. More important, these exercises are fueled by fat, not glycogen. To use fat, your body must have oxygen, which is why exercises involving continuous exertion are called aerobic (requiring "air"). Muscles can work by using fat for much longer periods of time than they can with glycogen, so you can burn off many more calories before you get tired. Aerobic exercise can release small quantities of fat from all over your body, particularly from the largest stores.

Walking, jogging, running, cycling, swimming, and surfing all qualify as aerobic sports. The most popular exercise among adults is walking. Walking is aerobic if done at a pace of about 3.5–4 miles per hour for thirty minutes. No slow strolls, please.

Many women find aerobic dancing fun, but some programs fall way below the minimum time necessary for aerobic benefits. Racquet sports do not require as much concentrated effort from the heart and lungs, especially the way most people play them. But if you play regularly over many years, you can get aerobic benefits. Golf and bowling, no matter how you play them, offer no aerobic benefits. Exercises that are worthless for the woman who wants to lose body fat include rubberized sweat suits, sauna belts, and other sweat enhancers; weight lifting; calisthenics; and spot reducing. "If spot reducing worked," quipped an author in *Weight Watchers* magazine, "people who chew gum would have thin faces."

Select an exercise that strengthens your entire body, is fun, and allows you to pace yourself. By working your large muscles and moving your body over a distance or against gravity, aerobic exercises improve blood circulation, strengthen the heart and lungs, and reduce fat deposits.

If you are not sure what type of exercise to try, look for resources available in your community. Check out newspaper ads and the phone book.

If necessary, choose an exercise that you can do at home. Cleaning the house or keeping track of kids, as tiring as they can be, do not count as exercises.

Weight Control: The Looking-Glass War

First steps toward fitness

Get the go-ahead If you are over thirty-five or have been fairly inert for five years, consult your doctor. This advice also goes for anyone with chronic obstructive lung disease, orthopedic problems, diabetes, or other metabolic disorders.

Warm-up You should begin with a five- to ten-minute warm-up of stretching and strengthening exercises. Yoga, walking, jumping jacks, and skipping rope all qualify. These will prepare your joints and muscles for a vigorous workout, prevent soreness, and slowly build up the workload on your heart.

Burn fat Next comes the aerobic component. Aim for fifteen to twenty minutes, gradually lengthened to thirty to forty-five minutes. Work out at least three times a week. (Better yet, alternate different aerobic activities. Run one day, swim the next.) Do not let more than two days go by without exercising, but allow yourself one or two days of rest each week. If you exercise four or five times a week instead of three, you will lose weight three times faster. Energy expenditure should be about three hundred calories a day. For an untrained person, this means forty minutes of exercise.

Check your pulse During the first two to three weeks, stop every five to ten minutes to take your pulse rate. To do this, place your first two fingers on the base of your neck near your Adam's apple or on the thumb side of your wrist. Immediately after you stop exercising, count your first pulse as "0" and continue counting for six seconds. Add a zero to get the number of beats per minute. You can determine the best target range for your heart rate from this formula:

Training heart rate range

Upper level $(220 - \text{your age}) \times 0.85 = \text{beats/minute}$
Lower level $(220 - \text{your age}) \times 0.70 = \text{beats/minute}$

For example, if you are thirty years old, you should keep your exercising heart rate between 133 and 161 beats per minute. If your heart rate falls below the lower limit, you are not getting a "training effect." If it is above the upper limit, you will get fatigued before you have achieved a training effect, and you may experience cardiovascular or orthopedic problems.

Cool down After you exercise for twenty to thirty minutes, cool down for five to ten minutes more. Walk, stretch, swing your arms, and relax with deep breathing. These exercises let blood return from the exercised muscles to other organs, such as the heart and intestines, and help prevent soreness. Without a cool-down period, blood can pool in the legs and cause irregular heartbeats, dizziness, fainting, and nausea. Use your cool-down to stretch and improve your flexibility.

Check your pulse at least once while you are cooling down, and make sure it is below your target zone. Your total fitness package, including warm-up and cool-down periods, should take forty to sixty minutes a day, for at least three days a week.

Do not overdo it You should not exercise too strenuously. If your partner adheres to the idea of "no pain, no gain," get a new partner. The intensity of exercise is actually less important than its regularity and duration. You also need to let your body rest to repair its damaged muscles, get rid of metabolic wastes, and rehydrate. Injuries often result from overexertion.

Life-style changes A regular workout is essential to a shape-up program. Try not to forget why you may have become out of shape in the first place—lack of exercise. In addition to whatever program you choose, make small changes in your everyday routine that will keep your body active:

- Park your car a block or more from the store and walk the extra distance. Get off the bus a few blocks before your destination and walk the rest of the way. Foot it everywhere you can.
- Take the stairs instead of an elevator.
- Instead of a morning coffee break, go for a quick morning stroll.
- At lunchtime, take half an hour to eat and half an hour to go for a brisk walk.
- Be kind to your pets and take your dog for an extra turn around the block.

Weight Control: The Looking-Glass War

- Turn off the television and go dancing in the evening.
- On weekends, plan bicycling trips, or explore your area on foot.
- Plant a garden, then get out in it and vigorously pull those weeds.

Combining diet and exercise If you start a workout program, you do not need to add special foods to your diet or take supplements. But be sure to get adequate iron because any exercise that involves pounding of the feet can cause iron losses. By keeping your food intake constant or by slightly increasing it to cover the extra calories you are burning, you can get all the nutrients you need. This is especially important because the average British woman eats only about 1900 calories daily. At that level, she may not get enough vitamins and minerals, especially iron and calcium. The more you exercise, the more you can eat before you gain weight.

A sound way to lose weight is to take your calculation from table 7-3 (see page 137) and do two things:

- Consume 500 fewer calories a day.
- Increase your activity so you are burning at least 300 extra calories a day.

You will average, over time, a weekly loss of one to two pounds. You may plateau at a certain weight for a few weeks because your fat cells, after losing their fat, temporarily fill up with water. In time, the cells will shrink, the water will be pushed out, and your weight will begin to drop again. Increase your food intake gradually over a year's time, so that after a year you are no longer restricting calories.

So begin moving your body by getting up, turning off the television, putting on some music, and waltzing around the room. Or to update an earlier suggestion: Become a human food processor and start twirling while fixing dinner.

A summary of dieting guidelines

The Dos:

- Do eat three meals a day.
- Do choose a diet that cuts no more than 500–1,000 calories

from your daily needs, unless you are under medical supervision.
- Do serve yourself moderate, not skimpy, portions of food during meals.
- Do eat a variety of foods.
- Do eat nutrient-rich foods, and limit fats, sweets, and alcohol.
- Do follow a regular exercise program.

The Don'ts:

- Don't skip meals, saving all your calories for one monstrous meal in the evening.
- Don't follow a very low calorie diet (fewer than 1,000 calories).
- Don't follow fad diets that eliminate entire food groups, such as carbohydrates.
- Don't try to lose weight by substituting liquid or powdered supplements for real food.
- Don't consume large amounts of diet products (sodas, sweeteners) that have few, if any, essential nutrients and may contain substances that long-term studies could prove harmful.
- Don't try to lose weight by dieting without increasing your physical activity.

By adopting a positive approach to weight control, you will feel better about yourself, and you will have a much better chance of getting and staying in shape. If you actually enjoy planning diets, counting calories, and adding and subtracting imaginary pounds, try to wean yourself from these behaviors. Develop a common-sense approach to food and eating that frees you from obsessive thoughts about weight—and lets you enjoy your food.

If you need to weigh yourself to keep up morale, do so once a week at most. Fluctuations in body water can cause your weight to go up and down and leave you discouraged. Work toward being fit rather than reaching a certain weight. If possible, toss your bathroom scale out the window (several times a day is great exercise). Remember, muscle weighs more than fat, so you may find yourself slimming down, toning up, weighing more, and looking more attractive than ever!

For those of you who would like a more controlled shape-up plan than the simple suggestions above, I offer a structured approach in chapter 8.

SPECIAL CONSIDERATIONS

Help for the seriously obese

If you are moderately obese (between 41 and 100 percent over your recommended weight) or severely obese (more than 100 percent over your recommended weight), you should diet only under medical supervision. You are likely to lose and gain weight quickly without finding a permanently stable weight.

Because extreme obesity can lead to serious health problems, doctors are likely to try more drastic measures than they would for the mildly obese (28–40 percent over the recommended weight). They sometimes give a patient who is moderately obese a very low calorie diet—four hundred calories supplemented with vitamins and minerals—and then closely monitor her. Problems with the heart, blood pressure, and acute gout can occur, so this treatment should be given only in a medical setting. The patient should also exercise and learn behavioral techniques to avoid gaining weight once she resumes normal eating.

Surgery is available for those whose weight is at least one hundred pounds over or double their recommended weight and who have not responded to other forms of treatment. One technique is the stapling or stitching of certain parts of the stomach, limiting the amount of food the stomach can hold. Obviously, these treatments are for people whose obesity is so severe that the risks to health are greater than the risks from treatment.

The shrinking woman—adjusting to a new body image

Successful dieters often have trouble adjusting to their new slimmer bodies. Many overweight people, after losing weight, imagine that they are still heavy. As the once fat character in Margaret Atwood's novel *Lady Oracle* put it: "The outline of my former body still surrounded me, like a mist, like a phantom moon, like the image of Dumbo the Flying Elephant superimposed on my own."

Simple techniques to ease the adjustment include taking "before" and "after" photos, keeping a running series of photos as weight is lost, and buying smaller-sized clothing as weight comes off.

Some women believe that their weight has kept them from reaching their potential. They are convinced that once they lose weight, everything in their lives will change. With a large weight loss, a woman may feel less socially isolated, but with smaller losses, life often goes on as before. If you fail to attain what you think is your perfect weight, you may end up feeling guilty and hating yourself. The solution to your unhappiness may not be a diet but learning self-love and self-respect.

Accepting a bigger body

Despite the many suggestions for losing weight, the number of overweight women who successfully reach and maintain their desirable weights is quite small. No method of weight control has a very enviable success rate. Women have used any number of methods—behavioral techniques, low-calorie diets, exercise, weight-loss organizations, fads—and either failed to lose weight or regained whatever they lost.

If parts of your body are naturally fatter than you want, you may have to learn to adjust to them. Eating well and exercising regularly may make you healthier, but they may not mold your body into what you consider your ideal shape. At some point you will have to decide either to accept your body as it is or to be miserable for the rest of your life. You may be reassured to know that, as women age, they become more comfortable with their bodies and are more likely to separate their body images from their successes and failures in life. So when you gain a pound, you are less likely to blame it on a personality defect as you are to admit that you ate too much on vacation.

When friends, colleagues, or family tell you that you are getting too fat, make an honest appraisal of your body and decide for yourself if you weigh too much. Do not rely on well-intentioned but sometimes uninformed opinions. Find out if you have a family history of diabetes, heart disease, or hypertension, and talk to your doctor about whether your weight poses a risk to your health. Be sure to discuss any of your past weight-loss efforts and decide what the chances are for success should you decide to start on a weight-loss program.

Underweight

Some women weigh too little. Underweight is defined as weight less than 90 percent of the recommended weight and results from many of the same factors as overweight: genetics, metabolism, and psychological and social factors.

Though some women who weigh slightly less than average may actually be healthier than those who weigh more, being *too* thin can be physically uncomfortable and can place you at risk of a serious deficiency should you get sick, particularly if you are an older woman. If you get pregnant, you are more likely to deliver an infant with a low birth weight. If your fat levels are too low, you may stop menstruating and possibly begin to show signs of bone loss, the long-term consequences of which are unknown.

Before you decide to gain weight, be sure nothing is physically wrong with you. Loss of weight is often a symptom of a number of serious disorders. If you have been underweight most of your life, you probably need to change a few habits in order to add pounds. Cut down on nervous activity and make sure you have enough rest. Be sure to get daily exercise to ensure a good night's sleep, but don't get fanatical about working out.

Neither side of this coin—too fat or too thin—is really a bargain. But with careful attention to your physical and psychological needs, eating can still be—and should be—one of your most satisfying experiences. To gain weight, eat nutritious snacks between meals, but not so much as to ruin your appetite. Snacks can include whole milk, peanut butter, grape juice, puddings, oatmeal cookies, half a sandwich, ice cream, cheese, and avocadoes. Eat six small meals instead of three large meals a day. Try eating more rapidly than usual so that you can get a few extra bites in before you get full. Eat your entree before your salad so you have your higher-calorie foods before your high-fiber, low-calorie greens. A little wine before dinner may help to stimulate your appetite. You can purchase special high-calorie liquid supplements such as Sustacal or create your own milk base to add to soups (homemade and reconstituted), casseroles, puddings, custards, baked goods, cereal, and hot beverages. Simply add 1 cup of skim milk powder to 3½ cups of whole milk. If you desire more calories, add any of the following: an egg, fruit nectar, ice cream, or chocolate syrup. If you smoke cigarettes, cut back or give them up. Just as dieting can lower your metabolism, eating extra food can raise it and make it difficult to gain weight.

RESOURCES

Overeaters Anonymous, Manor Gardens Centre, 6–9 Manor Gardens, London N7 6LA. This is a self-help organization that offers counseling to overweight people. It helps dieters overcome emotional roadblocks to weight loss and bingers to understand their compulsion.

Weight Watchers (UK) Ltd, 11 Fairacres, Dedworth Road, Windsor, Berkshire, SL4 4UY. Members are given a high-protein, low-calorie diet and meet weekly for pep talks and encouragement.

8
The Shape-up Plan: How to Make Food Behave

> Habit is habit, and not to be flung out of the window ... but coaxed downstairs a step at a time.
>
> Mark Twain, *Pudd'nhead Wilson*

When you shop at the grocery, do you find the chocolate-chip cookies jump into your cart and, once home, mysteriously disappear? Does ice cream vaporize into thin air while in your freezer? Does commercial magnetism pull you toward a chocolate vending machine? Although it may seem impossible to make food behave and stop exercising its powers over you, let me assure you that you can do it. Begin by accepting responsibility for your eating behavior and stop blaming it on food. Then take action.

Investigating your eating habits

First, I would like to introduce two hypothetical characters: Jeanne, the woman with admirable eating habits; and Helen, the woman with every eating problem imaginable. Jeanne eats only when she is hungry and, when she eats, she takes time to enjoy her meals. Helen is an emotional eater who responds to anger, frustration, and boredom by turning to food. To help you understand how such feelings can interfere with eating, I asked Helen to fill out a food and exercise diary (figure 8-1). Notice how quick, sugary foods grab her attention until lunch. She gets bored, so she snacks. When Helen has a fight with her husband, she binges. Later, she feels so badly about overeating that her husband comes over to cheer her up. Helen has found a subtle way to get attention from her husband after a fight, but it is at the expense of her weight and health. She also avoids dealing with the real issues behind their fights. But what about your situation?

Eat Beautiful!

HELEN
DAY:
DATE:

FOOD DIARY

Time	Feelings & Events Before Eating	Food Eaten	Amount	Where	Feelings & Events After Eating
8 am	running late, anxious, tired	coffee, english muffin, butter, jam	1 c, 1 whole, 1 oz, 1 tbsp	bedroom (while dressing)	rushed, jumped in car
10:30 am	hungry, tired, bored	coffee, pastry	1 c	coffee shop with Carol	hyper from coffee
12:30 pm	hungry, tired	wheat bread, pastrami, potato chips, mayo, coke	2 sl, 3 oz, 1 sm bag, 1 tbsp, 8 oz	diner	full, did a little shopping before returning to work
3:30 pm	frustrated with boss	coffee, chocolate cake	1 c, 1 piece	coffee shop with Carol	still frustrated with boss, feeling calmer, talked problems over with Carol
6:30 pm	still frustrated from afternoon	dinner: soup, tomato salad, lettuce, tomato, French dressing	1½ c small, 1 large	living room in front of TV	still hungry, beginning to relax
9 pm	hungry, argued with Bob	ice cream, chocolate sauce	2 c, 4 tbsp	living room in front of TV	hate myself for pigging out, and Bob didn't come over to console me

EXERCISE DIARY

Time	Activity	Duration
	no exercise	

Figure 8-1 Food and exercise diaries

The Shape-up Plan: How to Make Food Behave

Draw a chart as shown in figure 8-1. Take one full week to record your observations in a meal-by-meal, snack-by-snack report. Write down the time of day, what happened before you ate, what you ate and where, and what happened afterward. Fill out the record as completely as possible. The more information you put down, the better. Take the record with you during the day so you can jot down items you may forget later on. And remember—this is not the time to start changing your eating habits. You are recording your current habits, so do not try to put on a good show. No one needs to see this record but you. If you find it too bothersome to keep detailed records, write down as much as possible. Some information is better than none.

At the end of the week, go over your notes and look for certain eating patterns. Do you habitually eat in front of the television? Do you eat when you are under stress or depressed? Does a fight with your boss lead to frustration, goading you to binge? Does anger immediately cause you to grab a chicken leg? Do you eat most of your food after five o'clock? Do you skip breakfast? Analyze your record for these habits that promote overeating. Also, observe what happens after you eat. Do you feel good because you have indulged yourself? Do you feel self-loathing or guilt? Do people try to comfort you or pay more attention to you?

During this week, also keep track of your physical activity. Are there certain times of the day when you are more likely to exercise? Are you getting any exercise at all?

Record observations of your eating and exercise patterns for at least one week. Continue it for two weeks if the first week is unusual—if, for instance, you had a lot of parties and ate leftover party food all week.

Gaining control over your food

By examining your food and exercise diary, you should have some idea of why and how you eat, and whether or not you exercise. Are you snacking a lot during the day? Do you set aside time to work out? What about the quality of the foods you are eating? Do they bellow "Fattening!"

Being overfat and out of shape robs you of vitality and adds to your risk of certain diseases. But it is not easy to keep your eating habits from being buffeted about by your emotions and everyday circumstances. The shape-up plan helps set your sights on the possible. You will have just three goals.

THE SHAPE-UP PLAN—GOALS

1. Eat three meals a day.
2. Exercise for at least thirty to fifty minutes, three days a week.
3. Eat a balanced diet, low in fats and sweets.

Try to meet each goal in the order given above. Now what if you already eat only three meals a day and you do not snack? Great, go on to goal 2 and then to goal 3. If you already exercise for forty minutes three days a week, start with goal 1, and when you achieve it, skip to goal 3. Your progress may be gradual. After all, you are trying to learn new habits. And that takes time. Following is an explanation of each goal. You will be charting each goal; filling in your charts daily will keep up your motivation and allow you to see your progress.

Goal 1: *eat three meals a day*

Nothing is magical about eating three meals a day. In fact, some women find it easier to maintain desirable weight by eating five or six minimeals a day; once you gain control over your eating, you may want to do this. The shape-up plan calls for three meals a day—neither more nor less—for several reasons. For a woman whose weight problem stems not simply from overeating but from using food as an emotional crutch, it is easier to gain control of eating by having only three meals a day.

Many women are obsessed with eating. Having more than three meals may make you think about food too often. It is difficult to restrict your eating when you have snacks between meals. Snacks are usually consumed at an office desk or on the run and get you out of the habit of trying to control where, when, and how much you eat. Without great effort, you may find yourself snacking on fatty, sugary foods—the kind usually available in vending machines.

Women under stress often grab food for release. If you know that snacking is not a part of this program, you are more likely

The Shape-up Plan: How to Make Food Behave

to learn better ways to deal with pressure. Once you have gained control over your eating, feel free to include nutritious snacks in your day's meal plan. But for now (unless your doctor tells you otherwise)—hold off.

Before you read further, let me explain that in this program I make no distinction between a meal and snack. You are trying to limit the number of times you eat to three a day. (The exceptions here are certain "free foods" that you can have any time.) If you have a bowl of cereal at four p.m. and you think of it as a snack, you must still count it as one of the three times you ate that day. Eat moderate portions; don't limit your meals to skimpy amounts of food.

Women who eat fewer than two meals a day often find themselves hungry at inopportune times, such as when the only food around is pale, hardened pastries stuck to their plastic wrappers or candy canes left over from last year's Christmas party. Eating three meals can keep you satisfied so you are not forced to scrounge for crumbs.

Figure 8-2 shows how to chart your progress on limiting yourself to three meals a day. This chart illustrates how Helen worked her way down from eating forty-two times a week (three meals plus three snacks daily) to twenty-two.

Design a chart like that shown in figure 8-2. At the end of the day, fill in the number of times that you ate. Better yet,

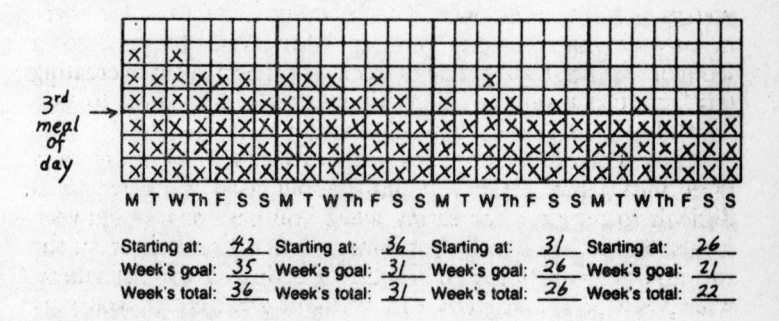

	Starting at:	Starting at:	Starting at:	Starting at:
	_42_	_36_	_31_	_26_
Week's goal:	_35_	_31_	_26_	_21_
Week's total:	_36_	_31_	_26_	_22_

Figure 8-2 Charting three meals a day Above is Helen's chart for one month during which time she was able to limit her eating from six times a day to three times.

mark down each time you eat as you are doing it. Each week, figure out your total and compare it to that week's goal. If you met your week's goal, reward yourself (see list p. 167), and move on to planning goal 1 for the following week. Once you have successfully limited yourself to three meals a day for an entire week, move on to goal 2—exercise—but continue charting goal 1.

It may take some time for you to move from goal to goal, but stay with it. On the other hand, do not get too comfortable at one level—keep trying to improve. What's important is keeping a constant pace. Do not be discouraged if you slip occasionally. If you are rigid with yourself or punish yourself, you will be doomed to failure. If you slide back into your old habits, keep trying. Eventually you will succeed.

Goal 2: Exercise for at least thirty to fifty minutes, three days a week

You cannot get fit and be healthy without exercise. Yet some women find this the hardest life-style change to make. The secret is to start out slowly doing things that you enjoy and build up to a program that promotes flexibility, strength, and aerobic benefits.

Before you start, you need to get in the right frame of mind. Listen to Jeanne and Helen preparing to launch into goal 2:

Helen: "But things are always coming up. I never know when I'll be free to exercise."

Jeanne: "Schedule a time for exercise. Taking care of yourself is as important as any other priority. So don't be flexible about your exercise time. Think of it as the last thing to come off your list when unexpected events pop up. And you'll have more energy to do other things after you exercise."

Helen: "I want to lose weight before I exercise. I'd die of embarrassment if anyone saw me like this."

Jeanne: "You are not going to get in shape unless you start now—with exercise. During your first week, your worst fears may be confirmed. If you take a dance class, you may not be able to keep up. Everyone may be better than you. But so what? You've got to start somewhere, right? If you're worried about what others will think, you'll be surprised to find out how much they respect you for your efforts. Besides, since you're starting out in bad shape, you'll see lots more improvement."

The Shape-up Plan: How to Make Food Behave

Eavesdropping on Jeanne and Helen, do you find that you tend to take one argument over another? Do you sound more like Jeanne or Helen? Before you start a workout program, take some time to acknowledge your phobias and anxieties about exercise. Throughout your program, remind yourself why you are doing this. Notice the positive changes in yourself, not just the fact that you may have a long way to go. Write them down and read them when you need some emotional support to keep going.

If you are uncertain what sort of exercise to do, refer back to chapter 7. Figure 8-3 shows how Helen tracked her progress. To determine what your starting week's goal will be, refer back to your food and exercise diary and see how much you are currently exercising. The chart indicates how many days and how long you exercised each week.

Set up a chart like that shown in figure 8-3. Fill it in daily and try to work your way up to a minimum of thirty to fifty minutes a day, three days a week. (Exercising for ninety minutes in one day does not count.) Remember, you should spend five

Day	Activity	Duration (min)
Mon	walk-jog	10
Tue		
Wed	walk-jog	15
Thur		
Fri		
Sat	began swimming class	30
Sun		

Minutes
Starting at: __0__
Week's goal: __40__
Week's total: __55__

Figure 8-3 Charting exercise Above is Helen's chart for one week during which time she was able to meet her goal of 40 minutes of exercise.

Eat Beautiful!

to ten minutes warming up, at least twenty minutes exercising aerobically, and five to ten minutes cooling down.

At the same time, eat three meals a day. Continue to chart both goals. Regularly list the positive changes you are experiencing (exercise is easier, you are more limber, lovemaking is more exciting . . .). If you reach goal 2 for two consecutive weeks, move on to goal 3—eating a balanced diet.

Goal 3: eat a balanced diet

Before you move on to this goal, assess your weight. Are you overweight? underweight? or just right? Now look at the first chart in appendix C, which offers eating plans at five different calorie levels. Choose the plan according to your personal weight goals:

- To stay at your current weight, choose a plan that meets your daily calorie needs (refer back to table 7-3, p. 137, if necessary).
- To lose weight, choose a plan that offers 500 fewer calories than your daily needs.
- To gain weight, choose a plan that offers 500 more calories than your daily needs.

Under this program, you are allowed a specific number of portions from each of seven food categories: "free foods," vegetables, fruits, starches, proteins, milk, and fats. These portions provide important vitamins and minerals, yet keep your diet within a designated calorie range. The list of foods appears in appendix C.

You can chart your progress on this goal as shown in the last chart in appendix C. Your weekly goal will be to work up to eating the specific number of portions from each food category. After you succeed for two weeks, you have met this goal.

Once you are comfortable with the eating plan, try to make the most nutritious choices from the selections in each category. For instance, one starch exchange can be used for either a slice of wholewheat bread or a small doughnut. But the bread has more nutrients and less sugar and fat than the doughnut.

Though it is smart to cut down on fats, sweets, and alcohol, you do not have to consider them forbidden. Banning your favorite foods could spell the downfall of your diet. People who

The Shape-up Plan: How to Make Food Behave

are the strictest with themselves about what they can eat are the ones who tend to lose control when stressed or under the influence of alcohol.

HOW TO REACH YOUR GOALS
Designing your environment

Old habits are hard to change. One way to make getting in shape easier is to arrange your living and work areas so food is not always jumping up and beckoning you to indulge. Following are ways to design your environment to promote sensible eating.

Buying food

- Buy only small amounts of food at a time.
- Plan your meals ahead of time and have a list of necessary ingredients.
- If you want to buy snacks for your family, buy ones that you do not like.
- Buy foods that need to be prepared before they are edible, even if they are convenience foods that simply need to be heated. (Do this especially if you are a binger.)

Storing food

- Keep food only in the kitchen and keep it out of sight.
- Get rid of candy or nut dishes that may be scattered throughout your house. Clear the jar of jelly beans off your office desk.

Preparing food

- Force yourself to stay out of the kitchen until it's time to fix meals. If you habitually head to the kitchen when you arrive home, do something else to keep yourself occupied.
- Preplan individual meals for the whole week's menu to avoid impulse eating.
- Avoid generous tasting as you cook. Some women find chewing sugarless gum helps.

Eating at home

- Restrict your eating to certain places inside your home. Do not eat anywhere else.

Eat Beautiful!

Okay for Eating	*Off Limits*
Kitchen	Living room
Dining room	Bedroom
	Bathroom
	Car

- Limit yourself to three meals a day, preferably at the same time each day.
- Do not eat while you are involved in other activities, such as watching television or reading.
- Make mealtime a ritual. Sit down and relax when you eat. Make your environment special. Use a favorite tablecloth and place setting. At night, light a candle.
- Place food on plates in the kitchen and keep serving dishes off the table during meals.
- Curb your appetite by beginning your meal with broth or clear soup, followed by a salad with a light dressing. The warm liquid plus the fiber in the salad will dampen your appetite.
- Eat full portions. Do not try eating as little food as possible. You will only end up snacking or bingeing later. Use smaller plates and bowls to make the portions look larger.
- Cut your food into small pieces and eat slowly enough to taste each bit. Put your fork down between bites. It takes about twenty minutes after eating before you begin to feel full.
- Do not go back for seconds.

Eating at the office

- Eat enough food at lunch so you will not be starving by the time you get home. Bring a variety of foods so you do not get bored.
- Do not eat at your desk. Going out will make you feel more like you have had a meal. Eat for half an hour and take a walk for the other half.

After eating

- Record what you eat if you are in the beginning stages of the plan.

- Put all food away after meals. Cover leftovers in opaque dishes so you cannot see them.
- Brush your teeth.
- Eat dinner at least a few hours before bedtime and take a walk afterward. Research shows that your body burns calories more efficiently if you exercise after eating.

Eating in a restaurant

- If you are in a restaurant that serves generous portions, either leave some food on your plate or ask for a doggie bag and take the extra food home. If you are with a friend, order two salads and split the entree. Avoid all-you-can-eat restaurants. Any money you save on these "deals" you will probably spend later on diet aids.
- Order single glasses of wine rather than a carafe.

Eating at a party

- Stay as far away from the hors d'oeuvres table as possible, and spend your time talking rather than eating.
- If you overindulge, cut back a bit on your portion sizes during the following week.

Rewarding yourself

Working toward the three shape-up plan goals will help you gain mastery over your eating, improving your diet, and getting out and exercising. *Do not gear rewards to weight loss, which does not indicate much about body fat or fitness.*

Draw up a list of balancers—activities or things that you greatly enjoy that serve as rewards for caring for your health.

Some balancers include:

- Spending some time alone doing something you enjoy
- Getting a haircut
- Buying a new book
- Meeting a friend
- Going on a trip
- Going to see a movie or play
- Buying special bath products
- Taking music lessons
- Taking dance lessons

Eat Beautiful!

- Going out to dinner with a friend or partner
- Buying new clothes (if you buy something on sale before you meet your goal, do not wear it until you have reached your goal)

Note: Specific foods should not be used as balancers.

Reward yourself with smaller balancers when you meet a weekly goal. Reserve "special" rewards for those times when you meet one of the three program goals. Some women, when the meet a weekly goal, like to put an "allowance" away in a clear jar (seeing the money can help motivate them). The money accumulates as they meet their weekly goals; then, when they have met one of the three major goals, they take the money and spend it. For other women, saving an allowance and buying special things is not rewarding. They prefer to have their husbands take the children out for the day to give them a chance to have some free time. Be sure to take the reward if you earned it. Postponing it will only hinder your progress. If you begin to tire of your old rewards, make a list of new ones.

Checks for weak moments

We all have moments when our minds are bent on doing one thing and are closed to any rational thought. Bingers know the feeling: you are suddenly overcome with a desire to stuff in enormous amounts of food, and your brain seems to be void of any arguments against it. For times like these, you need to stop long enough so you can regain control of yourself. It will help if you make a list of activities that you personally do not engage in while eating or that check your desire to eat. This list will vary for each woman. Sample activities include:

Sewing	Jogging
Taking a shower	Brushing your teeth
Playing favorite sports	Dancing
Practicing an instrument	Working in a garden
Reading in a library	Going somewhere special
Making phone calls	Chewing a stick of gum
Cleaning the house	Playing cards

When you feel an uncontrollable urge to eat and you are not hungry, quickly do one of your checks to give you time to think clearly. It may take fifteen to twenty minutes for the eating urge to pass. If you are at work and cannot get involved in one of these activities, tell yourself that you can eat—if you still want to—only after twenty minutes have passed.

Coping with others

People around you will have different attitudes toward your desire to get in shape. Some may feel threatened. Others may try to sabotage your efforts. A few may simply not understand how they can help, particularly if they can eat large amounts of food without gaining weight. You may go to a party where the hostess says to you, "I made these great goodies [cookies, stuffed mushrooms] myself. You can't tell me you're not going to even try them!" You should have an idea what your response will be. Are you going to politely decline? (You can even request that your hostess help you by not forcing the issue.) Or maybe you decided beforehand to sample everything and make up for it the next week. Just be sure you know what your plan of action will be.

Coping with yourself

Friends are not the only ones who may sabotage your fitness goals. You may be right up there with the worst of them. What you tell yourself can make the difference between the success or failure of your program. When you pass by the ice cream cabinet do you whine, "How can I possibly deny myself a taste of chocolate-chocolate chip?" or, "Why can't I be like everyone else and eat what I want?" Or do you take a more positive approach: "I'm on this program to get healthier," or, "I decided to follow this program because I want to do something good for myself." Your mantra should be one of hope, not self-pity. Practice reciting these positive statements, even if at first you don't believe them.

9
Eating Disorders: When Thin is Not Enough

Of course I had breakfast; I ate my Cheerio.

A defiant anorexic to her psychiatrist. From
The Golden Cage, Hilde Bruch

Angie works long hours for an advertising agency. The pressure in her job is constant, softened a bit by the pay. Though she is on an interminable diet, she is quite heavy. Her feet spread over the tops of her high heels, and her face is sallow and broken out. Her colleagues notice that she never eats a meal but is always sipping a diet soda and she seems to spend a lot of time in the bathroom. Everyone keeps telling her to eat some real food. No one can figure out how she can eat like a sparrow and look like a butterball.

On a coffee break, two of the women in the office entered the restroom right after Angie had left. One of them opened the door to the last stall and couldn't believe her eyes—the floor was littered with crumbs from tortilla chips.

Angie is a closet eater. By trying to fill up on diet sodas, she is allowing herself so little food that her body sends out distress signals for nourishment. She finds herself secretly bingeing on vending-machine snacks. Because she has made a big deal about being on a diet, she feels uncomfortable eating in front of her office mates. Her bathroom binges are not only creating nutritional problems but are also chipping away at her self-esteem.

Angie may have started with a simple diet, possibly one very low calories. She may have decided to skip certain meals. Then she may have skimped on portions for those meals she ate. Diet soft drinks worsened her problem because her body, begging for food, was getting a no-energy, no-protein, no-carbohydrate, no-fat, no-vitamin substitute. Her brain heard distress signals from her stomach and triggered her overwhelming desire to gorge. Unless she can start to eat normally, her denial–desire cycle will become a preoccupation, then grow steadily into an obsession.

Many women behave like Angie. They diet, not to be thin, but to gain control over their lives. A survey of college women found that quite a few saw hunger as obscene and constantly fought the impulse to eat.

The dieting done by most women is an all-consuming passion of self-abuse. Some women can stay slender only at the cost of being depressed and obsessed with food—and continually starving. Unless a woman is willing to choose a realistic goal for her weight and then make lifelong changes in her eating and exercise habits, she is better off remaining overweight. Simple dieting and full-blown eating disorders lie on a continuum, and between them is only a slender thread of control.

Anorexia nervosa—dying to be perfect

On February 4, 1983, Karen Carpenter, a pop singer whose records sold over 80 million copies, died as a result of anorexia nervosa. She had suffered from the disorder for about nine years, and during that time her weight dropped to eight-five pounds on a five-foot-four-inch frame. Her death at the age of thirty-two brought anorexia to the attention of millions of people. Though the public reacted with disbelief, confusion, and curiosity about this bizarre eating disorder, thousands of young women read the account and privately recognized their own obsession.

Anorexia nervosa, described as a "relentless pursuit of thinness," is a condition of drastic dieting or self-starvation that leads to severe weight loss. Society's overemphasis on thinness has greatly increased the number of women obsessed with dieting as a way to achieve an unrealistic weight. Anorexia is twenty times more common in British girls than boys. The highest risk period is just before or just after puberty when girls add body fat and become overconcerned about looks and body image.

Anorexia often begins after a stressful event, such as a death, parental divorce, broken romance, a sexual encounter, or simply being ribbed about being fat. The beginning of anorexia often coincides with the start of high school or college, when feelings of failure or loneliness are common.

Eat Beautiful!

Older women also become anorexic. This happens in part from their desire to control their lives and in part from the demands on them to be slim to attain professional success. Attempting to balance the roles of wife, mother, and career professional can force some women to set such unrealistic goals that they can never achieve them. Rigid dieting gives them control over one area of their lives. Some women find that after an illness they have lost weight. Pleased with the loss, they decide to continue losing weight without any reasonable goal.

The pressure for slenderness is causing a less severe form of the disorder in young dancers and athletes. The late George Balanchine may have been indirectly responsible for ballerinas flirting with the idea of self-starvation. Balanchine's ideal was a bony dancer who could move swiftly and change directions smoothly. He insisted, though, that this look came from vigorous training, not dieting. Sometimes dancers and athletes can be persuaded to eat more food once they learn that starving will compromise their performance.

Most anorexic girls come from good homes, are well behaved, and get good grades in school. They are often from families that are preoccupied with outer appearances more than inner worth. Their parents expect them to be obedient and to excel in their activities, but may withhold praise. Their parents may also give mixed messages: "Clean your plate" but "Don't be overweight." These girls find themselves futilely trying to earn approval.

The anorexic learns to be overcritical of herself and finds it difficult to develop self-esteem. Her parents may have overprotected her and further contributed to her feeling that she lacks control over her life. Rigidly controlling her weight provides her with a sense of power and direction.

A girl does not become anorexic overnight. She may start out a little overweight, just a little too plump. So she goes on a diet, and being a perfectionist, she follows it faithfully. As the weight comes off, her friends and family begin to notice her. The attention keeps her dieting, but she goes a step further and starts to manipulate the diet—to gain control over herself and others. Her eating patterns become more rigid and confined, and her body image more distorted.

An anorexic sees herself in ways that others view as bizarre. Even when she weighs a mere sixty pounds, she continues to think of herself as fat. A twenty-year-old patient of psychiatrist Hilde Bruch admitted, "I really cannot see how thin I am. I look into the mirror and still cannot see it; I know I am thin because when I feel myself I notice that there is nothing but bones." Another patient tied a ribbon around her waist to remind herself not to gain weight beyond its bounds. The ribbon, of course, made a small circle.

The anorexic's loss of weight is tragically complemented by a loss of reality. Depression, anxiety, and preoccupation with death are common. Sexual feelings disappear, and any desire for a romantic partner tends to be fanciful.

The anorexic is hyperactive and exercises frantically, all the while denying fatigue. Compulsiveness extends beyond exercise. Studying, cleaning, working—everything is done to excess. The anorexic also denies any desire for food, yet holds an all-consuming interest in it. She dreams about it, talks about it, and stares at it in supermarkets. She prepares rich dishes for others in which she would never consider indulging. Elizabeth Kaye, writing in *Family Health* magazine, described a fifteen-year-old, seventy-two-pound anorexic girl who "was amenable to hospitalization, on one condition: that she be allowed to bring a file box with her, which, it was learned upon inspection, contained many hundreds of recipes, including 14 different ones for making pecan pie." Besides will-power, the anorexic relies on appetite suppressants and amphetamines to prevent herself from eating. Even when she does eat, she underestimates her body's need for food. One patient claimed that two stalks of celery drenched in catsup was a meal; another lived on one chicken liver each day.

The anorexic may resort to ritualized eating: counting every calorie, eating only a limited number of bites at a time, arranging and rearranging bits of food on a plate, or not allowing food to touch her lips. Once she has reached a certain level of starvation, even small amounts of food can cause abdominal bloating and nausea. Though the term "anorexia" means loss of appetite, only in the advanced stages of this disorder does a true loss of appetite occur.

The physical symptoms are no less severe than the psychological ones. Menstrual periods stop. A girl may even stop menstruating before she begins to diet, possibly as a reaction to emotional stress. In many cases, this is the first sign of the disorder and leads some researchers to believe that the anorexic girl is struggling to delay the physical onset of maturity. Extreme weight loss leaves her painfully sensitive to cold. Even a moderately warm environment is uncomfortable. Her pulse rate slows, blood pressure drops, and she may suffer from insomnia and constipation. Her hair may fall out, and what remains becomes dry and straggly. An odd growth of fine hair called lanugo may spread over her cheeks, neck, forearms, and thighs. Her skin itself may become dry and pimply. A girl who turns to vomiting, diuretics, or antidepressive drugs, all of which cause the mouth to become acid, may do irreversible damage to her teeth.

When her weight reaches its absolute minimum, the result is permanent brain damage, invalidism, or death. There are few statistics on death rates, but they are believed to be high. Death usually results from cardiac arrest due to fluid and electrolyte imbalances, particularly potassium. The other major cause of death among anorexics is suicide.

In severe cases, treatment may begin with restoring nutrients to the malnourished victim by feeding her directly through a tube in her stomach. Behavioral techniques are helpful. A patient may be required to gain a certain amount of weight before she will be allowed to continue her much desired exercise. But weight gain alone will not cure the disease. A girl must have a realistic body image before she can recover. Body-image therapy may take the form of drawings, mirrors, photographs, or videotapes. Individual and group therapy can give the patient a better understanding of her body weight and nutritional needs and can improve family interactions. She can learn assertiveness through self-help groups, training courses, and books.

Anorexia nervosa is curable. The earlier it is detected, the greater the chance for recovery. Some patients do not regain normal body functions for many years. While menstrual periods can take up to ten years to return, they generally resume one year or more after weight returns to normal. But the periods may never be regular. Even without the return of menstrual periods, anorexics can have children as long as their ovaries are active. Researchers have not yet established the long-term effects of anorexia on offspring, but most babies seem to be healthy if the mother is a recovered anorexic who keeps her weight at an acceptable level. Proper nutrition can also restore the gloss and fullness to hair, but this may take a long time even after normal weight is reached.

Recovered anorexics may still have trouble managing their eating and weight. Relapses are common, and over one-third of anorexics return to the hospital within two years of their initial recovery. Others go on to become compulsive eaters or bulimics (discussed in the next section, "Bulimia").

Because anorexics do not consider themselves ill or abnormal, few seek help on their own, and most view a therapist as just one more person who wants to make them gain weight. Detection often occurs when the anorexic tries to obtain diet pills or seeks help for insomnia or severe constipation. Some early-warning signs of anorexia nervosa are: loss of menstrual periods; preoccupation with dieting; defiance when confronted with questions about weight or dieting; compulsive exercising; feeling bloated after eating normal amounts of food; bingeing; complaints of being fat regardless of actual weight; refusal to maintain minimum body weight for age and height; severe weight loss with no known physical illness as the cause; withdrawal and isolation from friends; complaints of being constantly cold.

If you suspect someone has a problem, you can do one of several things:

- If you are close to the person, be open and honest with her and let her know that you care. Instead of focusing on her weight, focus on her feelings. She will not seek help for an eating disorder that she does not even realize she has, but she will seek help if she believes someone can lift the depression, loneliness, and hurt she feels inside. Do activities together that you both enjoy to feel positive about living.
- If you are not close to the person, speak to someone who is, someone from whom she seeks love. Encourage the two of them to talk.
- If the person is in a severe stage, talk to her parents or partner about immediate hospitalization.

If you suspect you may have the disorder, the following suggestions may help you deal with it. (These suggestions were made by a woman who has recovered from anorexia and who counsels women with eating disorders.)

- Remember that it is okay to seek professional help to work out an emotional problem. Don't believe it when you find yourself thinking, "Oh, you're always making things so serious, trying to draw some attention to yourself," or, "It's not that serious. You can work it out for yourself—if you're really strong, you won't ask for help." Anorexia can be life-threatening. It requires immediate treatment.
- Remember that you are worth taking care of. You are not being selfish when you take care of your own needs. You are as worthwhile a person as anyone else and have no reason to be self-destructive.
- Losing weight is not going to make you less lonely or less depressed. If you look at it honestly, you are controlling your weight because you feel ineffective in living with others and uncomfortable with your life. If you are really strong, you will fight to find your identity, become satisfied with yourself and love yourself, and learn to love others without seeking unrealistic expectations.
- Recognize that recovery is slow and be patient with yourself. Avoid setting limits on recovery ("I'll be better by . . ."). Be gentle with yourself—you are trying.

Those of you who have toyed with the idea of becoming anorexic just until you lose those few pounds should not be fooled. Anorexia nervosa is a painful and dangerous condition. To avoid it, all weight-conscious women should strive to take the following steps:

- Do things that make you feel good about yourself.
- Take responsibility for your actions.
- Be aware of stressful times and learn relaxation techniques so you can deal with tension.
- Talk to your colleagues, friends, parents, or teachers about your problems, or seek professional counseling, if necessary.
- Exercise moderately to stay in shape and to help you feel positive about your body.
- When you decide to diet, be realistic. Find out what a good

weight is for you, and learn the basics of nutrition (this book is a good place to start). Set a goal that you can reach without literally killing yourself.

Bulimia—the endless (but terminal) binge

Thirty-six-year-old Cecilia spent eight exhausting hours working on a magazine layout, arrived home at six in the evening, and started cooking dinner—seven hamburgers. While these were frying, she curbed her appetite by starting her evening binge: one quart of mint chip ice cream, three pounds of chocolate, two dozen iced doughnuts, and several quarts of milk (low-fat). The amazing thing about Cecilia is that she is five feet five inches tall and weighs only 120 pounds. Her secret? She spends her after-dinner hours throwing up.

Cecilia is not alone. These vomiting and starving behaviors are becoming so widespread that many young women consider them normal. Sixty percent of sixth-form girls are now or have been on severe reducing diets. They may simply be trying to lose a few pounds, but before they know it, some of them will have a full-blown eating disorder.

While anorexia nervosa is characterized by drastic dieting or self-starvation, bulimia is the consumption of enormous quantities of food followed by purging with laxatives and/or vomiting. These two disorders can overlap. About 50 percent of anorexics, usually those who develop the disorder at an older age, binge and purge during the course of their illness or after gaining weight during recovery. Bulimics occasionally show an anorexic pattern.

About 80 percent of Americans with eating disorders are bulimics. Most are women. (In Britain, there are more bulimics than the estimated 5,500 anorexics. Between a tenth and a quarter are male.) The victims, in their teens, twenties, and early thirties, tend to be from the middle and upper classes, and most have attended college. As many as 20 percent (some researchers say almost 80 percent) of American high school and college women may have occasionally binged and purged, while 8 percent practice it on a regular basis. Many students find that bingeing allows them to forget their personal problems with academics, life goals, and their love lives. The most likely candidates for bulimia are dancers, models, actresses, and athletes such as gymnasts.

A bulimic is likely to have a history of weight problems. She may become bulimic at the end of a weight-reducing diet. Or her first experience with vomiting may have followed an infraction of her diet, often during Thanksgiving or Christmas. A bulimic, like an anorexic, often feels as if she has no control over her life. She is obsessed with being thin and reaching that state of physical perfection where life is supposed to be wonderful. She tends to be compulsive, depressed, and anxious. Though she maintains high standards, she has little self-esteem and becomes particularly disgusted with herself after a binge.

A binge usually consists of large amounts of "forbidden foods." Some women have been known to consume as much as 55,000 calories in one binge. For a bulimic, bingeing releases tension, much as cigarettes, alcohol, drugs, and exercise do for others. By throwing up, she can get rid of the "bad feelings" she hid by overeating.

The relief is short-lived. Bingeing feeds on itself: anxiety, to another binge. Sometimes the vomiting can give a temporary physical and emotional relief and leave the bulimic convinced that she can eat whatever she wants and not gain weight.

A bulimic can get so absorbed in her bingeing and purging that she has little time for other matters. These large amounts of food can run into hundreds of dollars, and like the drug addict, she may resort to stealing to maintain her habit. One bulimic woman in the US went bankrupt from her food bill of $100 a day.

A bulimic is usually aware that her eating pattern is abnormal but fears that she will be unable to stop eating. Actually, by vomiting two to three times a day over many months, she may find that she cannot stop the vomiting. She knows her behavior is abnormal and experiences depression, shame, and guilt similar to that of young alcoholics. To keep her vomiting undetected, she starts to avoid friends and family. Living alone is a necessity. Unlike the anorexic, a bulimic is sexually active, though she often feels misused.

Bulimia can cause a woman serious medical complications. Continual vomiting can tear the lining of her stomach and esophagus, cause dehydration, and create electrolyte imbalances so severe that she has muscle spasms, kidney problems, and possibly cardiac arrest. Urinary infections are common. The continued pressure from vomiting can cause the blood vessels in her eyes to break. Vomiting erodes the enamel on her teeth and permanently damages them. Sore throats are common, as are swollen salivary glands that make her cheeks puffy. When a bulimic woman relies on laxatives and diuretics for long periods of time and then discontinues their use, her body may bloat until her intestinal muscles can respond in a normal way. Sometimes she permanently damages her colon. Her menstrual periods may cease even if her body weight is normal. She can die from bulimia, but it is less life-threatening than anorexia. Suicide tops the list as the cause of death for bulimics.

Treatment for bulimia is different for each patient but usually involves individual and group therapy. The patient needs to admit to herself that her behavior is dangerous and needs changing. Many patients must address feelings of worthlessness and depression before they can deal with their eating behavior. For some, even career planning can help.

During recovery, a bulimic may find she spends enormous amounts of time planning her meals and diet. Food dulls the emotional lows, and she may find that after she gives up her bingeing habits, the resulting free time leads to feelings of depression and anxiety. By filling this time with finicky meal planning, she is able to keep her thoughts on positive matters. Eventually she needs to wean herself away from planning every second of her life, but initially it can be therapeutic.

Here are the warning signs of bulimia: unrealistic concern over weight; rapid consumption of a large amount of food, usually high-calorie sweets, in a relatively short period of time (less than two hours); strict dieting followed by bingeing; preoccupation with food and calories; guilt or shame over eating; disliking to eat in restaurants (may first check out bathroom to see if there are private stalls); disappearing after a meal; overeating in reaction to depression or stress; frequent weight fluctuations greater than ten pounds due to bingeing and purging; fear of being unable to control eating; repeated attempts to lose weight by vomiting, diuretics, and severely restricting calories; discomfort around food.

If you suspect someone you know is bulimic, state your concerns and be willing to share information on the subject or help the person seek treatment. Many times a bulimic is relieved to find someone to whom she can talk about her secret bingeing and purging. If she is not ready for help, reassure her that you will be available if she needs you. Sometimes it takes a while for bulimics to muster the courage to confront their eating behavior. Even when they do, it may be difficult to break the habit. Some older women have suffered from it for more than twenty-five years.

Those of you who feel you might be at risk for this condition may find the following steps helpful:

- Admit to yourself that your problem is serious. It means seeking professional help to change not only your eating habits but your feelings as well. The right therapist can help you learn to increase your self-esteem. You might want to begin by recognizing what you and others like about you and by doing things that make you feel good about who you are. You can really help yourself by deciding on a direction for your life.
- Learn relaxation techniques to help you keep calm under high-stress situations. When you feel stressed, try to sit or lie comfortably, and consciously relax your body. Slow, rhythmical deep breathing sometimes helps.
- If the urge to binge bites, do something else for twenty minutes and see if the urge passes. Exercise is a positive way to relieve tension, but do not become compulsive about it.
- Do not keep cookies, cakes, potato crisps, and other binge foods around the house. Instead, have popcorn or cut-up raw or marinaded vegetables for those times when you feel compelled to grab lots of food.
- Establish regular meals and daily routines. These can give you a certain emotional and physical satisfaction and prompt you to do other "good things" for yourself. Instead of ending the day with a snack, try a hot, candle-lit bath or steamy shower.
- Look for patterns in the times you eat. Are you actually bored? If most of your bingeing occurs during free time, plan activities to keep yourself occupied during these times.

- If you do binge, forgive yourself and get back in control by eating moderately. Do not follow a binge with a fast. Strict dieting and fasting will only lead to another binge.
- Avoid fad diets, which will only worsen your problem. In *The Beverly Hills Diet*, authors Judy Mazel and Susan Shultz actually promoted a form of bulimia: they suggested that after a binge, you should eat enormous amounts of raw fruit in order to produce diarrhea. Sadly, it was the best-selling book for 1983.
- Try not to label certain foods "forbidden." If you eat one of these foods, the ensuing guilt can trigger a binge. Occasionally eat foods that you tend to think of as forbidden so you will lose your craving for them. Feel free to go out at times for dessert. It is easier to limit how much you eat if you are at a restaurant than if you decide to bake at home.
- Eat meals with other people. Take time to enjoy and savor your meals as well as the company. Appreciate the love and care that goes into preparing food; take your time to eat. Remember, food is not the enemy.

RESOURCES

For further information on anorexia nervosa or bulimia, write:

Anorexic Family Aid National Information Centre
Sackville Place, 44 Magdalen Street, Norwich,
Norfolk NR3 1JE

Anorexic Aid
The Priory Centre, 11 Priory Road, High Wycombe
Buckinghamshire, HP13 6SL

Anorexia and Bulimia Nervosa Association
Annexe C, Tottenham Town Hall, App Road,
London N15 4RX

The Maisner Centre for Eating Disorders
PO Box 464
Hove, East Sussex, BN3 2BN
(Private treatment centre for compulsive eating and related disorders.)

10
The Athlete: Sharpening the Racer's Edge

> For my feedings during the race from the boat, I drink a hot powdered liquid that provides me with thirteen hundred calories and more protein per tablespoon than a four-ounce steak.... A cup of this stuff every hour barely helps. Before the hour's up my sugar is way down, I can feel it. I feel depressed.
>
> Diana Nyad, long-distance swimmer, in *Esquire* magazine

Marathon runner Joan Benoit thinks nothing of having a cone of pistachio ice cream and calling it "lunch." Hollis Stacy, pro golfer, loves to eat Mexican food that is so hot it makes her ears burn. Cynthia Woodhead, a world-class swimmer, eats whatever she wants as long as she does not gain weight. If there is such a thing as a winning diet, you would not know it by looking at what most champions eat.

Performance depends at least as much on your genes, conditioning, and coaching as it does on nutrition. But although a good diet cannot strengthen rubbery legs or speed up a snail's pace, a poor diet can dull a top athlete's winning edge. What follows is advice to the woman who is a professional athlete or who trains and competes just for fun.

The energy crisis

Like everyone else, an athlete gets energy from three nutrients: carbohydrate, fat, and, when these are unavailable, protein. With all these energy sources, your body can choose how to drive itself. It selects a specific fuel depending on what exercise you are doing, how much oxygen is available, and how well conditioned you are.

Using carbohydrates and fats for energy Carbohydrates run

The Athlete: Sharpening the Racer's Edge

through your bloodstream as glucose. When glucose levels rise, insulin directs both the liver and muscles to store the glucose as glycogen. Because glycogen contains a lot of water, it is bulky, and you can store only limited amounts. An athlete may have about 2,000 calories available as glucose and glycogen but have 140,000 calories' worth of stored fat.

Your body can burn fat only when enough oxygen is on site (it is an aerobic, or "air"-requiring process). You burn fat when you are at rest or during long, slow, moderate exercise like strolling. To exercise aerobically, you must be able to breathe comfortably, without gasping for air.

During short, intensive activities like springing, in which you have no chance to slow down or relax, your muscles begin to feel leaden. What happens is this: Your body needs quick bursts of energy, so it burns almost all glucose. By staying in shape and regularly working out, you can actually condition muscles to burn fat along with glucose, thus sparing your glycogen stores.

Running on empty If your liver's glycogen is depleted, your brain will inform you with dizziness, confusion, weakness, and shakiness. You may break out in a cold sweat. Known as "bonking," this condition is quickly relieved by eating carbohydrate-rich foods such as sandwiches, fig bars, and grapes.

When you run out of muscle glycogen, you "hit the wall." Depending on which muscles you have been using (legs for runners, legs and arms for swimmers), your limbs will feel too heavy to move. Unlike bonking, you have no immediate way to recover from hitting the wall. You will need at least forty-eight hours and a carbohydrate-rich diet to bring muscle glycogen back to its initial level.

Stocking up on fuel

Your calorie needs depend on your age, weight, height, body size, sport, and training. You require more calories if your sport exposes you to cold temperatures, as swimming, skiing, or skating do, or if it requires repeated, rather than sustained, muscle contractions. Swimmers and runners need more energy than gymnasts. Equestriennes do not require nearly as many calories as their horses.

Eat Beautiful!

If you expend a lot of energy, you have to eat more food to maintain your weight. Usually, your appetite will rise to the occasion. Always eat at least three meals a day (or even five or six) because skipping meals can hinder performance.

Though you may be able to indulge in sundaes, cream puffs, and pork pies without gaining weight, smarter choices would be fruits, vegetables, whole grains, lean meats, dairy products, and dried beans. To break down carbohydrates, fats, and proteins for energy, you need vitamins and minerals—nutrients present more in whole, unprocessed foods than sugary sweets, fluffy pastries, and fatty meats.

Carbohydrate For intensive work, your body derives energy from carbohydrates. (You also need some carbohydrate to break down fat.) Because you can store only a limited amount of glycogen, you must replenish these supplies from carbohydrates in the diet. At least 50 percent of your calories should be carbohydrate, mainly starches, not sweets. As marathon runner George Sheehan says, "How can one play and think and find truth when stuffed with jelly doughnuts?"

Fat For exercise lasting more than a couple of minutes, your body reverts to fat for energy, gearing up after four or five minutes. You have this fat to burn even if there is no fat in your diet because excess carbohydrate and protein are transformed and stored as fat. Of course, you do not need to avoid fats altogether. Linoleic acid is an essential fat that you must obtain through your diet. Also, flavors usually ride in the fatty part of foods, so cutting out all fats can make meals very bland.

Protein Muscles are made of protein, so many athletes believe they need extra protein to build muscles or stay strong. The average adult requires about 0.4 grams of protein per day for each pound of desirable body weight. To determine your own protein needs, multiply your desirable weight in pounds by

0.4 if you are well conditioned and not in heavy training
0.45 if you are in the early phases of training
0.9 if you are in heavy training

Note: This formula uses your desirable weight because you

The Athlete: Sharpening the Racer's Edge

require protein only for your lean tissue, not for any extra fat cells.

Chances are good that you already eat more protein than this. Compare your meals to these estimates to determine your daily protein consumption:

- Meat and other rich protein foods: 7 grams of protein each for

    1 ounce meat, fish, poultry
    1 egg
    ¼ cup tuna fish or 1 ounce canned salmon
    ½ cup lentils, dried peas, baked beans
    2 tablespoons peanut butter
    24–30 walnut halves, 15–20 cashews, 2 teaspoons peanuts
    1 ounce sunflower seeds

- Dairy products: 8 grams of protein each for

    8 fluid ounces milk
    1 cup yogurt (1 cup = 8 fluid ounces)
    1 ounce cheese
    ⅓ cup cottage cheese
    2 cups ice cream

- Bread and cereals: 2 grams of protein each for

    1 slice bread
    ½ cup rice, noodles, pasta, potato

- Starchy vegetables: 2 grams of protein each for

    ½ cup peas, carrots, beets

- Fruits, vegetables, juices: small amounts of protein (may contribute a total of 5–10 grams)

- Butter, margarine, oil, sugar, coffee, alcohol: 0 grams of protein

To increase protein, eat larger portions of high-protein foods, or add powdered milk to your regular milk or any dish—casseroles, baked goods, desserts, soups. Avoid buying special (and costly) protein supplements.

Most athletes would be better off thinking about the consequences of too much protein. High-protein diets decrease endurance, demand extra water to flush out the kidneys, pull calcium from the body, and can cause ketosis, dehydration, diarrhea, and loss of appetite. Protein also replaces the more critical fuel, carbohydrate. The only reason to eat the traditional monstrous steak dinner is if you believe it will give wings to your feet or power to your stroke. The psychological boost may overcome your sluggish digestion.

Ergogenic aids—shortcuts to success?

Ergogenic means "tending to increase work," so ergogenic aids are practices or substances that supposedly give the athlete extra zip. Theoretically, dietary aids work by either renewing or boosting energy stores, accelerating biochemical reactions, delaying fatigue, or maintaining optimal body weight. Some of these aids work, others do not. Following are descriptions of the more popular ones.

Carbohydrate loading The more muscle glycogen you have, the longer you can avoid fatigue. This has led to what is dubbed "the thinking marathon runner's secret weapon"—carbohydrate (or glycogen) loading. As with many weapons, you run risks as well as the race.

Normally, you have enough glycogen for two hours of continuous exercise, but by carbohydrate loading you can double this store. The traditional regimen calls for one day of exercising to exhaustion to deplete your glycogen stores. This is followed by three days of eating few carbohydrates but loading up on proteins and fats (a diet that suspiciously resembles one designed to promote heart disease). During this so-called bacon-and-egg phase, you may experience fatigue, dizziness, irritability, and nausea. For the next three days, you eat plenty of starches and do not exercise. During this time, you are replenishing your glycogen stores.

New research shows that the regimen does not need to be so rigid. One week before the event, try the following:

Day 7. Eat normally. Train for about ninety minutes.
Days 6–4. Eat normally. Train for progressively fewer minutes.
Days 3–1. Eat high-carbohydrate foods. Rest.

Carbohydrate loading works only for marathons, for high-altitude sports, and for sports that last over one hour. The better trained you are, the less likely it is that your endurance will improve at all. Probably the best method for achieving peak performance is to go into a competition well rested.

Vitamin supplements Vitamins help enzymes speed up metabolic reactions, including those that release energy. If you do not get enough vitamins, you show deficiency symptoms, such as lowered performance. But unless you are vitamin deficient, supplements will not improve performance, endurance, productivity, strength, cardiovascular function, or resistance.

Because the B vitamins (thiamin, riboflavin, and niacin) are needed for the release of energy, an athlete may require larger amounts. (Your requirement for these vitamins parallels your requirement for calories.) Women who exercise vigorously and regularly, but who keep their weights constant by eating more food, may need almost two times as much riboflavin. And those who lose weight because of regular exercise may require even more than this. Instead of taking riboflavin supplements, eat extra dairy products, fortified breads and cereals, lean meat, eggs, and leafy greens. In fact, your extra needs for any B vitamin should be met by food because supplements can work against you.

Megadoses of niacin inhibit your body from using fats during exercise, so you burn up your glycogen stores faster than necessary. Vitamin B_{12} supplements are supposed to cure chronic fatigue, but they work only if you are B_{12} deficient (a rare condition unless you have a malabsorption disorder or have been a careless, strict vegetarian for years). If you are chronically fatigued, chances are greater that your body potassium is low. The solution? Have a banana.

Many athletes believe in megadosing with vitamin C to improve endurance and performance and to speed up healing. But the evidence for taking extra vitamin C is far from convincing. After examining the research, Dr. Emily Haymes wrote in *Ergogenic Aids in Sport*: "For every study that has reported a beneficial effect from supplementing vitamin C, there appears to be at least one study that found no beneficial effects."

And what about vitamin E? Tests comparing athletes who took vitamin E with those who did not found no differences in performance, strength, speed, or endurance. Some faint evidence suggests that vitamin E may help in high altitudes and may protect the lungs against air pollutants, particularly ozone.

Wanton pill popping of vitamin supplements, particularly for vitamins A and D, can cause severe side effects (see appendix A). If you insist on supplementing your diet, stick with multivitamin-mineral pills that fall within recommended daily amounts.

Iron supplements Taking iron supplements is supposed to ensure that you have adequate hemoglobin to carry oxygen to your muscles. Though an endurance athlete may exhibit low hemoglobin levels, some physiologists call this a "pseudoanemia" and believe it to be a normal adaptation to training.

If you are an athlete, your hemoglobin level can actually be in the normal range but be too low to allow for optimal endurance. (Also, your iron stores may be deficient.) Anemia can be a chronic problem for athletes who are poor eaters, who are weight conscious, or who experience constant bruising or trauma from their feet pounding on the ground. Iron losses from menstruation and sweat may make it worse. Unless you have been diagnosed as iron deficient, avoid large iron supplements. Instead of improving your performance, they may cause nausea, stomach upset, and constipation.

Women athletes who have heavy menstrual losses may need to take extra iron in recommended amounts of 18 mg daily. Consult a doctor before taking large doses. All athletes should have their blood values checked and include iron-rich foods in their diets (lean meats, poultry, dried beans, iron-fortified cereal, and dried fruit).

Special foods and supplements To get more energy, athletes have taken just about everything—lecithin, yeast, alfalfa, dextrose tablets, phosphates, ginseng, bee pollen, royal jelly (honey)—even sand (marketed as "silica"). Pangamic acid, which is supposed to keep muscles operating at peak efficiency, is a meaningless term chemically because manufacturers can put anything they want into the product. Ingredients in some pangamic acid preparations are mutagenic (they alter genes) and carcinogenic. The US Food and Drug Administration has made it illegal to sell as a drug or supplement.

The Athlete: Sharpening the Racer's Edge

Bioflavonoids ("vitamin P") are a group of substances first found in the white segments of citrus fruits, now commonly found in sport supplements. Particularly popular are hesperidin, rutin, and citrin. No evidence exists to suggest any benefit may be obtained from consuming them. Kelp tablets are supposed to give muscles definition, while garlic purifies the blood. Gelatin is said to give you high energy. Raw eggs are supposedly better than cooked eggs. But not one of them gives you an edge.

If any foods can improve your performance, they are pasta, rice, potatoes, waffles, pancakes, breads, oatmeal, raisins, and fruit—your basic high-carbohydrate fare.

EATING FOR COMPETITION

Precompetition

First, the science behind the precompetition meal. When you start to exercise, and as your exercise becomes progressively more intense, your blood begins to flow away from your liver, kidneys, and stomach toward your muscles, supplying them with as much oxygen as possible. Think about what this means.

When you choose a precompetition meal, you do not want food in your stomach competing with your muscles for blood. The meal should clear your digestive hurdles by the time you start competing. Fats empty from your stomach in about five hours, or more, proteins in about three hours, and carbohydrates in about two hours. Though protein takes only an hour more to empty than carbohydrates, its nitrogen must be excreted by the kidneys—yet during exercise little blood flows to these organs.

Once I was in a diner eating breakfast when the conversation from the booth behind me began to waft over. Three young wrestlers, along with their fathers, were talking excitedly about loading up on carbohydrates before the Big Meet that was scheduled within the next two hours. I noticed that drifting along with the conversation was the distinct aroma of sausage and bacon. When I rose to pay my bill and glanced at their plates, staring back at me were partially ravaged stacks of pancakes (drenched in butter and syrup), heaps of sausages, rashers of bacon, mounds of greasy eggs, and glasses of whole milk. Rather than filling up on carbohydrates, these ravenous wrestlers and their fathers were in the middle of *fat* loading. To avoid this common mistake, follow these guidelines for a precompetition meal (three to four hours before competing):

1 serving of meat or poultry (roasted or broiled)
1 serving of mashed or baked potato or ½ cup pasta or noodles (1 teaspoon butter or margarine, optional)
1 serving of vegetables
1 cup skim milk
1 serving fruit
Dessert of sugar cookies or plain cake plus 2 teaspoons of jelly or other sweet
1–2 cups extra beverage

Consuming enough water is the most important step you can take to fight exhaustion. Without enough water, the activities of cells are impaired, you produce less urine, toxic wastes build up in the blood, and your body temperature rises. Drinks at refrigerator temperature empty from the stomach faster than warm beverages. But be careful: iced drinks delay digestion and can cause cramping.

Some athletes prefer liquid meals to solid food. Liquid meals leave your stomach faster, reduce mouth dryness, and help avoid the indigestion, nausea, vomiting, and muscle cramping caused by nervous tension. You can purchase special liquid meals like Ensure, Sustagen, or Sustacal, but the homemade variety is cheaper and often more nutritious (see recipe 6 in appendix D).

Avoid sugar in the last hour before competing. Taking sugar solutions thirty to sixty minutes before an event can cause early muscle exhaustion for cyclists, marathon runners, and long-distance swimmers. Sugar stimulates insulin, which causes your muscles to remove glucose so quickly that your blood sugar drops. Insulin also inhibits the use of fats for energy, so you have to rely on your limited stores of glycogen.

Now you know the science behind the precompetition meal, but don't ignore the reality. You should eat whatever foods you believe will make you perform better. One world-class swimmer consumed a lunch of two hamburgers, french fries, a root-beer flat, three brownies, and a candy bar two hours before setting a new world record in the 200-meter butterfly.

The Athlete: Sharpening the Racer's Edge

During competition

Endurance athletes can avoid fatigue by nibbling small bits of sugar every hour—no more than the equivalent of three rounded tablespoons each time, however: too much sugar draws fluid into your stomach, causing dehydration, cramps, nausea, gas, and diarrhea. If you are participating in shorter events, you do not need to eat sugar. If you will be competing on and off over a prolonged period of time, eat sandwiches (heavy on bread), cake without icing, or nut breads, or drink fruit juices.

Long gone are the days when an athlete, parched from perspiring, was told to suck on an ice cube (fluids during exercise supposedly caused cramps). Now it is recognized that restricting water during performance can cause serious dehydration. If you do not replace large sweat losses with water, your body cannot circulate blood and regulate body temperature. You may not feel hot, but you require more effort to perform. To keep your body cool and your performance hot, replenish lost fluid with plain water or one of the beverages suggested in table 10-1. If you show signs of heat intolerance (heat stress, cramps, exhaustion), stop exercising, move to a cool spot, and drink lots of water. Get medical treatment as soon as possible.

For some events it is impossible to replace water as you lose it. During marathons, runners may sweat out eight to thirteen pounds (sixteen to twenty-six cups) of water. Unless the loss is greater than 2 percent of your body weight, you will not suffer harmful side effects. (The average adult loses less than one percent of body weight daily.) After that, losses become progressively more dangerous.

To avoid a serious loss of water, replace fluids according to the guidelines set down by the American Dietetic Association:

Time	Fluid Consumption
2 hours before event	2½ cups (1 pint)
10–15 minutes before event	2 cups
10–15 minute intervals during event	½ cup (not to exceed 1 quart each hour)
After event	Replace weight loss with fluid

Postcompetition

After competition, you may not feel like eating for a few hours. During this time, drink fruit juices, lemonade, water, or beverages from table 10-1. When you can eat, have a light, balanced meal (about 600–1,000 calories). To replace glycogen as quickly as possible, avoid the high-protein, high-fat meal of a steak and fried potatoes. Instead choose chicken, rice or a baked potato, and vegetables.

Your thirst response is blunted during and immediately after vigorous exercise, so weigh yourself before and after competition and drink enough fluids to replace the lost weight. Two pounds of body weight equal about 1 quart of sweat. For instance, a loss of 5.2 pounds from a 130-pound woman represents a 4 percent loss of body water, or 2.6 quarts. It may take twenty-four to thirty-six hours to replace large water losses (4–7 percent of body weight).

But sweat is more than just water. It contains sodium, potassium, and magnesium. The concentration of sodium in sweat is less than in blood, so as you sweat heavily and lose water, your blood actually becomes saltier. Replacing water is your first priority. Then you can replenish sodium by eating a balanced diet.

If you have sweated heavily, put extra salt on food or have some broth or bouillon. However, if you lose more than six pounds (six pints of water), drink a solution of one-third teaspoon table salt in one quart of water, or drink a commercial electrolyte solution diluted with equal parts of water. Avoid taking salt tablets unless you have lost four quarts (eight pounds) of water, and then only on the advice of a doctor. Such large water losses usually occur only with heavy exercise in very hot weather and over several days. Salt tablets are harmful if consumed with too little water because they draw water from tissues into the intestines. By taking them, you increase the risk of getting blood clots and bringing on a heart attack, a stroke, or kidney failure. You also can deplete your body of potassium.

Potassium deficiency is more common than most athletes realize. When you are low on potassium, you feel tired and irritable. No warning bell clangs "Get more potassium!" The best way to avoid a deficiency caused by rigorous exercise is to consume

The Athlete: Sharpening the Racer's Edge

Table 10-1 What to drink before, during, and after exercise*

Drink	Before	During	After	Reason
Tap water	Yes	Yes	Yes	The basic liquid your system needs.
Carbonated mineral water	Yes	No	Yes	Carbonation can cause problems during event.
"Athletic" drinks e.g. Gatorade, ERG	Yes	Yes**	Yes	Only if 10 to 15 minutes before because of possible insulin reaction to sugar.
Cola	No	No	Yes	Has twice as much sugar as athletic drinks and may retard emptying of fluids; good after for carbohydrate replacement.
Diet cola	Yes	No	No	Carbonation is a problem during and lack of carbohydrates limits value after.
Defizzed cola	No	Yes	No	Properly diluted, a good fluid during but lack of palatability may make it undesirable at other times.
Beer	No	No	Yes	Controversial; alcohol does not help performance; mellowing effect after.
Wine and liquor	No	No	No	Alcohol content is undesirable.
Fruit juices	No	No	Yes	Sugar concentration is high; after, when fluid emptying speed not a factor, okay.
Coffee	Yes	No	No	Caffeine may provide pre-event stimulation.
Iced tea	Yes	Yes	Yes	Plain (without sugar) iced tea is a good source of fluid, plus its caffeine content can be pre-event stimulant.
Milk	No	No	No	More a food than a drink.

*"Before" means less than a half hour prior to events; "during" means at any time during the event; "after" means soon after the event.

**Qualified "yes" during the event because if not well diluted, sugar may retard the emptying of fluid from stomach to intestine.

Source: Compiled by William J. Fink, physiologist at the Ball State Human Performance Laboratory. Reprinted with permission of *The Runner*.

potassium-rich foods, such as orange juice, bananas, dried fruits, and potatoes.

Magnesium helps control muscle contractions and the conversion of carbohydrate to energy. Too little magnesium results in fatigue and muscle cramps. Be sure to eat rich sources of magnesium, such as legumes, nuts, cereals, leafy greens, seafoods, and cocoa.

THE ATHLETE'S BODY

Body composition

In sports, body fat content is much more important to performance than weight is. Many athletes step on a scale, check a height–weight table, and discover that they are too heavy—yet they may have normal or even below normal amounts of fat.

Most young women have body fat in the range of 20–26 percent of weight, though fit women usually have body fat under 23 percent. Women athletes have less, averaging between 12 and 18 percent. (Male athletes have levels closer to 7–12 percent.)

Your ideal fat level is the one at which you perform your best. It will depend on your age, health and sport. Women runners, for instance, generally have less than 12 percent body fat, yet the runner who held most of the American middle-distance records had over 17 percent fat. Having more fat gives women in endurance sports an edge over men because, in these events, the body draws on fat for energy. Still, a serious runner should keep below 20 percent body fat because excess fat creates a drag on the body.

In one sport, the extra fat serves women particularly well. Women dominate long-distance, open-water swimming because their extra fat gives them buoyancy and better insulation, a plus in cold water. Few swimmers with less than 30 percent fat make it across the English Channel. In downhill skiing, sheer mass or weight gives skiers the momentum to speed down the slopes. While strong, well-developed muscles are a must, skiers can afford slightly more body fat than, say, sprinters.

For most sports, though, agility, speed, and coordination come first, and fat only creates extra weight and a greater work-

The Athlete: Sharpening the Racer's Edge

load for the heart. Though you may want to reduce your body fat to a low level, refrain from falling below 10–12 percent.

Paring down body fat Trying to force your body to have too little fat is as hazardous as trying to reach a ridiculously low weight. If you already have low fat stores and lose weight, it will be at the expense of your muscles. To reach your ideal level, figure out your current body fat percentage, either by getting weighed underwater or by being measured with skinfold calipers.

If you are unsure what your goal should be, gradually reduce your body fat. If your performance begins to slide, you may have overshot your ideal. There is no scientific formula to determine your best body composition; ultimately, it comes down to trial and error. Once you have decided on your ideal percentage of body fat, figure out your competitive weight according to table 10-2.

To lose fat, combine a reducing diet with exercise. Your diet should provide 500 fewer calories a day than you need to maintain your weight. For a rough guide to your maintenance needs, multiply your desired weight by:

Table 10-2 Determining competitive weight

Suppose you currently weigh 140 pounds and have 19 percent body fat, but you want to lower your fat content to 12 percent. Figure out your goal weight as follows:

Current Weight: 140
Current Body Fat: 19%
Desirable Body Fat: 12%

Subtract desirable body fat from current body fat:
　19% − 12% = 7%
Multiply this figure by current weight:
　7% × 140 = 980
Divide the result by 100 to get recommended weight loss goal:
　980/100 = 9.8 pounds
Subtract this figure from current weight to get goal weight:
Goal Weight: 140 − 9.8 = approx. 131 pounds

Adapted from Wilmore, J. 1983. *Stay in Shape with the Champions*. Sunkist Growers.

18, if you're very active
23, if you're training intensively

Now subtract 500 from this number. Your diet should always provide at least 1,600 calories a day and lead to a weekly loss of no more than one to three pounds.

To eliminate 500 calories from your diet, first cut back on fats, sweets, and alcohol. Besides dieting, you should expend an additional 300–500 calories daily through aerobic exercise.

Make these diet and exercise changes gradually. Abrupt changes can impair performance. Diets promising faster losses than one to three pounds a week can cause fatigue, dehydration, and weakness. You will lose not only fat but reserves of protein, glycogen, and minerals vital for competition. Periodically, get your body composition reassessed to ensure that you are losing fat, not muscle.

To gain weight or muscle To gain weight, eat larger-than-normal portions of dairy products, lean meats, poultry, whole grains, dried beans, fruits, and vegetables. Plan snacks that are high in both nutrients and calories.

To gain muscle, eat more food and combine it with a program of progressive resistance exercises, like the Nautilus workouts. Consuming extra food, including supplements or protein powders, without stimulating the muscles will not build muscle tissue.

Eating disorders

All athletes try to perfect their bodies to improve performance. But often their goals are based on other athletes' bodies, not their own. Sometimes the pressure comes from parents or coaches, and sometimes it leads to eating disorders. These disorders not only impair performance but can slow growth. Because training requires a great expenditure of energy, an athlete's weight can drop remarkably fast. One way to detect excessive restriction of food is to weigh young athletes weekly.

The number of athletes who suffer from eating disorders is unknown. Some say the problem is widespread; others believe that few serious women athletes are truly anorexic because they are unwilling to tolerate the ensuing fatigue and weakness. Most will eat normally at the end of the season.

The thinning trend for athletes is beginning to change. At the 1984 Olympics, muscular Mary Lou Retton, at 4 feet 10½ inches and ninety-three pounds, stunned the Olympic audience with her powerful gymnastic style and returned to athletes the right to be chunky. (More on eating disorders in chapter 9.)

The Menstrual cycle

In the last ten years researchers have begun to study a physical phenomenon happening to women athletes: exercise-induced amenorrhea. Anywhere from 15 to 20 percent of them stop menstruating for some period of time. The reasons for this have so far eluded researchers, but theories include a disturbance in the brain's hypothalamus, too many endorphins, too few calories, too little dietary protein or cholesterol, and low body fat. It may be a few years before researchers figure out the exact mechanisms at work. In the meantime, what are the hazards, if any, to the athlete?

Infertility In some athletes, amenorrhea may be caused by a permanent imbalance in hormones (which could exist whether or not the women exercised). Others, though they have few periods, still ovulate occasionally and can become pregnant.

To date, evidence indicates that exercise-induced infertility is reversible. If an amenorrheic athlete wants to get pregnant, she can slow her speed or cut back on distance. If she has less than 17 percent body fat, she should gain weight. If her cholesterol intake is below 300 mg, she should increase it. (Basically, this means not completely cutting out eggs, cheese, and organ meats.) For some women, ovulation-inducing drugs are necessary.

Bone loss In 1981, Christopher Cann of the school of medicine at the University of California in San Francisco examined a woman in her late thirties who had a stress fracture in her pelvic bone and discovered that she had somewhat less bone mass than most women her age and height. A month later a slightly younger woman walked into his office with a stress fracture, and she, too, had thinner bones than the norm. Considering that both women had suffered fractures, it was not surprising that they had thinner bones. What was surprising was that both were long-distance runners who were amenorrheic.

Researchers were bewildered. Exercise, by stressing bones, tends to make them stronger: ballet dancers have dense bones in their legs, tennis players in their dominant arm. It seemed as if amenorrhea could override the advantages of exercise and pull calcium from the bone, perhaps because calcium migrates to areas under stress or that bear weight. A runner may lose bone calcium from her spine because it migrates to stress points in her leg bones. An oarswoman, on the other hand, will be stressing her back and arms. What was disturbing about this scenario was the possibility that amenorrheic athletes would be at greater risk of osteoporosis once they passed menopause.

Research is still preliminary, and treatments are at best speculative. Diet should be one of the first approaches. Make sure you are not restricting calories too severely. Be sure to get at least 1,000 mg of calcium each day. Eat rich calcium foods: skim or low-fat milk, yogurt, cottage cheese, tofu, and leafy greens. If you cannot get your daily quota of calcium from food, take a 500-mg calcium supplement. A slight change in your exercise workout may help. Runners, for instance, should consider adding activities that stress the entire body rather than just the legs.

Finally, amenorrhea can result from serious disorders that are unrelated to exercise; always get checked by a doctor if your periods stop.

RESOURCES

London Sports Medicine Institute,
c/o Medical College
of St Bartholomew's Hospital
Charterhouse Square
London EC1M 6BQ

11
Beauty: Beneath the Makeup

> Woman is nature. Her body is like lightning; it looks pleasing—and it can run a toaster.... The new beauty is possibility—what women can become.
>
> Carol Muske, New York poet

Forget about cucumbers on your eyelids, strawberry-honey pâté on your face, and lemon meringue in your hair. Nutrients do not squeeze through skin pores, nor do they sidle up shafts of hair to surprise your scalp. They enter your body by way of your mouth. So to be beautiful, look to your diet.

Hair—hair's what you need to know

Frustrated over the ten pounds of fat clinging to her waist, thirty-year-old Ann devised her own quick weight-loss diet. For one month she ate nothing but canned tomato soup, ritually ladled out in three daily portions. In twenty days she had dropped the ten pounds. But to her dismay, within a few months she not only regained all the lost weight, but her hair began to fall out.

Hair structure   A shaft of hair is only a pile of dead cells. Before they die, these cells grow deep in the skin pores, where they cluster at a hair follicle bulb. Needing room to multiply, young cells begin nudging out older ones, pushing them toward the surface of the skin. As the old cells move out, they stretch, huddle together, die, and harden into a hair shaft. In this way, your hair keeps lengthening.

Scalp hairs grow for about three years. When a hair reaches its length limit, the follicle (the only living part) enters a resting phase for a few months. At any given time, about one out of ten hairs is taking a break and resting; the other nine are growing.

Your diet, metabolism, and hormones affect when and how fast your hair grows. Of course, growth can be slowed much easier than accelerated. Any physical stress, such as rigid dieting, childbirth, blood loss, and major surgery, can force your hair into a temporary resting stage. You only notice this months later when the new growth pushes out the old hair.

Emotional stress creates dull hair. Two to three months after a stressful event, the sheen of hair fades because stress disrupts the hormones that control hair oil.

Illness or trauma can start you graying, but nothing can turn your hair white overnight. A shock can cause most of the hairs to enter a resting phase, then fall out. When the new growth comes in, the hair may be colorless. Graying is irreversible, so do not bother with vitamin or protein therapies "guaranteed" to restore your natural color.

Shampoos and conditioners Most shampoos are basically alike—water plus synthetic detergents. You can temporarily disguise thin, limp, or damaged hair by using shampoos with protein, balsam, egg, or beer. These shampoos glue together split ends and coat the hair to make it feel thicker. They can make oily hair look worse. A mildly acidic conditioner can brighten up dullness left after shampooing by flattening the cuticle scales so the hair looks shiny. Some conditioners, such as lemon juice, will dry out the hair.

No amount of protein or amino acids will repair damaged hair. Adding the nucleic acids DNA and RNA to conditioners does not reconstruct the hair, despite manufacturers' claims to the contrary. Nucleic acids are usually derived from yeast, so even if the DNA or RNA could reconstruct protein on your head, it would reconstruct yeast protein, not hair protein. No product can substitute for the hair that grows strong and healthy when you eat well.

Feeding your tresses Besides letting the world know that you lead a stressful life, hair screams out your nutritional problems. Because hair follicles are metabolically active, your hair will mirror any dietary deficiency. If push comes to shove, your body will neglect to "feed" your hair long before other, more vital tissues, like brain or nerve cells.

Crash diets, poorly planned vegetarian diets, and prolonged fasting can make your hair fall out or look like straw. Eating too few calories can trigger a resting phase. With too little protein, the body cannot make color pigments and the hair turns a strange reddish blond. With a zinc deficiency, you can easily pull out a cluster of hairs along with their bulbs. Hair loss can also result from iron-deficiency anemia.

To have great-looking hair, you must eat to supply your body with proteins, fats, vitamins, and minerals. Proteins make up hair, fats lubricate it, and vitamins and minerals strengthen it. These nutrients, along with oxygen, reach the hair through blood vessels near the bulb. So anything that slows circulation, such as heart disease or old age, will affect the hair. Although hair is very active and requires many nutrients, forget about taking special supplements, and eat a balanced diet instead.

Hair analysis   For up to £60 a private health centre will analyze your hair to determine your nutritional status. After a spectrographic analysis, they will give you a computerized listing of the minerals in your hair, often with advice that you take vitamin and mineral supplements to correct a deficiency.

What they do not tell you is that hair trimmings do not contain vitamins. They exist only near the bulb below the skin's surface. During hair growth, as dead cells accumulate and form the shaft, delicate vitamins are destroyed. The sturdier minerals survive, but no reliable standards exist for measuring normal concentrations of minerals in the hair.

Hair analysis is useful only when there is a case of suspected poisoning or exposure of a group of people to a toxic element, such as arsenic, chromium, cobalt, nickel, or lead. Even then, many factors, such as hair sprays, dyes (some contain lead), and shampoos (some for dandruff contain zinc or selenium), can distort the results.

Promoters will sometimes recommend natural chelation therapy to remove metal poisons (chelating agents bind to metals and pull them from the body). This therapy should only be done under the supervision of a doctor and only when the metals pose a severe threat to your health. Some chelating agents are toxic and can cause kidney injury and even death. In short, save your money.

Skin deep

"Nature gives you the face you have at twenty," said Gabrielle Chanel in a 1956 *Ladies' Home Journal*. "It is up to you to merit the face you have at fifty." The way to "merit" a good complexion is to understand how skin grows and what you need to nourish it.

Skin structure   One-fourth of your body's protein is reserved, not for muscles, but for skin. Your skin has two layers. The upper layer, or epidermis, is enmeshed in a protein called keratin that makes for a tough, waterproof surface. The epidermis gives rise to the hair, glands, and nails, and is where all skin problems show up. It is your first defense against microorganisms, change in fluid level, and injury. As thin as an onion skin, this versatile covering is entirely restored with new cells every fifteen to thirty days.

Below the epidermis is a layer packed with nerves, blood vessels, fat, hair roots and their muscles, sweat and lubricating glands, and the connective-tissue proteins, called collagen and elastin, that allow skin to be strong and elastic. In a sense, this layer, known as the dermis, is your real skin.

The dermis contains tiny projections that fit into depressions in the epidermis and hold the two layers together, like puzzle pieces. Scattered through the dermis are capillaries that act as waiter and busboy, delivering food and oxygen to nourish new cells and then dragging away their wastes. In women with poor circulation, the capillaries have to struggle to get food and oxygen to the cells. Aging, particularly after age fifty, decreases circulation enough to affect skin tone and appearance.

Dotting the skin surface are tiny pores through which hairs grow and oil is secreted. Your genes, along with diet and medications, affect how much oil your glands produce. Although no evidence supports the idea, many people believe certain foods such as chocolate, fats, citrus fruits, and hot spices make their skin more oily. Avoiding these foods will not do any harm, but consider other possible culprits: city pollution and hot, humid weather.

Beauty: Beneath the Makeup

Adult skin After age twenty-five, tiny lines and permanent wrinkles etch patterns in your face. They come from stretched collagen fibers, plus a loss of skin moisture, the pull of gravity, and damage from the sun, wind, heat, and cold. Not only is collagen breaking down, but fat slowly disappears from under facial skin. As it is lost, your skin begins to hang in folds. When you are young, this can happen from crash dieting, which does not give the skin time to shrink. Baggy skin may even appear under the eyes.

Dry or oily skin With a normal complexion, a waxy oil coats the skin and holds in water. With dry skin, too little oil is produced (the amount set by your genes and hormones), and the epidermis loses more water than it can replace from the underlying tissues. Dry skin does not cause wrinkles, though wrinkles will be more pronounced when the skin is dehydrated. Dry skin can result from fad dieting or anorexia nervosa.

Soaps and creams In an 1892 issue of *The Woman's Journal*, an ad for Dr. O. Phelps Brown's celebrated alabaster jar of tissue builder (from an old Roman oil formula) states that it "feeds the tissues, fills up wrinkles, and plumps the figure." The ad is sandwiched between two others: one for Dr. Hebra's Viola Cream and Professor I. Hubert's Malvina Cream. You could question what old Romans and violets have to do with skin care, and you could even smile faintly at the idea of a "celebrated alabaster jar," but today's eternal-youth claims are not much more enlightening than those of the 1800s.

Today women are told to fortify their skin with protein, placenta, and collagen, and to feed it strawberries, cucumbers, honey, and milk. For these remedies, Americans spend over $10 billion a year—amazing when you consider that the only thing cosmetics can do is close pores or disguise wrinkles. The best way to have good-looking skin is to follow a simple regimen of keeping it clean and moist and, again, eating well.

Nutrients added to creams to give special beautifying properties are worthless. Amino acids, the small components of protein, are supposed to rejuvenate cells. Processed collagen and elastin are added in the mistaken belief that they will give the skin strength and flexibility. Eggs are thrown in to provide

Eat Beautiful!

protein, minerals, and vitamins. The trouble is that only vitamins A and D can pass through the skin's surface. All others, including vitamin E, are not absorbed. Honey adds no special property to a cream, and both honey and vitamin E can cause allergic reactions.

Natural and organic cosmetics Natural cosmetics are usually based on some vegetable, fruit, or herb and are claimed to be hypoallergenic (less likely to cause allergies). But these products can irritate, clog, and photosensitize your skin as much as synthetic cosmetics. Not only can the basic ingredients provoke allergies, but adding vegetables, fruits, or herbs may cause further allergic reactions.

By definition, organic cosmetics are derived from plants or animals that have been raised without the use of hormones, pesticides, or synthetic fertilizers; but organic usually means whatever the manufacturer wishes. Herbal cosmetics tend to affect the skin according to the herbs added. Some herbs soothe the skin, others stimulate circulation, and still others may irritate. Be sure the herbs added to the cosmetics will not irritate your skin.

Feeding your face Your skin is nourished from the inside, not from the outside. If you want a great complexion, take the fruits and vegetables that you are told to smear on your face and instead—eat them. Like hair, skin is metabolically active, so a poor diet will quickly surface on your face. As Gloria Swanson so delicately phrased it, "No one can have skin like a baby's bottom if they're going to stuff that hole in their face with chocolate and banana splits." With too few or the wrong kinds of foods, your skin becomes pale, dry, and less elastic. It is more vulnerable to irritants and infections.

Severe deficiencies often show up as scaling or oiliness. If you eat too little food or have a long illness, you will look all skin and bones because your fat stores are gone and your skin has become thin and inelastic.

Because the skin stores about a quart of body fluid, drink about six glasses of water daily to keep your skin looking fresh. Try to maintain your desirable weight. Yo-yoing weight losses and gains can leave ugly stretch marks. Exercise can improve

Table 11-1 Effects of nutrition on skin

Skin Condition	Possible Cause
Acne	Too many androgens or androgenlike substances: Wheat germ, shellfish, organ meat (liver, kidney, sweetbreads)
	Too many iodides: Kelp, seaweed, sea salt, saltwater fish, cabbage, shellfish, spinach, peanuts, artichokes, franchise fast foods (iodine is used to disinfect machinery)
Allergies	Any ingredient; vitamin E common
Bruising	Deficiency of vitamin K, vitamin C
Dry, inelastic skin	Too few calories
Fatty tumors	High cholesterol levels in body
Frequent boils, itching, infections	Diabetes
Pale skin	Anemia; too little iron (possibly from ulcer, hemorrhid, cancer)
Rashes	Obesity
Red flushes or red, spidery blotches	Vasodilators (expand blood vessels): Chili, curries, hot peppers, Caffeine, Alcohol
Sunburn	Photosensitizers (taken internally): Artificial sweeteners.
	Photosensitizers (applied topically): Lime juice.
	Ingredients in some natural products: Figs, fennel, dill, parsley, carrots, celery
Wrinkled, droopy skin that will not heal well	Too little protein
Yellow skin (especially on palms, soles of feet, and ears)	Too much carotene (the vitamin A precursor in fruits and vegetables)

circulation and give you a glowing complexion. Just as stress affects the oiliness of hair, it also ruins the skin. Table 11-1 summarizes the effects of nutrition on the skin.

Nails

The shape and strength of your nails are set by your genes, but environment and diet can make a difference. If your nails are naturally soft, eating gelatin is not going to harden them. Though nails are built from protein in the diet, your body can use this protein only after it has been broken down to its amino acids. Compared with other protein foods, gelatin is low quality because it has too little of the sulfur-containing amino acids and tryptophan. Few Western women are deficient in protein, anyway, so adding more to your diet will not improve your nails.

Nails can reveal nutritional disorders: a slowing down of nail growth can be a sign of malnutrition, and pale, whitish nails that "spoon" (become concave) can indicate anemia. Blackened nails can result from a vitamin B_{12} deficiency, though the more common reasons are staining from hair dyes or photographic developer. There are no special foods to eat for strong nails, but because nails mirror your overall health, the best way to have great-looking nails is to eat well and stay healthy.

PART 3
Disease Prevention

As a woman, you are more likely than a man to be obese, diabetic, anemic, arthritic, and depressed. On the positive side, your risk of heart disease is much lower—but only until menopause. This section focuses on the three major killers of women—"Atherosclerosis," "Cancer," and "Diabetes." Each chapter discusses how the disease develops and in what ways diet can prevent or sometimes halt it. In "Gastrointestinal Disorders," you will read about some of the common mishaps that can occur in the stomach and intestines, such as constipation, appendicitis, hemorrhoids, and gas, and find ways to keep your digestive system functioning smoothly—and "regularly." Designing your diet to prevent such diseases and disorders will help you enjoy the years you have to the fullest.

12
Atherosclerosis: When the Heart Breaks

> The Heart asks Pleasure—first—
> And then—Excuse from Pain—
> —Emily Dickinson

She was only forty-two years old, yet she had not felt well for years. One day she was overcome by a "violent uneasiness" on her left side. Her left arm became numb, and she was gasping for breath. On a trip to Venice that year she was stricken with a similar moment of pain, and saying to her companions that she would die, she then died. The year was 1707, and her case was reported by the anatomist Giovanni Morgagni. It was the first account of a pre-menopausal women suffering from angina. The case was unusual because heart disease was—and is—so rare among women prior to menopause.

Though women in their twenties and thirties almost never have heart attacks, after menopause their risk suddenly jumps. Cardiovascular disease is the number-one killer of postmenopausal Western women. Most often, heart disease is fatal because of a heart attack. Stroke and hypertension are the next most frequent causes of death.

Cardiovascular disease is a broad term covering several disorders of the heart (cardio) and blood vessels (vascular). It includes high blood pressure, rheumatic heart disease, congenital heart disease, and atherosclerosis. Arteriosclerosis refers to any thickening, hardening, or loss of elasticity of the arteries, but the type that most often leads to serious problems is atherosclerosis, a thickening of the lining and narrowing of the channel in the arteries of the heart, brain, or legs. It is the main cause of heart attacks and strokes.

The development of atherosclerosis

One of the first changes in the arteries is that fat-filled cells embed themselves in the artery wall and form fatty streaks. These fatty streaks do not bulge into the artery lining and do not impede blood flow. Chances are that they do not signal anything about future heart disease.

After fatty streaks comes plaque buildup. Plaque forms where an artery branches, at points of high turbulence. Sometimes the artery lining has been injured, possibly by cigarette smoking or high blood pressure. Fat particles collect under the damaged lining, and little spheroid platelets, normally needed to coagulate blood, migrate to the site. This collection of cell debris is called plaque, and it begins to protrude into the artery channel. The artery wall thickens, becomes less elastic, and cannot easily handle the flow of blood. As the channel narrows, more pressure is required to force blood through at normal rates. If plaque continues to pile up, a crisis closes in, yet the person may suspect nothing. Now, one of several things can happen.

The plaque may narrow the affected woman's channel so much that if her system is overloaded, say, from exercise, not enough blood and oxygen will reach her heart. She feels pain, pressure, and tightness in the front of her chest—called angina. Over the long run, she may have to restrict her activity. Or if she has a mild case, she may be able to live with a partially blocked artery and never suffer a heart attack.

Another outcome is that her artery wall will spasm and squeeze off blood flow. The ventricles of her heart may fibrillate, beating hundreds of times a minute. At this point, it is crucial to get her to a hospital immediately where her heart can be electrically stimulated to beat normally.

Or a blood clot or thrombus traveling through the artery may get wedged in the narrow space left after plaque buildup. The narrowed channel itself can cause turbulence, loosening a clot, which then cuts off all blood flow. If the blocked artery feeds the heart, the woman has a heart attack. She may experience chest pain, nausea, and shortness of breath. She may break out in a cold sweat. The pain can radiate down the left arm or to her neck, shoulders, or jaw. As her heart muscle dies, scar tissue develops that cannot contract to pump her blood. As long as the damage remains minimal, her heart may continue to function.

If a clot blocks an artery leading to her legs, tissue will die and lead to gangrene. If a clot blocks an artery to the brain, she has a stroke. Her brain tissue dies, and if any of her nerve cells are damaged, the areas they control will no longer function. She may experience memory loss, dizziness, partial paralysis, extreme mood fluctuations, or difficulty in speaking. She may have double vision, or her vision in one eye may dim. A stroke can also occur when a diseased brain artery bursts. Brain cells fed by that artery then die.

What have studies shown us?

Researchers have approached the study of heart disease in two main ways: population studies and intervention studies. The most extensive population study of heart disease to date is one begun in 1949 in the Boston suburb of Framingham that involves more than 5,000 men and women of ages thirty to sixty-two years. Nearly all were healthy when the study began, and their subsequent diseases and deaths have been followed for thirty-five years. By collecting dietary information and the results of medical exams, researchers have discovered that lifestyle, much more than heredity or aging, is the determining factor in heart disease.

For an intervention study, researchers select a group of people and fiddle with certain factors to see if they can avoid or delay heart disease. One such study—the Coronary Primary Prevention Trial—began in 1973 and 3,806 healthy middle-aged men who had no history of heart disease, but who had high levels of cholesterol in their blood. Half were given a cholesterol-lowering drug and a moderately restricted diet. Half were given only the diet. In 1985 the results were published, revealing what some researchers thought was a surprising finding. By lowering the level of blood cholesterol, a person could decrease his chance of getting heart disease. The level of blood cholesterol was a powerful risk factor.

Risk factors

Heart disease has no single cause, but it does have a number of risk factors, personal habits or inherited or acquired traits, that predict who is most likely to succumb to a disease. In the United States, the most dangerous risk factors for heart disease are high levels of blood cholesterol, high blood pressure, and cigarette smoking.

Blood (serum) cholesterol "Atherosclerosis" comes from the Greek words "athera" for gruel and "sklerosis" for hardening, evoking the image of burnt oatmeal stuck to your artery walls. Actually, plaque along the artery lining looks more like a yellowish, fatty glob and is composed of fat, calcium, cell debris, and—most of all—cholesterol.

Your liver produces about 80 percent of your body's cholesterol, the rest coming from your diet. Cholesterol is essential to life and is needed to make hormones, vitamin D, and bile acids for fat digestion. It also forms the protective sheath around nerves. Like fats and oils, cholesterol does not dissolve in water, so to travel in blood, it must first bundle itself in a water-soluble protein coat. This coat, lined with fat, is known as a lipoprotein.

Several types of lipoproteins rove through your blood, but the two most often implicated in the development of atherosclerosis are low-density lipoproteins (LDLs) and high-density lipoproteins (HDLs).

LDLs have been dubbed the "bad" lipoprotein carriers because they cart cholesterol to cells for deposit. If they transport more cholesterol than your cells can use, the excess accumulates in your arteries. The more LDL cholesterol you have, the greater your chances of developing heart disease.

HDLs, the "good" lipoprotein carriers, are your body's garbage trucks, hauling cholesterol *away* from tissues (probably) to the liver, where the cholesterol is removed from the body. The higher your HDL cholesterol, the smaller your chances of developing heart disease. HDLs are higher in premenopausal women, thin people, nonsmokers, people who exercise regularly, and those who drink moderate amounts of alcohol.

A cholesterol reading of under 180 mg/dl is low risk for adults in their twenties. A reading of less than 200 mg/dl is desirable for those thirty years or older. Someone with a reading of 265 mg/dl or over has a four times greater chance of developing heart disease than someone with 190 mg/dl or below.

Having your total blood cholesterol measured does not tell

you much about whether your cholesterol is the "good" or "bad" kind. William Castelli, director of the Framingham study, suggests that the best single predictor of heart disease is the ratio of total cholesterol to HDL cholesterol. For instance, if you have a relatively low cholesterol reading of 200, but of that only 30 mg are HDLs, your ratio would be 200/30, or 6.7. Castelli recommends taking steps to improve a ratio greater than 4.5.

Giving further weight to blood cholesterol as a risk factor, the Coronary Primary Prevention Trial found that for every one percent drop in blood cholesterol level (presumably LDLs), your risk of heart attack drops 2 percent. People with initially high levels who lower blood cholesterol with drugs and diet can cut their risk of heart disease by as much as 50 percent.

High blood pressure As blood courses through your arteries, it exerts pressure on the artery walls. Blood pressure naturally falls during sleep and rises when your heart and muscles need more blood, such as during exercise or moments of excitement. But when pressure stays high, problems develop.

If you have high blood pressure, you may get headaches in the back of your head or upper neck, or you may suffer fatigue, insomnia, tension, or flushing in your face. But usually symptoms occur only after organs have been damaged, so hypertension is called a "silent killer."

When your blood pressure is measured, two numbers are taken. One is the systolic pressure, read when the heart is contracting; this is the maximum pressure the heart exerts to force blood through the arteries. The second is the diastolic pressure, measured between beats when the heart relaxes and fills with blood; this indicates how much work the heart has to do to overcome artery resistance.

If either the diastolic or systolic reading is consistently elevated, you may be in trouble. A high systolic pressure can tear the lining of an artery wall. A high diastolic pressure can increase the workload of the heart, enlarging it and wearing it out. It can injure and burst delicate blood vessels. In the brain, the hemorrhaging can lead to a stroke. In the eyes, the burst blood vessels can impair vision. The kidney may become so damaged that the hypertension worsens. If untreated, high blood pressure can cause heart attacks, strokes, or kidney disease. Table 12-1 shows normal and high levels of blood pressure:

Table 12-1 What blood pressure readings mean		
	Diastolic	*Systolic*
Normal	<85	<140
high normal	85–89	<140
Hypertension		
Borderline*	<90	140–159
Systolic hypertension*	<90	160+
Mild**	90–104	Any systolic reading
Moderate	105–114	Any systolic reading
Severe	115+	Any systolic reading

*If your diastolic pressure is normal (below 90), you may still have high blood pressure based on your systolic pressure.
**If your diastolic reading is above 90, you are considered hypertensive no matter what your systolic reading.

An estimated 60 million Americans have high blood pressure, and 15 million are at intermediate risk. Risk is higher in blacks, post-menopausal women, some women on the Pill, those who are overweight, or those with a family history of high blood pressure. Blood pressure increases with age, and since women live longer than men, they tend to have higher rates. Certain behaviors or habits, such as stress or frequent and heavy drinking, have been linked to hypertension. Nutritional factors include a diet high in sodium and low in potassium.

Drugs may be prescribed to dilate the arteries so they offer less resistance to blood flow. Diuretics pull water and sodium from the body, but they also pull potassium. If you are taking diuretics, eat high-potassium foods, such as leafy greens, dates, bananas, cantaloupe, dried peas and beans, potatoes, and peanut butter. (Avoid monosodium glutamate, or MSG, which contains sodium and counteracts the effectiveness of the drugs.)

The biggest problem with drugs is persuading people to take them. Because drugs have side effects and the long-term effects are unknown, greater emphasis is being placed on other therapies, such as dieting, exercising, and giving up cigarettes, particularly for individuals with mild hypertension.

Other risk factors

Cigarette smoking The Framingham study revealed that moderate smoking doubles the risk of heart disease. Generally, the risk increases with the number of cigarettes smoked: a two-pack-a-day smoker is at higher risk than someone who smokes only one pack a day.

Obesity Framingham showed that very obese people have high death rates from heart disease, while thin people (at least those who do not smoke cigarettes) have low death rates. Surprisingly, thinner individuals consumed more calories, fat, and sodium than heavier people but still retained their lower risk, possibly because they were more active.

Some research shows that fat above the waist is much more likely to be associated with heart disease than fat below. Not all researchers are convinced that moderate obesity, without other risk factors, increases the chances of developing heart disease. However, the obese are more likely to have high blood lipids (fats), low HDL levels, high blood pressure, and diabetes, and their risk may be increased simply because of these other factors.

Lack of exercise Exercise that produces cardiovascular conditioning (aerobic exercise) can both lower LDL cholesterol and raise HDL cholesterol.

Diabetes Diabetic women are over twice as likely to get heart disease as women who are not diabetic (in men, the rate is 50 percent higher). To reduce her risk, a diabetic should reach and maintain a desirable weight, take medication (if prescribed), exercise regularly, avoid cigarettes, and eat a diet low in saturated fats.

Blood (serum) fats Besides cholesterol, a fat called triglyceride floats through the bloodstream. Triglycerides come from fats in food and are produced in abnormally large amounts by some people. By itself, a high level of triglycerides does not seem to cause heart disease, but people with high levels usually have other risk factors (such as obesity or low HDLs). To reduce fat levels in the blood, reach a desirable weight, eat a diet low in fats and high in fiber, and get involved in a regular exercise program.

Stress and personality type One study found that women holding clerical jobs have almost twice the incidence of heart disease as homemakers. These women expressed hostility over having nonsupportive bosses, too little job mobility, and too much work. They reported more daily stress and marital dissatisfaction than either homemakers or men. They also reported a greater degree of stress if they raised more than two children and were married to a blue-collar worker (they were said to have repressed personalities). These women felt helpless, depressed, and wanted to give up.

Stress hormones raise blood pressure and blood cholesterol, narrow the arteries, and cause platelets to clump. Over a short period of time this poses no hazard, but in the long run it can damage arteries. Some researchers remain critical of this stress theory and point out that many people under pressure take up smoking cigarettes, overeating, or overdrinking, and that *these* practices raise the risk of heart disease.

Heredity Some individuals may have certain genetic defects that predispose them to early heart disease, even if they eat a nutritious diet, exercise, stay lean, and do not smoke. Dr. Jan Breslow at Rockefeller University in New York estimates that 5–10 percent of the US population fall into this group. An equal number, says Breslow, show the "Winston Churchill syndrome"—drinking, smoking, being overweight, and enjoying it all into old age.

A diet for a healthy heart

Probably nothing is so perplexing as trying to understand how nutrition affects the risk of heart disease. If you think that a diet for preventing heart disease is going to forbid all your favorite dishes or promote weird foods, you might be in for a surprise: following are some suggestions for changing your diet to reduce your risk.

Cut down on saturated fats One of the most misunderstood things about the relationship between heart disease and diet is that the strongest nutritional factor affecting blood cholesterol is *not* dietary cholesterol, but saturated fat. Your liver makes cholesterol from saturated fat, whether or not your diet contains any cholesterol.

Saturated fats raise blood cholesterol. They are present primarily in animal products and tend to be solid at room temperature. Check your diet for the following saturated fats:

butter	cheese	chocolate
coconut	egg yolk	lard
coconut oil	meat	milk
palm oil	poultry	dripping

Polyunsaturated fats lower blood cholesterol. These fats are present more often in vegetables, beans, and grains and are usually liquid at room temperature. However, do not start adding a lot of polyunsaturated fat to your diet; too much of *any* fat is linked to cancer and weight gain. New research indicates that eating fish may help prevent heart disease because fish contain so-called omega 3 polyunsaturated fatty acids, particularly one known as eicosapentaenoic acid (EPA), which may keep platelets from clotting. This does not mean you should drastically change your diet to include fish at every meal; researchers have not yet studied if large amounts of these fatty acids also increase risk of cancer or other diseases. Check your diet for these sources of polyunsaturated fats:

almonds	corn oil	cottonseed oil
hazelnuts	fish	margarine (soft)
mayonnaise	pecans	safflower oil
salad dressing	soybean oil	sunflower oil
walnuts		

Monounsaturated fats neither raise nor lower blood cholesterol. Check for these sources:

avocado	cashews	olives
olive oil	peanuts	peanut oil
peanut butter		

Close to 40 percent of all calories in the current British diet come from fat. The DHSS recommends that you limit fats to 35 percent of your day's calories, with less than half coming from saturated fat. Other researchers believe 25 percent of total calories would be even better, though such a diet would be more difficult to follow. To cut back on fat, eat dry beans and peas, low-fat or skim dairy products, lean meats, fish, and poultry. In addition, limit your intake of eggs, organ meats, butter, cream, and shortening. Trim excess fat from meats before you broil, bake or boil them. (For further details on cutting out fat, see chapter 16.)

Nathan Pritikin, a man self-taught in nutrition, devised an even stricter diet for preventing and treating heart disease, one that provides only 10 percent of calories from fat. On the Pritikin plan, all dairy products must come from skim milk, and only four to five ounces of very lean meat, fish, or poultry are allowed each day. No butter, margarine, oils, dressings, egg yolks, nuts, coffee, tea, alcohol, or sugar are permitted. Fruits are limited, and the bulk of calories is met by consuming vegetables, dried beans, and grains. This diet can lower blood cholesterol levels, but no more so than the DHSS recommendations, which most people find easier to follow. Recognizing that people may have trouble changing their diet so drastically, the Pritikin plan does suggest sensible ways to "cheat." Table 12-2 compares the level of fat in these three different diets.

Cut down on cholesterol A few years ago, the average American consumed about 700 mg of cholesterol a day. Now the amount is down to 300–500 mg. To keep your diet low in cholesterol, cut back on high-cholesterol foods (see table E-6 in appendix E). Eat only two to three eggs a week.

Cut down on sodium Only about 5 percent of people are sensitive to sodium and get high blood pressure from too much. But you have no way to know if you are one of them. Though sodium is the culprit, the main source of sodium in the diet is salt, a combination of sodium and chloride. The average Briton consumes about 12 g of salt a day, compared to the 3–8 g required. Most is added during processing or is sprinkled on at the dinner table.

To cut back on sodium, try getting in touch with your taste buds. Unsalted food may taste "funny" at first, but you can

Atherosclerosis: When the Heart Breaks

unlearn your taste for salty foods. Put your salt in a shaker with fewer holes or keep it off the table altogether. Substitute other spices for seasonings (see recipe 5 in appendix D). Rely less on convenience foods and find quick ways to cook from scratch.

Check this list of foods high in sodium to see if you are salting your diet too heavily:

- canned or dried soups
- cottage cheese
- processed meats
- olives
- frozen dinners
- ice cream
- soy sauce
- canned vegetables
- potato crisps
- tomato juice
- canned tuna
- instant pudding
- luncheon meat
- monosodium glutamate (a flavor enhancer)
- cheese
- pretzels
- dill pickles
- canned crab
- breakfast cereals
- kosher foods

Keep your overall sodium intake low for the day. If you have Chinese food for lunch, eat low-sodium foods for dinner.

Increase dietary fiber Certain types of fiber, particularly those from carrots, oats, fruits, soybeans, and chickpeas, can lower blood cholesterol. (Bran does not lower cholesterol.) Also, high-fiber diets help control obesity and diabetes, both risk factors for heart disease.

Drink only moderate amounts of alcohol and coffee Heavy alcohol drinking is associated with a greater risk of hypertension, but ironically, moderate drinking raises the levels of a type of HDL cholesterol. If you consume fewer than two drinks a day, you need not worry about cutting back; but then again, no one is suggesting that you take up drinking as a way to prevent heart disease, especially since alcohol raises the risk of death from other causes.

People with high cholesterol levels may want to keep their coffee consumption under two to three cups a day, and those with irregular heartbeats should cut back or avoid coffee altogether. (More information on alcohol appears in chapter 18 and on coffee in chapter 17.)

Table 12-2 Comparison of fat content in three 1,600-calorie diets

Type of diet: (calories from fat)	Typical Diet (40–42%)	Recommended diet (25–30%)	Pritikin diet (10%)
Breakfast	Grapefruit, ½ *Scrambled eggs, 2* *Bacon, 2 slices* Toast, white, 2 slices *Butter, 1 teaspoon* Coffee/tea	Grapefruit, ½ Oatmeal, 1 cup Yogurt, skim, ½ cup Raisins, 1 tablespoon Toast, whole wheat, 2 slices *Margarine, 1 teaspoon* Coffee/tea	Grapefruit, ½ Oatmeal, 1 cup Yogurt, skim, ½ cup Raisins, 1 tablespoon Toast, sprouted wheat, 2 slices Decaffeinated coffee
Lunch	Sandwich: Bread, whole wheat, 2 slices *Swiss cheese, 1 ounce* *Mayonnaise, 1 tablespoon* Lettuce Apple Diet soda	Sandwich: Bread, whole wheat, 2 slices *Swiss cheese, 1 ounce* Mustard, 1 teaspoon Lettuce Apple Carrot Milk, skim, 1 cup Cookie, date-nut	Sandwich: Bread, whole grain (not fat, sugar), 2 slices Cottage cheese, dry curd, 6 tablespoons Cucumber, slices, ¼ medium Apple Carrot Milk, skim, 1 cup Tomato–vegetable soup, 8 ounces Vegetable salad (lettuce, radishes, tomato) Dressing, lemon/apple juice, 2 ounces

Dinner	Roast beef, 2 slices Baked potato *Sour cream/chives, 1 tablespoon* Peas, 2/3 cup *Butter, 1 teaspoon* Salad (lettuce, tomato) *French dressing, 1 tablespoon* Sauterne, 3½ ounces Fruit salad: Oranges, bananas, cantaloupe, blueberries	*Chicken, baked, 2 slices* Baked potato Yogurt (skim)/chives, 1 tablespoon Peas, 2/3 cup Salad (lettuce, tomato) *French dressing, 1 tablespoon* Sauterne, 3½ ounces Fruit salad: Cantaloupe and blueberries	Chinese vegetables with bits of chicken, 16 ounces Brown rice, 3/4 cup Salad (lettuce, tomato, radishes, carrot, cucumber) Lemon-mustard dressing, 1 tablespoon Milk, skim, 1 cup Fruit salad: Oranges, bananas, cantaloupe, blueberries
Total grams of fat:	75	45	16
Fat as percentage total calories:	41%	25%	10%

Italicized foods are those providing the most amount of fat.

A summary of guidelines

- Cut down on cholesterol, sodium, and dietary fats, particularly saturated fats.
- Eat a variety of foods to ensure that your body gets an adequate supply of all the nutrients.
- If you are on birth control pills, have your blood pressure checked every six months.
- If your blood pressure is high, see your doctor about ways to lower it.
- If you smoke, the choice is not easy: cut down or, better yet, quit.
- Reach and stay at your desirable weight.
- If you sit a lot, begin a sensible exercise program.
- If you drink alcohol, do so in moderation.
- If you have one or more of the risk factors previously listed, talk to your doctor about ways to lower your risk.

RESOURCES

Food Should be Fun. Order from the British Heart Foundation, 102 Gloucester Place, London W1H 4DH.

Wright, M. *The Salt Counter*. Pan, 1984.

13
Cancer:
The Diet Connection

> Let's forget the morbidity too long linked with
> cancer and start celebrating survival and triumph
> instead.
>
> Maura, twenty-three, a cancer victim at age
> eight, *Newsweek*

A diagnosis of cancer was once believed to be a death sentence, but things have changed drastically. An increasing number of people with cancer are surviving for at least five years without any recurrence: in effect, they are cured. Not only are better techniques now available for treating cancer, but researchers are unraveling the mystery behind what causes it and are beginning to find that prevention may lie well within our reach.

The development of cancer

Cancer refers to a number of diseases in which abnormal cells grow uncontrollably. A single cell or a few cells may mutate and reproduce rapidly, sucking nourishment from normal cells and forming a mass called a tumor or neoplasm. Benign tumors are not neoplasms, for their cells are confined in a capsule and grow slowly. Once removed, they tend not to recur. Yet they can harm surrounding tissues, sapping their blood supply, and should be surgically removed. Cancer refers to malignant tumors. With no boundaries, these cells multiply rapidly, compress and kill neighboring cells, then break away into the lymph and blood to destroy other parts of the body. Once embedded in a new site, these secondary tumors metastasize and further spread the disease until it is eating away the entire body.

A substance that causes cancer is called a carcinogen. Closely related to carcinogens are mutagens. A mutagen actually alters genetic material and damages the "gene pool" of future generations. If a substance can cause mutations, chances are it may also cause cancer.

Cancer kills more women between ages fifteen and fifty-four than any other disease. For other age groups, it hovers ominously in second or third place. Since the risk of cancer rises with age, its prevalence increases as people live longer. The only truly dramatic rise in recent years is for lung cancer.

Over one hundred kinds of cancer exist, though only thirty are fairly common. The death rate is highest for those cancers whose symptoms are hidden or whose mutant cells spread quickly to other parts of the body. For British women, these are cancers of the breast, lung, colon, ovaries and stomach.

Can cancer be prevented?

Consumers, ever wary of the food supply, have sometimes devised their own theories about cancer. One person wrote to the US Food and Drug Administration: "You may think I'm nuts, but I think that a heck of a lot of the 'cancer epidemic' is due to the preservatives that are put in bread . . . both rich and poor get cancer, and we all eat bread."

Researchers have looked at what everybody does in like fashion, but they have been more puzzled by just the opposite—why does cancer strike different groups at different rates? In Japan the rate of stomach cancer is one of the highest in the world, but rates of breast and colorectal cancers are low. In the United States and Britain, the opposite is true. Also, as people from one country migrate to another, they acquire the rates of their new homeland.

The question that naturally comes to mind is, What is different about these groups that makes one prone to certain cancers and the other not? If it has something to do with the way they live, then by changing certain factors, we should be able to reduce the risk of cancer. In fact, some researchers believe that 90 percent of cancers are environmentally determined, with over half of all cancers in women related to diet. This places diet second only to cigarette smoking as a determinant of cancer, and some researchers believe diet should rank first.

Most often linked to diet are cancers of the mouth, esophagus, stomach, colon, rectum, liver, bladder, and, indirectly, cancers of the breast and uterus. Some nutrients or other substances in food may promote the growth of tumors, while others may inhibit them. Many of these relationships have been shown statistically—that is, comparing the diets and cancer rates among different groups of people. But no one can predict who will or will not be protected by making certain dietary changes. Following are some of those factors that you need to watch out for.

Cancer promoters in the diet

Excess weight Cancers of the uterus, gallbladder, kidney, stomach, and colon are higher for women who weigh 40 percent or more above the average. Some researchers speculate that rather than body weight, it may be a high-fat diet (which also happens to cause the obesity) that is at fault.

Breast cancer rates are higher for obese women who have reached menopause, but not for younger women. Fat cells can produce the female hormone estrogen, a known cause of breast cancer in laboratory animals.

It may be some time before researchers fully understand the association between excess weight and cancer, but until then you would be smart to reach and maintain a desirable weight and get involved in a regular, aerobic exercise program to lower your level of body fat.

Fat and cholesterol Diets high in fat (particularly when combined with low fiber) have been linked to colon cancer. Both Japan and Chile, where diets are low in fat, have little colon cancer, yet Belgium, New Zealand, the United States and Britain where diets are fatty, have high rates. In the digestive tract, fat stimulates the body to produce bile acids that are believed to promote colon cancer. (Fiber is thought to dilute these acids.) Large amounts of fat may prod bacteria in the colon to produce carcinogens.

Some researchers suspect that the culprit is processed polyunsaturated fats. When polyunsaturated fats are hydrogenated to make them solid at room temperature (margarines and shortening, for instance), unusual fatty acids called trans-fatty acids are formed. If these strange fatty acids become incorporated into cell membranes, according to this theory, the membranes may be ineffective at shielding the cell from carcinogens.

Breast cancer rates are strongly associated with the total

amount of fat in the diet. Fats may raise hormone levels, which in turn alter breast tissue and render it susceptible to carcinogens. (For information on how to cut fat intake, see chapter 16.) Evidence relating to high and low levels of blood cholesterol and cancer is inconclusive.

Protein Several epidemiological studies correlate high-protein diets and cancers of the breast and colon, but this data could be muddied because foods rich in protein tend to be rich in fat, too.

Alcohol Heavy alcohol drinkers, particularly those who also smoke cigarettes, are at much greater risk for cancers of the mouth, larynx, and esophagus. Moderate drinking (one or two beers or drinks of wine or spirits a day) is linked to a slight increase in risk. Beer drinking in particular has been linked to colorectal cancer.

Alcohol itself may not be a carcinogen, but it may harbor substances that are. Wine contains over 1,500 congeners, such as nitrosamines and fusel oil, that can produce cancer in laboratory animals. Alcohol may also damage cell membranes, allowing carcinogens, say from cigarette smoke, to penetrate. Alcohol abuse can cause liver cirrhosis, which sometimes leads to liver cancer. Finally, alcoholics may be malnourished, a condition that increases their risks of esophageal cancer. To lower your risk of cancer, cut back on beer, wine, and hard liquor, and substitute club soda, tonic water, and fruit juices.

Coffee The relationship of coffee to cancer is about as murky as a day-old cup of coffee with cream. Some epidemiological studies have associated coffee drinking with cancers of the bladder, ovary, pancreas, and colon. Yet experimental animals that were fed coffee developed no tumors. To date, research findings do not justify giving up coffee. Moderate use does not seem to pose a risk. Remember, the factor in question here is coffee, not caffeine. (More information on coffee and cancer appears in chapter 17.)

Food preparation Flames and smoke contain carcinogens that contaminate food while it cooks. Also, high temperatures can create carcinogens or mutagens within the food. The theory is that these substances in fried and broiled meats initiate cancer and that high-fat diets further promote it.

Benzopyrene is a powerful carcinogen that forms from the burning of wood or charcoal and is carried to food in the smoke and flames. To avoid benzopyrene in smoked foods, cut back on smoked sausages, chicken, turkey, ham, and pork; smoked seafood (salmon or lox, oysters, cod, whitefish); and all smoked cheeses. Instead, eat fresh meat, poultry, and seafood and unsmoked cheeses.

To minimize benzopyrene in barbecued foods, avoid cooking fatty meats or basting with oil or fat. Do not cook meat close to coals, and try to keep flames and smoke away from meat by using foil or a pan. Do not eat the skin of charcoal-broiled chicken or fish.

Cook food slowly at cooler temperatures or grill in a stove with gas or electric heat, under (not over) the flame.

Cooking hamburgers at high temperatures (above 300 degrees F) can form mutagens, though some evidence indicates hamburgers contain substances that block the effects of mutagens. To minimize your exposure, cook hamburger in a regular or microwave oven without a browning plate or fry at temperatures under 300 degrees.

Food additives Usually the first word that comes to people's minds when they hear "food additive" is cancer, but most additives have not been shown to increase cancer rates. Food additives would most likely affect the stomach, yet rates of stomach cancer have been dropping over the past twenty-five years. (Some additives, such as BHA and BHT, may even help prevent cancer.) However, three additives known to cause cancer in laboratory animals—nitrate, nitrite, and saccharin—are still on the market.

Nitrate and nitrite are preservatives added to processed meats, poultry, fish, and certain imported cheeses to prevent botulism and sometimes to impart a distinctive color and flavor. When you eat these foods, the nitrates or nitrites combine with amines (a breakdown product of protein) to form potent carcinogens known as nitrosamines. Nitrosamines can also form when you fry these foods at high temperatures. Manufacturers often add vitamin C and related chemicals, such as sodium ascorbate to cured meats to prevent nitrosamines from forming and are gradually phasing out the use of nitrates and nitrites altogether.

Nitrates exist naturally in carrots, lettuce, celery leaves, and drinking water (as well as human saliva), but these do not form nitrosamines when cooked or consumed. Nitrosamines were once present in beer, formed when the barley malt got too hot. Brewers now know how to prevent this from happening. To reduce your exposure to nitrosamines in meats and seafood, choose fresh meat, poultry, and seafood and cut back on

bacon	sausage
ham	luncheon meats
corned beef	smoked seafood

At high levels, saccharin can cause bladder cancer in rats, but this does not seem to happen in moderate amounts. Few efforts are being made to get saccharin off the market because it is gradually being replaced by aspartame.

Natural carcinogens in food "Nature is not benign," writes Bruce Ames, chairman of the department of biochemistry at the University of California at Berkeley and father of the Ames test, a laboratory technique for identifying mutagens. Plants often protect themselves from insects by synthesizing toxic chemicals. Natural carcinogens or mutagens are present in such common foods as mushrooms, black pepper, grains, nuts, alfalfa sprouts, celery, and rhubarb.

By law, natural carcinogens cannot be added to food but are allowed in their natural sources. Safrole, for instance, is a known carcinogen that occurs naturally as a component of nutmeg, mace, wild ginger, laurel, and black pepper. One very powerful carcinogen—aflatoxin—is produced by molds that grow on nuts, grains, and seeds. To reduce your exposure to aflatoxin, avoid eating these foods if they are moldy or have not been kept dry.

You do not have to give up food to lower your risk of cancer. As Ames points out, sunshine is a carcinogen, but who puts up an umbrella every time she goes out? Nature may not be benign, but it is also not malicious. It gives your body the means to detoxify these substances. The cells of your digestive tract that are constantly exposed to dietary carcinogens are sloughed off every few days and replaced by new ones. The liver defends you against many of these toxins, and running through your body are antioxidants and enzymes that shield you from much damage. Finally, nature, ever inventive, has endowed other plants with substances to protect you.

Cancer fighters in the diet

"I have yet to know a single adult to develop cancer who has habitually drunk a quart of milk daily," wrote maverick nutritionist Adelle Davis, a cancer victim herself at age seventy. The idea was appealing—but wrong. Yet today's research seems to be telling us something similar: rather than attempting the impossible task of eliminating every carcinogen in the food supply, we would be better off protecting ourselves against these substances by eating certain foods that may fight cancer.

Carotene Carotene is the form of vitamin A present in fruits and vegetables. Carotene has been found to lower cancer risk for the larynx, esophagus, and especially the lung. It also tends to inhibit cancers that have already begun and enhances the effectiveness of breast-cancer chemotherapy. No one is sure how it works, but it may strengthen the immune system or limit damage to DNA.

Taking massive doses of vitamin A or carotene supplements does not seem to lower cancer risk. It is even possible that the anticancer agent in fruits and vegetables is something other than carotene. But to be on the safe side, eat plenty of

- Dark leafy greens (kale, broccoli, swiss chard, spinach, green peppers)
- Yellow-orange vegetables (red peppers, carrots, sweet potatoes, pumpkin, winter squash)
- Yellow-orange fruits (peaches, cantaloupe, apricots)

Vitamin C Studies have shown that where diets are low in vitamin C, stomach and esophagus cancer rates are higher. Theoretically, vitamin C would work by strengthening the immune system, encapsulating the tumor, blocking nitrates in the stomach from converting into carcinogens, preventing damage to DNA, and helping the body to absorb selenium. To date, there is little solid evidence that vitamin C—particularly beyond that present in the diet—protects against cancer in humans. However, it is still smart to get enough vitamin C by eating

- Fruits, such as oranges, grapefruit, lemons, strawberries, cantaloupe, and other melons
- Vegetables, such as broccoli, cabbage, green peppers, fresh chili peppers, leafy greens, and kale

Vitamin E There is no evidence that vitamin E protects against cancer. But because other antioxidants (carotene, selenium) seem to, it would be prudent to get adequate amounts of vitamin E in your diet by eating

- Whole-grain breads and cereals
- Nuts and seeds
- Vegetable oils, especially corn, safflower, and soybean oils

Selenium In some countries where the trace element selenium is scarce, there are higher rates of breast and colon cancers. Like carotene and vitamin C, selenium is an antioxidant and can prevent damage to cell membranes. In this way, it may protect against cancer. Because selenium is toxic, supplements are not recommended. However, it is naturally present in meat, whole grains, and fish.

Fiber Dr. Denis Burkitt, a British physician, has amassed an enormous amount of evidence supporting his claim that Western societies have eight times more colon cancer than developing countries because of their low-fiber diets. He observed that in areas of Africa where diets are high in fiber, colon cancer hardly exists at all.

Fiber may dilute a carcinogen by pulling water into the stool; may bind to the carcinogen, rendering it powerless; or may alter the bacteria in the colon that would normally convert substances into carcinogens.

High-fiber diets may protect against breast cancer by trapping estrogen that would normally be stored in bile and released into the intestines and by pulling it out of the body in the feces. This could explain why vegetarian women have lower rates of breast cancer than women who eat meat. According to another theory, fat in the diet is a cancer promoter, while fiber is an inhibitor. Scientists point to the Finns, who eat more fat than almost any other group studied, but who have low rates of colon cancer because, researchers say, they get plenty of fiber from wholegrain breads and cereals, brown rice, legumes, fruits, vegetables, seeds, and popcorn.

Cruciferous vegetables Cruciferous vegetables contain "indoles," which may strengthen your body's natural defense against carcinogens and reduce risk of cancers of the gastrointestinal and respiratory tracts. These include cabbage, cauliflower, broccoli, brussels sprouts, kale, turnips, and kohlrabi.

One easy way to increase your consumption of these cancer fighters is to eat more vegetables and grains. Try a weekly stir-fry meal with broccoli, onions, green and red peppers (and any other vegetables you like) served over brown rice. (See recipe 7 in appendix D.)

Cancer quackery

No one knows exactly how many charlatans from the eighteenth century on have become rich off people's fear of cancer. The number of bogus cancer remedies is astounding and ranges from cobwebs saturated with arsenic powder to zinc-lined boxes in which the patient sits to absorb "orgone energy."

One of the most popular scams in recent times is Laetrile (also called amygdalin, aprikern, or vitamin B_{17}), a chemical present in the seeds of peaches, apples, almonds, plums, and apricots. In the presence of certain enzymes, it releases cyanide.

In the United States Laetrile has been extensively studied in animal tests by the National Cancer Institute, New York City's Memorial Sloan-Kettering Cancer Center, and independent researchers. None has found any evidence that Laetrile is effective. A 1982 study on humans by Dr. C. G. Moertel and colleagues showed no benefit in terms of "cure, improvement, or stabilization of symptoms related to cancer, or extension of life span."

Laetrile itself can be dangerous. If the body breaks it down to cyanide, it causes symptoms of itching, dizziness, headache, vomiting, diarrhea, high fever, and weakness. Cases of both cyanide poisoning and deaths have been documented. Small amounts of cyanide can be converted to a goitrogen, and all goitrogens are potentially carcinogens. So Laetrile may actually cause cancer. The fact that a few American state legislatures have approved the manufacture and distribution of Laetrile does not make it any more effective in treating cancer, and it is banned in Britain.

A diet for the cancer patient

While undergoing cancer treatment—surgery, radiation, or chemotherapy—a patient often loses a lot of weight. With chemotherapy she may complain of nausea or vomiting. An antinausea drug may be the most effective solution, but she may find some relief by avoiding fatty foods, drinking liquids only between meals, sipping ginger ale, or sucking juice bars. Any food that brings on nausea should be avoided. Also, fasting for a few hours before therapy may prevent the patient from associating food with the unpleasant sensations.

A patient who loses her appetite or feels full after only a few bites should eat smaller meals more often and chew foods slowly. Only beverages that provide nutrients as well as calories should be consumed. These include juices, milk, milk shakes, or liquid supplements. By saving beverages until after the meal, she can delay feelings of fullness. Anything that boosts the amount of calories or protein in food will help keep her from wasting away. Try the following:

- Use powdered milk whenever possible (in soups, puddings, casseroles, baked goods, and cereals).
- Add bits of meat, poultry, fish, or cheese to sauces, soups, casseroles, or vegetables.
- Serve fruits and vegetables with high-calorie dips made from sour cream or yogurt, or smear peanut butter on them.
- Use cream instead of milk with cereal. Stir whipping cream in coffee, hot chocolate, or use it to top off desserts.
- Always have snacks available. Include nuts, dried fruits, slices of bread with margarine, butter, or cream cheese.

A patient who complains of a bitter or metallic taste in her mouth may find meat unpleasant to eat. Usually it will taste better if marinated in sweet-and-sour sauces or sweet wines, prepared in casseroles or soups, or served cold instead of hot. Strong seasonings (oregano, basil, tarragon, mint) may disguise the meaty flavor. Some patients find brushing their teeth before eating makes the meal more pleasant.

The best advice for preventing cancer is to reduce your risks by changing your life-style and by getting early detection and treatment. The best advice for the cancer patient is to stay under the care of competent doctors and avoid unproven methods of treatment.

RESOURCES

Diet and the Cancer Patient. Free booklet.

BACUP Cancer Information Service, 121 Charterhouse Street, London EC1M 6AA.

14
Diabetes:
The Sweetest Scourge

> I am five feet five inches tall, and when I found out sixteen months ago that I had diabetes, my weight was up to 336 pounds. [My doctor] told me that I had high blood pressure on top of diabetes and that I had to lose weight "or else." ... All my life I had been putting my diet off "until tomorrow"—tomorrow had finally come.
>
> Margaret, a diabetic, *Diabetes Forecast*

After heart disease and cancer, diabetes with its complications kill more Americans than any other disease. In Britain over a million people are diabetic. To make matters worse, half do not even know they have it.

When cells refuse to eat

Behind your stomach sits the pancreas, an organ that contains beta cells, which produce insulin. When you eat, your pancreas secretes insulin, which courses through your bloodstream to your liver, muscle, and fat cells. At the surface of each cell, the insulin comes face to face with thousands of special receptors. By activating these receptors, insulin informs the cell that glucose (blood sugar) and amino acids are on their way and will need to be taken in. Insulin also tells fat cells to take up the fat and the liver to store glucose as glycogen. The receptors are like footmen at a grand ball who check invitations, announce new arrivals, and bounce unwanted guests. Insulin is the caterer.

Normally after you consume a meal—even a large one—your blood sugar stays within a narrow range because the more you eat, the more insulin is released. But with diabetes, something goes wrong. After each meal, blood sugar rises and stays high. Instead of being admitted into the cells, glucose is banned to the bloodstream. Some is forced to pass through the kidneys, dragging water with it and spilling into the urine. Your blood becomes a veritable ocean of nutrients that, like bored delinquents, can get into nasty trouble.

Before you read what this trouble is, consider how such an unpleasant scenario can happen. In Type I diabetes, your body cannot produce insulin, either because the pancreas is damaged (from infection, for instance) or has been surgically removed. The tendency to develop diabetes is also strongly gene-related. Your immune system may go haywire and attack the beta cells or allow viruses to attack the cells. Once 90 percent of the beta cells are destroyed, you get diabetes. Type I diabetes was once called juvenile-onset diabetes because it typically strikes before adulthood, often around the time of a girl's first menstrual period. Only one third of known diabetics in the United Kingdom has Type I.

In Type II, or maturity-onset diabetes, your pancreas may pump out enough insulin—even too much—but the cells have too few receptors and ignore it. Glucose floods the blood and triggers the release of yet more insulin. All this excess insulin makes the situation worse because the cells, sensing this barrage of insulin, defensively shut down many of their receptors.

Though Type II diabetes is striking an increasing number of children and young adults, it usually occurs in adulthood. One-third of the victims have a family history of the disease, and the majority have a diabetic parent. A Type II diabetic may inherit defects in body cells or pancreatic cells that cause resistance to insulin. Such individuals may sidestep the disease for years until their bodies become overstressed from obesity or too little exercise.

Close to 600,000 people in Britain may already have Type II diabetes and not know it, according to the British Diabetic Association. Every year about 40,000 new cases are identified, and the rate is increasing slightly.

How diabetes damages the body

Type I diabetes is usually believed to be the more severe form, but either one, if untreated, can cause debility and death. Diabetics have twice the risk of heart disease and are seventeen times more likely to develop kidney disease. High blood sugar wreaks havoc on the nerves, particularly those in the legs and feet. The nerves swell and cannot signal sensations of temperature and pain. Because of poor circulation, reduced sense of touch, and impaired healing, the diabetic is prone to foot injuries and infections, which, if untreated, can cause gangrene. The limb may have to be amputated.

Diabetics are twenty-five times more likely to suffer eye problems, and diabetes is the main cause of new cases of blindness in adults. A diabetic's skin may be prone to pimples, boils, and lesions because the high level of blood sugar hinders the white blood cells from attacking bacteria and preventing infection.

The scary part is that all of this damage can happen and you may still be unaware that you are diabetic. But these complications are not inevitable. They develop in people who do not keep their condition under control and who allow high blood sugars to remain in their bloodstream for too long. Many diabetics find that by controlling their diets, by exercising, and by reducing the stress in their lives, they end up healthier than their nondiabetic friends.

Symptoms

The onset of Type I diabetes is sudden. Because no insulin exists, symptoms become acute within weeks—sometimes days. The child or young adult may become incredibly thirsty and drink lots of fluids, urinating frequently. Bedwetting is common. The Type I diabetic may be constantly hungry, sometimes nauseated, but she may also be losing weight rapidly. She feels tired, weak, and irritable. If her condition is not caught early enough, she may experience rapid breathing and drowsiness, and then go into a coma. If you have any of these symptoms, see a doctor immediately.

These same symptoms, plus others, may occur with Type II diabetes. You may feel tingling or numbness in your legs, feet, or fingers. Your vision may change or blur. Your skin may itch or become infected frequently, and cuts and bruises may heal slowly. You may have constant vaginal infections. Sometimes, however, you may experience none of these symptoms. Type II diabetes may go undetected for years. Many diabetics are unaware of their condition until they have a routine blood test or suffer a heart attack, kidney disease, or eye problems.

Who is at risk?

For Type I diabetes, boys and girls are at equal risk. Most are lean, and many have a family history of the disease. Type II diabetes, some researchers say, is a disease of affluence. They blame overeating, lack of exercise, and stress. Obesity is certainly the number-one risk factor. A fat person is eight times more likely to get diabetes than a thin person.

Recent research indicates that the *distribution* of fat on your body affects the risk of getting diabetes. Fat on your waist, abdomen, chest, and neck is much worse than a cello body, in which fat settles on your hips, buttocks, and thighs. If you are obese and unsure where your fat is, use this formula:

Waist measurement divided by hip measurement is	*Then you have*
Less than 0.76	Lower-body obesity
About equal to 0.76–0.85	Generalized body fat distribution
Greater than 0.85	Upper-body obesity and a high risk of diabetes

About 25 percent of all obese women have upper-body obesity; their fat cells are enlarged, like balloons stretching outward. These overstuffed cells have few insulin receptors to pull in glucose or metabolize it once it gets inside. Because of the resulting high levels of blood sugar, these women are at greater risk of diabetes. Researchers speculate that fat cells in the upper body become enlarged when you overeat as an adult.

The fat cells of women with lower-body obesity are normal size, but there simply are too many of them. These cells are responsive to insulin. Such women may have inherited these cells or inadvertently revved up their production by overeating during critical periods of childhood or at puberty.

Luckily for the diabetic, it is easier to lose fat from the upper body: you simply have to shrink the overstuffed fat cells. There is little to shrink on the lower body, so there you actually have to get rid of existing cells.

The risk of Type II diabetes increases with age, usually striking after age forty. Part of this increased risk is due to aging. Your cells become less sensitive to insulin as you get older; in addition, people tend to become less active and neglect their diets with age.

If you are over forty, overweight, have a family history of diabetes, or have given birth to a baby who weighed over ten pounds, get screened for diabetes about once a year.

Controlling diabetes with diet

In the past, diabetics have been given diets very low in carbohydrates and told to eat heavy cream, steak, eggs, and butter (but not bread). Such diets may have inadvertently raised the risk of heart attacks and strokes. Today, recent studies on two fronts may soon change the way diabetics are routinely advised to eat. First, Dr. James Anderson of the University of Kentucky found that he could take dozens of Type II diabetics off their insulin by getting them to eat a diet high in fiber and carbohydrate, but low in fat. All fiber foods are not alike; the ones that keep blood sugar down are present in legumes, fruits, and oats, but not in whole grains.

The second set of data punched a hole in the well-accepted theory that sweets, because they are rapidly absorbed, send blood sugar soaring, while starches take more time to digest because their sugar chains must first be split apart. It all made perfect sense until someone decided to actually measure these effects. Nutritionist Phyllis Crapo and her associates at the University of Toronto worked independently on the same problem. By feeding volunteers everything from spaghetti to Mars bars, they studied how different foods affected blood sugar. Jenkins created a "glycemic index," which compares the rise in blood sugar caused by each food with the rise caused by pure glucose (rated as 100). Foods that rated high (80 or more)—and that cause high levels of blood sugar—included carrots, parsnips, instant potatoes, cornflakes, and honey. Those with low scores (50 or under) included spaghetti, dried beans and peas, oranges, apples, dairy products, and peanuts. Surprisingly, potatoes created higher blood sugar levels than did table sugar, higher even than a Mars bar.

Even in the face of this evidence, a diabetic should not use the glycemic index as the sole guide to choosing foods: dining on Mars bars is still not a great idea. It is important to realize that some foods slow the blood sugar response because they contain a lot of fat (fat tends to delay digestion). Ice cream and pastries may not cause blood sugar to jump, but eating such fatty foods can increase the risk of obesity and heart disease, common complications of diabetes. Though cooked carrots rated a high glycemic score (92), they are still a nutritious food. Instead of eliminating carrots from the diet, the diabetic should eat them as part of a meal, so that the digestion of other foods with low glycemic scores will slow the rise in blood sugar from eating foods with high glycemic scores.

Exercise Exercise offers a double bonus to the diabetic. For the short term, muscles burn glycogen (stored inside the cells) and glucose and gradually lower blood sugar. After exercise, the muscles restock their glycogen supply by continuing to pull glucose from the bloodstream. Cells are more sensitive to insulin during exercise and for several days afterward, so with regular exercise, the diabetic may show a "permanent" sensitivity to insulin. After six weeks, diabetic college students who exercised vigorously for an hour daily had lowered their blood sugar levels from 220 to 115 (normal is from 80 to 100). Exercise also lowers the risk of heart disease by reducing body fat and making platelets less sticky so they are less likely to clump.

Hypoglycemia (Nondiabetic)

Everyone experiences low blood sugar to some degree throughout the day. Three to four hours after a meal, when your level of blood sugar is at its lowest, you will experience mild hypoglycemia. You may get hungry and weak, and your head may pound. Your body reacts by releasing the hormones glucagon, epinephrine, and norepinephrine (adrenaline), which raise blood sugar levels by breaking down stored carbohydrate, fat, and protein. So far, everything is normal.

If any part of this system fails, true hypoglycemia may result. Two types of hypoglycemia exist, and though neither is a disease, one type, called fasting hypoglycemia, can signal that disease is present. Fasting hypoglycemia can occur if a tumor on the pancreas is secreting excessive amounts of insulin. This type of hypoglycemia is unrelated to what and when you eat and is generally severe because blood sugar may fall too low for your

Eat Beautiful!

brain to function normally. Symptoms include fatigue, confusion, amnesia, headache, convulsions, and loss of consciousness.

The second type, called reactive hypoglycemia, is controversial, partly because the symptoms are vague and partly because no one knows how to measure it accurately. Reactive hypoglycemia usually occurs a few hours after eating. It can also be brought on if you do not eat any carbohydrate for a few days, then have a dose of sugar, or if you consume a sweet alcoholic drink on an empty stomach. You may experience irritability, palpitations, shakiness, and anxiety.

Symptoms like irritability and anxiety are not much different from those caused by stress, which also triggers the release of epinephrine and norepinephrine. It is easier to blame such feelings on a physical problem such as low blood sugar than to admit that you are under too much pressure.

Also, reactive hypoglycemia is difficult to measure. No one is certain how far blood sugar can drop and still be normal. Sometimes the results of two or three tests are inconsistent. If you experience some of the symptoms, consult your doctor. Never diagnose yourself.

If you are hypoglycemic, here are some ways to slow the rate at which sugar enters the bloodstream:

- Avoid simple sugars. Instead, eat starchy foods such as pasta.
- Eat five or six small, high-protein meals a day rather than a few large, sugary meals.
- Eat slowly.
- Include plenty of fiber from legumes, fruits, and oats.
- If you feel dizzy, weak, or faint when working out, try exercises that are longer and slower rather than brisk and intense. Eat a high-protein dish before exercising. Over time, regular aerobic exercise helps to even out blood sugar swings.

If you experience a hypoglycemic reaction in spite of these measures, drink a glass of fruit juice for a quick sugar surge, then follow it with a snack of protein and starch (like crackers and cheese). Symptoms usually abate on their own after fifteen to twenty minutes.

RESOURCES

The British Diabetic Association
10 Queen Anne Street, London W1M 0BD

15
Gastrointestinal Disorders: Gut Reactions

> Part of the secret of success in life is to eat what
> you like and let the food fight it out inside.
>
> Mark Twain

In the sporting arenas of your stomach and intestines, foods may pummel themselves into a mishmash, as Twain suggested, but you will not be a cheering spectator. Eating habits and diet are linked to many gastrointestinal disorders, from the mildly annoying to the life-threatening. About 20 million Americans are chronically ill because of these disorders, and 200,000 a year die. To understand how to lower your risk, you first need to visualize the digestive system (figure 15-1).

Anatomy of the gut

From your mouth to your anus stretch thirty feet of pouches, organs, and convoluted tubing through which food shuffles along, getting churned, mashed, mixed with acid, neutralized, partially absorbed, and finally expelled.

Digestion begins in your mouth, where chewing breaks up food and mixes it with enzymes in saliva. Starches begin to dissolve into sugars. Once you swallow, the food enters your esophagus, where a few seconds and ten inches later it lands in your stomach. Like an old-fashioned washing machine, the stomach churns and mashes the food, tears it into smaller pieces, and mixes it with hydrochloric acid and the enzyme pepsin. When everything is thoroughly mashed into a mushy "chyme," a valve at the lower end of the stomach relaxes and squeezes a small amount into the intestine. Because carbohydrates are digested quickly, they are first to arrive. (This is why you feel hungry so soon after eating Chinese food.) Proteins and fats are broken down at a slower rate, from which comes the mistaken notion that they are "hard to digest."

Gastrointestinal Disorders: Gut Reactions

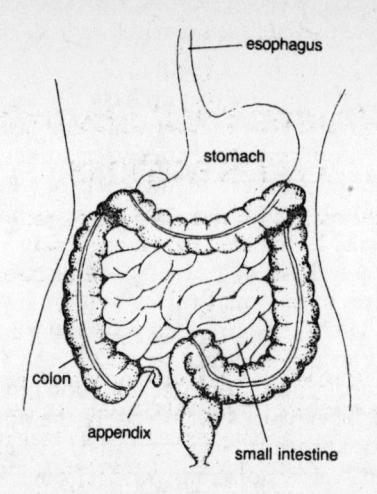

Figure 15-1 The gastrointestinal tract

In the small intestine, carbohydrates, fats, and proteins are broken into even smaller pieces and most of the nutrients absorbed. The remaining chyme moves into the large intestine (or colon), where water and mineral salts are absorbed. Three bands of muscles run the length of the colon. Because they are shorter than the colon, they draw it into sacs or segments, like elastic pulled through the casing of a waistband. Wastes remain in the colon until they are excreted. While there, they provide a banquet for billions of microorganisms. Most of these microorganisms are harmless. Some even produce vitamins, such as vitamin K and vitamin B_{12} (in humans, vitamin B_{12} is produced below the site where it can be absorbed). Others such as *Escherichia coli*, *Streptococcus*, *Clostridium*, and yeast can cause disease, but they are usually thwarted by the far greater number of beneficial microorganisms. If disease, diet, or antibiotics upsets this natural balance, problems develop.

In large part, fiber determines the types of bacteria that will thrive because it passes through the stomach and small intestines virtually intact. For instance, in the small intestine, fiber can bind to the milk sugar lactose and drag it to the colon, where *Lactobacillus acidolphilus* will convert it to lactic acid. This makes the colon acidic and hostile to harmful microorganisms.

Eat Beautiful!

Fiber: the undigestible, uncontestable wonder

On June 23, 1965, Alice Farnsworth had the Most Embarrassing Moment of Her Life. In line to purchase her week's groceries, she was forced to wait at the register while the cashier yelled to a stockboy: "Fifteen-ounce box of Sunsweet prunes, how much?" Alice could hear the snickers in the checkout line. Of all the items she was buying, why did the unpriced box have to be filled with *prunes*!

By 1980, the purchase of prunes no longer caused a chain reaction of giggles; in fact, half the carts in line were filled with All-Bran, whole-wheat fig bars, and coarse dark bread. At last Alice could glory in her foresight.

Fiber is not exactly food. To do its job, food must be absorbed by the body. But fiber works for precisely the opposite reason: your body cannot absorb it. So it swooshes through your intestines, sucking up water, softening wastes, then hurrying them through the colon.

Fiber is the undigestible cell of walls of plants. There are five types: cellulose, hemicellulose, pectins, gums, and lignin. (Intestinal bacteria do digest some of this fiber, particularly pectin, producing volatile fatty acids that are absorbed through the intestinal lining.) Each type of fiber performs differently in your body.

When you eat plants with cellulose and hemicellulose, you digest the inner part of the cell, leaving empty spaces in the cell wall. Water fills in these spaces and makes stools softer and bulkier so that they speed through the colon. This relieves constipation (reducing risk of diverticulosis and possibly hemorrhoids), dilutes carcinogens (reducing risk of colon cancer), and pushes fats through the digestive system so they have less time to be absorbed (reducing risk of obesity and heart disease). Foods high in cellulose include

whole-wheat flour	bran	cabbage
young peas	green beans	cucumber skins
broccoli	brussels sprouts	carrots
peppers	apples	

Those rich in hemicellulose are

bran	corn	cereals

Gastrointestinal Disorders: Gut Reactions

whole grains   brussels sprouts   greens
beet root

Gums can bind to bile acids and remove them from the body. Because bile acids are formed from cholesterol, the body has to pull more cholesterol from the blood to replace the lost acids. Not only can this reduce risk of heart disease, but since bile acids are sometimes converted into carcinogens, it can also reduce the risk of colorectal cancer.

Both pectins and gums slow the emptying of food from the stomach. Instead of being walloped with a rush of sugar, the bloodstream receives sugar in smaller, gradual doses. This offsets the need for large amounts of insulin—a plus for diabetics. Pectins and gums are often added to food as thickeners. Sources of gums include

oatmeal
other rolled-oat products
dried beans

For pectin, eat

cauliflower   apples   citrus fruits
dried peas   green beans   cabbage
potatoes   carrots   strawberries

Lignin gives you many of these same benefits: it speeds food through the intestines, binds bile salts, and so lowers blood cholesterol. Lignin is present in

breakfast cereals   bran
strawberries   aubergines
green beans   radishes
older vegetables   pears

Table E-7 (see appendix E) lists dietary fiber values of some common foods. As consumers began to demand more fiber in their foods, some manufacturers got a little carried away. One bakery began marketing loaves of bread with added wood fiber. Dr. Dean Oliver, professor at the Food Research Institute of the University of Wisconsin at Madison, amused with the high price the manufacturer was charging, jokingly suggested that a cheaper way to get wood fiber would be to eat paper napkins. Not only could people simply eat their napkins after a meal, but "a blender puree of napkin and fruit preserves has something of the character of a milk shake."

Westerners could probably offset some of today's health problems by increasing their current fiber intake of 20 grams daily to 30 grams or more with

- A variety of fresh fruits and vegetables
- Unfiltered fruit and vegetable juices
- Brown rice
- Nuts, seeds, popcorn
- Lentils and dried beans and peas (recipe 8 in appendix D gives one way to serve lentils)
- Whole-grain breads, cereals, and pasta.

If you eat bran and other bulk producers dry, they can obstruct the esophagus and even be constipating, so be sure to drink plenty of fluids. Also, add fiber gradually to your diet, so your intestinal bacteria can adjust to the change. Otherwise, they may retaliate by giving you gas and diarrhea.

Too much fiber is not the answer, either. Excess pectin cuts vitamin B_{12} absorption. Other fibers interfere with minerals such as iron, zinc, calcium, phosphorus, and magnesium. (You absorb less iron from whole-wheat bread than white, even though the whole wheat may contain more iron.) To its credit, fiber does not discriminate in what it chooses to bind. It drags both drugs and heavy metals such as lead out of the body, too. To minimize fiber's interference with nutrients, eat a variety of fibers rather than sprinkling bran on everything you eat. Unless recommended by your doctor, avoid fiber supplements (bran tablets, purified cellulose).

Disorders related to too little fiber

Constipation Your gastrointestinal tract normally sweeps itself clean of wastes by a series of motions. The contraction of a muscle in one segment of the intestine pushes the food into the next segment, and so on. As you age, these muscles lose their tone and contract less efficiently. Wastes move more slowly, and water has more time to be absorbed, so the stool gets harder, denser, and more stubborn.

Eating high-fiber foods, particularly those with lots of cellulose and hemicellulose, can keep water in the stools so they are softer and bulkier (corn, by the way, is better at this than wheat bran). Drink plenty of fluids, and exercise. Do not rely on laxatives.

Diverticulosis and diverticulitis With chronic constipation, your colon muscles must contract more to expel wastes. Over time, they thicken from the strain. The colon is segmented, and if the area where two segments join thickens, pressure builds up until the colon blows out or protrudes through the overlying muscle layer. These protrusions, called diverticulosis, affect more than 2 million American women over seventy years old.

If feces get trapped in these pockets, the area becomes infected, causing diverticulitis, a condition more common in men than women. Symptoms include acute abdominal pain, nausea, and vomiting. Sometimes attacks will go away without treatment. Other times, the patient receives intravenous fluids to rest the colon. Antibiotics are prescribed to fight the infection, and in chronic cases, surgery may be required.

Appendicitis The appendix hangs off the cecum, the pouch where the colon begins. Perhaps a remnant from earlier days of the species, the appendix serves no known purpose. The cause of appendicitis is still clouded, though one theory links it to diets low in fiber. What supposedly happens is that the opening between the appendix and the intestine becomes blocked by a small, hardened mass of feces or by a muscle spasm in the wall of the appendix. (Both could result from firm feces caused by a low-fiber diet.) As long as the opening remains blocked, the appendix swells and pressure rises. If the pressure becomes too intense, the appendix bursts, throwing bacteria into the abdominal cavity. A dangerous infection can ensue.

Evidence against the fiber theory is statistical. In the United States from 1955 to 1975, the incidence of appendicitis dropped by 40 percent at a time when the average American was eating very little fiber.

Hemorrhoids If you are constipated, you may have to strain during a bowel movement. When you do this, you stretch the veins in the rectum, and over time hemorrhoids form. They can be above the sphincter muscle (internal) or below it (external). Hemorrhoids can develop from pregnancy, and infection, rectal cancer, and from sitting all day at a desk job. Rectal bleeding may occur from a ruptured hemorrhoid and should be checked out by a doctor.

Other disorders (not directly related to fiber)

Indigestion What do you do about those feelings of heartburn, nausea, abdominal discomfort, no appetite, belching, and gas? Indigestion, common during or following a meal, results from bolting your food, overeating, chewing too little, swallowing air, or eating foods that are poorly cooked, very sweet, or fat. Foods that irritate the stomach lining, such as onions, lettuce, and cabbage, can also cause indigestion. In some people, coffee relaxes the ring of muscles at the end of the esophagus so it allows food to flow backward and cause heartburn. Another likely cause of indigestion is "nerves."

To avoid indigestion, eat well-cooked foods and stay clear of anything spicy or rich (or any foods that cause you trouble). Also, have relaxed meals. Unless prescribed, avoid enzyme products (papain from papayas, betaine hydrochloride, pepsin) that are promoted as digestive aids. Enzymes vary in activity and even when coated are likely to be deactivated by stomach acid. If indigestion occurs frequently, have it checked out. It could indicate a more serious illness.

Excess gas Excess gas is not produced by your body but by bacteria living in your colon. If carbohydrates and proteins are not completely digested in the small intestine, they arrive in the colon, where bacteria attack them.

The main foods that cause this are wheat, beans, and dairy products (especially in people who lack the enzyme lactase to break down milk sugar). Baked beans are the worst. They contain sugars that cannot be split by enzymes in the small intestine, so they pass into the colon. Undercooked beans contain raw starch that also end up in the colon. To lessen the effect of beans, soak them in water for several hours before cooking, then discard the water and cook the beans in fresh water. To avoid gas from milk, eat foods with partially digested lactase,

Gastrointestinal Disorders: Gut Reactions

such as yogurt, ripened cheeses, and buttermilk, or add the enzyme Lact-Aid to milk before you drink it. For gas problems with wheat, switch to gluten-free wheat.

Food allergies Your head is stuffed up, your nose is runny, and you are feeling as if you just got smacked with the latest flu bug. Maybe you have the flu, or maybe you are reacting to something you ate. Allergy symptoms can include a head cold, bad breath, nausea, headache, hives, dizziness, bloody urine, and painful joints. Because these symptoms mimic so many other disorders, food allergies are commonly misdiagnosed. But they are real and can be dangerous.

Allergies are not exactly gastrointestinal problems, but food allergens enter through your mouth, and some have been linked to intestinal disorders, such as ulcerative colitis. An allergy develops when you ingest, inhale, or somehow encounter a substance—usually a protein—that your body labels "foreign." About 95 percent of food allergies are the delayed type, in which symptoms take more than four hours, sometimes days, to appear. Usually, each time you eat a specific food, you will experience the same symptoms.

Many people with food allergies will react only if they eat certain foods frequently or in large amounts. An athlete may take to guzzling milk, or a dieter to a bizarre reducing diet of tomato juice. If these foods are eaten only occasionally or in smaller amounts, no reaction occurs. Other people react violently to a tiny bit of an offending food.

Physical and emotional states can affect your reaction to a food. Some hay fever sufferers or those which bronchial asthma may have no problem eating foods like peaches, melon, sweet corn, chocolate, or seafood until hay fever season, when they experience severe reactions. Other people who show sensitivity to certain foods can eat them with no reaction unless they are under stress. One woman would break out in hives on the first of the month. Her attacks always occurred if she ate celery and was also worrying about paying bills.

Usually a doctor will take your family and personal medical history. Allergies tend to run in families, so if other members are allergic to a food, there is a chance you are, too. If you had a food allergy as a child, you may still be sensitive to the food, only display different symptoms.

Next, you are asked to keep a food diary to see what kinds of things (including toothpaste, mouthwash, vitamin pills, chewing gum, medicines) you normally eat. An elimination diet is prescribed, in which you exclude all possible food allergens from your diet for a few weeks, then add them back one at a time to see if they cause a reaction. Usually the culprit can be caught this way. If your symptoms persist, your problem may not be with food at all but with something less easy to eliminate, like your cat's fur. Once a food allergen is identified, you may be able to eat it in small amounts without a reaction.

Common food allergens include milk, eggs, wheat, seafood, nuts, mustard seeds, chocolate, oranges, and tomatoes. If you are allergic to one food, you may react to foods in the same botanic family. For instance, if you break out after eating oranges, you probably will break out after eating grapefruit and lemons, too. One way to avoid food allergens is to check the labels on the products you buy. However, because spices, flavors, and colors do not have to be listed by name, you may not know if the ingredient to which you are sensitive is present. Some people live in constant fear of attack from invisible ingredients in food. One US color additive, Yellow No. 5, causes allergies in at least 50,000–90,000 Americans, particularly those allergic to aspirin.

A popular but controversial method of testing for allergies is called cytotoxic testing, in which white blood cells are extracted, centrifuged, and exposed to extracts of 150 or more foods. Within ninety minutes (the amount of time varies with each lab), technicians measure which food extracts damage the white blood cells.

Proponents explain that by eliminating these foods, you can cure fatigue, arthritis, migraines, and an array of other ailments. Critics argue that, unlike the test, whole, undigested food does not enter your bloodstream. You may not be allergic to the food at all but to a product formed during its digestion, so the extract may not even contain the allergen. Also, the way the extract is prepared or stored will sometimes render a true allergen harmless and it will not show up on the test. Because test results are often inconsistent and subjectively interpreted, people have complained that different labs give you totally different results. Some allergy specialists believe that too little data exist to support the current usefulness of this test.

Lactose intolerance Some people may suffer symptoms similar to allergic reactions when they drink milk. They have lactose intolerance and lack the enzyme lactase, which breaks down the milk sugar lactose into its two component sugars, glucose and galactose. Without this enzyme, lactose remains in the intestines, pulls in large amounts of water, and fosters the growth of bacteria that form irritating acids. People who cannot digest milk sugar get abdominal cramps, gas, and watery diarrhea.

A few people cannot have any milk at all, including a tablespoon or two to lighten coffee. But most can handle small amounts, particularly when consumed slowly with other foods. Many can eat foods in which the lactase has been partially digested from bacteria—yogurt, ripened cheeses, buttermilk, sour cream, and acidophilus milk, for example. Also, you can buy the enzyme lactase (marketed as Lact-Aid) and add it to milk products about twenty-four hours before you consume them. By the time you drink the milk, all that remains are harmless simple sugars.

If you cannot consume dairy products, be sure to include other rich sources of calcium in your diet, such as soybean curd (tofu), nuts, kale, broccoli, and greens. Check with your doctor about taking a 500-mg calcium supplement daily.

Cleaning out the intestinal tract

Laxatives Laxatives flush out the intestine by irritating the lining of the colon and leaving it inflamed. They can be used occasionally but should never be depended on for "regularity" or for treating symptoms of abdominal pain or vomiting. (Having a bowel movement only every three days or so is still considered "regular.") Overuse of laxatives can speed nutrients through your intestines so quickly that there is no time for absorption. Avoid using mineral oil in particular, which has no redeeming value and prevents the absorption of carotene, a vitamin A precursor. Though it can relieve constipation, it pulls fat-soluble vitamins out of your body. Loss of vitamin D is especially a problem for women at risk of osteoporosis. Other

Eat Beautiful!

laxatives such as methylcellulose, psyllium seed, Epsom salts, and castor oil prevent the absorption of the minerals calcium, iron, magnesium, potassium, and zinc. Finally, muscles need to work to stay in shape; by continuously taking laxatives, your intestinal muscles will lose their tone.

Enemas Enemas work by flushing the rectum with fluid and are commonly used before surgery, delivery, and X-ray exams. Lately, people have taken to using them on a routine basis to stay "regular." What they do not realize is that prolonged, continued use of enemas can lead to a dependence because your colon eventually loses its cleansing savvy.

Practitioners of colonic irrigation or high colonic enemas use a tube that stretches from twenty to thirty inches (an ordinary enema tube measures three inches long). They insert this tube, then flush the colon with warm water, often adding coffee, herbs, enzymes, wheat, and grass extracts to the solution. There is no evidence to support claims about colonic therapy; in fact, the procedure itself can be hazardous. Deaths have occurred from imbalances in body salts, tearing of the bowel lining, bowel disease, and toxic colitis.

The best way to keep your colon healthy and to stay "regular" is to eat plenty of high-fiber foods, drink lots of water, exercise regularly, and find ways to cope with stress.

PART 4
Life-Style

When women eat out in restaurants, the most popular item is not salad or pasta or even white wine, but "I-just-want-a-bite-of-yours." Such delicate appetites result from the desire of many women to stay slender when their frenetic everyday pace prevents them from getting regular exercise. This section will help you avoid such a rut; it is about food choices. "In the Kitchen" offers practical guidelines for buying, storing, and preparing foods to get the most nutrients for your money. Suggestions for eating well, whether you spend most of your day working behind a desk or over a bassinet, appear in the chapter "In the Workplace." Finally, because everyone harbors some nutritional "vice," be it chocolate, pastries, or alcohol, "On the Town" explains how to enjoy such indulgences, yet keep them in perspective. After all, as Julia Child says, "Life itself is the proper binge."

16
In the Kitchen: the Politics of the Pantry

> Cooking is like love. It should be entered into with abandon or not at all.
>
> Harriet Van Horne, in *Vogue*, October 15, 1956

Like love, cooking is enhanced with a dollop of knowledge, a pinch of awareness about health, and a dash of skill. Because you are already reading this book, I assume you are health conscious, so what follows is the knowledge you will need to shop for, prepare, and serve nutritious meals. And the dash of skill? As in all endeavors, that comes with persistence and practice.

The Western diet

As societies become richer, their people eat more meat, dairy products, refined flour, sugar, and highly processed foods. They skimp on whole grains and fresh fruits and vegetables. Many Americans, for instance, adhere to the three B's: bacon for breakfast, bologna (luncheon meat) for lunch, and burgers for dinner.

On the plus side of the affluent diet is plenty of high-quality protein. Weighing down the minus side is too much fat, cholesterol, sodium, sugar, and calories, too few trace minerals and vitamins, and too little fiber. This diet is associated with a greater risk of heart disease, cancer, diabetes, obesity, and gastrointestinal disorders. Obviously, it has a few shortcomings.

Various guidelines exist for improving the Western diet. The four food groups guide has long been the standard for judging diets, but you can follow this guide and still eat poorly. A fatty burger with french fries, a milk shake, and coleslaw contains items from each food group, but the combination is far from a sterling example of a nutritious meal. In the United States the Center for Science in the Public Interest has created its own version of the basic four, which gives more guidance on choices within each group (see table 16-1).

The alternative diet—vegetarianism

At one time, nutritionists and doctors categorized vegetarians as faddists and seriously questioned whether a meatless diet could sustain human life. Such questions have been put to rest—we now know that vegetarians were on to something.

In general, vegetarian diets are low in saturated fat, total fats, and cholesterol, and high in fiber and certain vitamins. Partly because of this, vegetarians as a group have lower risk of cardiovascular disease and colorectal cancer, and possibly diabetes, osteoporosis, urinary stones, gallstones, and cancers of the breast, pancreas, and ovary. Avoiding meat may not be the only factor. Many vegetarians typically do not consume coffee, tea, alcohol, or highly refined foods and are health conscious and active.

To be a healthy vegetarian, you must do more than simply give up red meat. The more foods you restrict or give up, the harder time you will have getting all the essential nutrients. If you subsist on peanut butter or cheese sandwiches, your diet will still be high in fat.

What poses a problem for the vegetarian is getting enough *high-quality* protein. All plant and animal foods contain the same twenty-two amino acids. Of these, eight are essential for adults and must come from the diet in the proper amounts and proportions. But legumes, grains, nuts, and seeds are low in one or more of these essential amino acids. (Soybeans are the exception.)

A lacto-ovovegetarian gets high-quality protein from dairy products and eggs. But if you are a strict vegetarian or vegan (you eat no animal products whatsoever), to get the right proportions of amino acids, you must combine vegetables, grains, legumes, nuts, and seeds so that the amino acid deficient in one will be compensated for by another (see table 16-2). Or use textured vegetable protein (meat analogs) made from grains or legumes.

Besides combining proteins, a vegan must find reliable sources of vitamin B_{12}. A vegan should be sure to eat foods fortified with vitamin B_{12}, such as soy milk, some cereals, meat analogs,

Table 16-1 The revised four food groups

	Anytime	In moderation	Now and then
GROUP I: Beans, grains and nuts Four or more servings/day	Barley Beans Bread & rolls (whole grain) Bulgur Lentils Oatmeal Pasta Rice Whole-grain cereal	Nuts Peanut butter Soybeans White bread and Cereals	
GROUP II: Fruits and vegetables Four or more servings/day	All fruits and vegetables except those listed on right Unsweetened fruit juices Unsalted vegetable juices Potatoes, white or sweet	Avocado Fruits canned in syrup Salted vegetable juices Sweetened fruit juice Vegetables canned with salt	French fries Olives Pickles
GROUP III: Milk products Children: 3 to 4 servings or equivalent; adult: 2 servings (favor *anytime* column for additional servings)	Buttermilk Low-fat cottage cheese Low-fat milk with 1% milkfat Skim-milk ricotta Skim milk	Frozen low-fat yogurt Ice milk Low-fat milk with 2% milkfat Low-fat (2%) yogurt, plain or sweetened Regular cottage cheese (4% milkfat)	Hard cheeses: blue, camembert, cheddar, (note: part-skim mozzarella and part-skim ricotta are preferable but still rich in fat) Ice cream Processed cheeses Whole milk Whole-milk yogurt

GROUP IV: Poultry, fish, egg and meat products

Two servings (favor *anytime* column for additional servings. If a vegetarian diet is desired, nutrients in these foods can be obtained by increasing servings from Groups I & III.)

Poultry:
Chicken or turkey (no skin)

Fish:
Cod
Flounder
Haddock
Halibut
Perch
Pollock
Rockfish
Shellfish, except shrimp
Sole
Tuna, water-packed

Egg:
Egg whites

Fish:
Herring
Mackerel
Salmon
Sardines
Shrimp
Tuna, oil-packed

Red meats:
Flank steak
Ham*
Leg of lamb*
Loin of lamb*
Plate beef*
Round steak*
Rump roast*
Sirloin steak*
Veal*

Poultry and fish:
Deep-fried and breaded fish or poultry

Red meats:
Bacon
Salt beef
Minced beef
Hotdogs
Liver
Liver sausage
Pork: loin
Salami
Sausage
Spareribs
Untrimmed meats

Egg:
Egg yolk or whole egg

MISCELLANEOUS (Note: snack foods should not be used freely, but the middle column suggests some of the better choices.)	Fats: (none) Snack foods: (none)	Fats: Mayonnaise Salad oils Soft (tub) margarines Snack foods: Fig bars Gingerbread Ginger snaps Digestive biscuits Popcorn (small amounts of fat and salt) Sherbet	Fats: Butter Cream Cream cheese Lard Sour cream Snack foods: Chocolate Coconut Commercial pies, pastries and doughnuts Potato crisps Soda pop

*Trim all outside fat.

© 1979 CSPI. Adapted from *The New American Eating Guide*, published by the Center for Science in the Public Interest.

Table 16-2 Combinations of high-quality protein

PROTEIN FOODS

Legumes

peanuts, roasted	red beans	lentils
soybeans	black beans	mung beans
split peas	white beans	black-eyed peas
kidney beans		soybean curd (tofu)

Grains

wheat	rye	buckwheat, dark
bulgur wheat	cornmeal (maize)	millet
barley	brown rice	oats (oatmeal)

Nuts and seeds

walnuts	cashews	sunflower seeds
brazil nuts	pecans	sesame seeds
almonds	pumpkin seeds	

Vegetables (A)

kale	swiss chard	yam

Vegetables (B)

peas	asparagus	green beans
brussels sprouts	okra	cauliflower
spinach	greens	broccoli

Vegetables (C)

spinach	soybeans
broccoli	greens
okra	sweetcorn

PROTEIN COMBINATIONS AND SERVING SUGGESTIONS

Grains and legumes

Tabouli and peas	Brown rice and lentils
Barley and lentil soup	Falafel
Whole-wheat pita bread with hummus	

Legumes and nuts or seeds

Raw peanuts and sunflower seeds	Lentil-walnut salad
Bean casserole with sesame seeds	Split-pea soup with sesame roll
Stir-fry tofu with almonds and broccoli	

In the Kitchen: the Politics of the Pantry

> *Legumes and vegetables (A)*
> Kidney beans with stir-fry vegetables
>
> *Protein combinations and serving suggestions*
> Chick peas with tomatoes and courgettes stuffed in chard leaves
> Stir-fry combination: peas, beans, chard, onion, celery
>
> *Grains or corn with vegetables (B)*
> Corn and peas
> Bulgur wheat pilaf with brussels sprouts
> Brown rice with steamed broccoli and sweetcorn
> Bulgur wheat salad with green beans
> Stir-fry combination: sweetcorn, peppers, onions, asparagus
> over brown rice or bulgur wheat
>
> *Potatoes with vegetables (C)*
> Potato-spinach salad
> Casserole with potato, broccoli, onion, and mushroom
> Diced potato and soybean casserole
> Sauteed diced potatoes, corn, green onions, and peppers
> Potato leek soup with okra
> Potato salad with corn and slightly cooked broccoli spears
>
> Adapted from Pemberton, C., & Brown, M. 1983. *The Creative Eater's Handbook: Better Nutrition Through Vegetarian Eating*. Oakland, Calif: American Heart Association. Information used by permission of The Regents of the University of California

and yeasts (nutritional, brewer's, torula), or take a vitamin B_{12} supplement. Even if you show no deficiency signs for vitamin B_{12}, you may be draining your stores (body stores of vitamin B_{12} can last for years).

Other vegetarian diets, such as the highest levels of the Zen macrobiotic diet and the fruitarian diet, are so restrictive that they pose serious health hazards.

Should we all become vegetarians? Just because vegetarians have lower rates of certain diseases does not mean you have to give up meat to be healthy—just cut back on the amount. If you want to cook steak, cut your normal portion size in half and serve it with lots of vegetables and a salad. If you have a meal high in fats and sugars, cut back for the other two meals of the day. Be creative with salads. Iceberg lettuce alone does not make a salad: it makes a plate of iceberg lettuce. Try spinach or red leaf lettuce and top with tomatoes, cucumbers, green peppers, mushrooms, carrots, and spring onions. Also, include more legumes in your diet (see recipe 9 in appendix D). Toss them into soups, salads, or casseroles, or make sandwich spreads and vegetable dips.

Experiment with some vegetarian staples. Tofu, for instance, is a soybean curd that is a good protein source, is high in calcium, and as a legume has no cholesterol. (Women can never have too many calcium sources.)

BUYING FOOD—PART 1: WHERE TO GO?
Health food stores

Among nutritionists, health food stores have mixed reputations. They usually offer a wide variety of bulk foods and specialty items for vegetarians or people with allergies. Where else are you going to find amazake (rice nectar), kefir (cultured dairy drink), dulsem kiwi-apple juice, tempeh, "soysage," millet, buckwheat noodles, vitamin B_{12}-fortified soy milk, or special flours (barley, oat, potato, rice, rye)? The drawbacks to these stores are their promotion of "health" foods, "organic" foods, and diet supplements, and their dispensing of inaccurate nutrition information.

Health foods Not surprisingly, "health" foods are claimed to promote health. They are supposed to be so high in certain nutrients that they help you resist stress, infection, and disease. When you label something a health food, you imply that it can perform functions beyond those of other foods. Yet no one food or nutrient taken in addition to an adequate diet is going to perform miracles.

The mystique enveloping health food has led more than one believer to shun medical advice about potentially life-threatening illnesses and opt instead for various regimens of nutritional supplements and special foods, none of which has been shown to be effective or safe.

At various times, rice, bran, yogurt, wheat-germ oil, and honey have been promoted as health foods. Here are descriptions of some of the most popular:

Amino acids The amino acids arginine and lysine are sold in combination as a "natural weight-loss supplement." Claims for the product are based on research that shows obese persons have low levels of growth hormone and that certain amino acids—arginine, ornithine, and lysine—raise growth-hormone levels in persons of normal weight. What goes unstated is that only arginine has been tested on obese persons—and it failed to raise these hormone levels.

Bee pollen Pollen does not contain any extraordinary nutrients and, despite the claim, does not confer any advantage on athletes or ward off allergies. It is high in nucleic acids, so individuals at risk of gout or who show signs of renal disease should avoid this particular panacea, as should asthma or hay fever sufferers.

Brewer's yeast Brewer's yeast is high in the B vitamins thiamin, riboflavin, pyridoxine, and niacin and in the minerals potassium, phosphorus, iron, and chromium. Recently, some yeast has been introduced on the market that is fortified with vitamin B_{12}, so it is a good supplement for strict vegetarians (unfortified brewer's yeast does not provide much B_{12}). Supplementary yeast can add extra amounts of certain nutrients, but it is not a magic food and will not improve athletic performance. Make sure that the yeast you take is dead; individuals have experienced yeast infections from daily supplements of brewer's yeast that contain live organisms.

"Health" snacks Snacks promoted as more healthful than regular candies or chips include carob candies, yogurt-coated dried fruits, "natural" corn crisps, potato crisps, soy crisps, and banana crisps. These are just as high in sugar and fat as regular snacks, only more expensive. Raw nuts are not better for you than roasted nuts and may even contain toxic substances normally destroyed with roasting.

Wheat germ Wheat germ is the heart of the wheat berry and is high in polyunsaturated fats, vitamin E, B vitamins, iron, and the amino acid lysine. Besides this, wheat germ does not have any special nutritional value, but it makes a good topping on cereals; use it sparingly, however, because of its fat content. (Also, keep it refrigerated.)

Spirulina Spirulina is a blue-green alga high in protein that is promoted as a health tonic, a strength builder, and an aid for weight loss. Spirulina offers no special benefits to the health seeker, body builder, or dieter. Many varieties of spirulina exist, and at least one (*S. subsalsa*) is toxic. Spirulina is often sold combined with other substances of questionable safety (comfrey root, for example, which causes cancer in laboratory rats). Though it contains large amounts of vitamin B_{12}, much of this is in the form of B_{12} analogs that may not have any vitamin activity in humans.

Pastas Pastas colored with vegetable dyes contain only an insignificant amount of extra nutrients because very little dye is added. Pastas with soy flour contain more protein and are recommended for vegetarians. Whole-wheat pastas, like the whole-wheat flour from which they are derived, contain more nutrients and fiber, but some consumers find the taste too strong for tomato or white sauces. Whole-wheat pastas are not the only way to increase nutrients and fiber. Cook regular pasta and make a sauce filled with vegetables, or serve vegetables as a side dish.

Organic foods "Organic" food is actually a misnomer: all foods are organic, meaning they come from living things and contain carbon. A more accurate term is "organically grown" foods, meaning the food was grown without synthetic fertilizers, pesticides, or antibiotics, and processed without additives. Many people claim these foods are more nutritious and tastier. But are they?

No matter what type of fertilizer a farmer uses, a plant will contain the same amount of protein, carbohydrate, fat, and vitamins (set by the plant's genes). Only certain minerals—iodine, zinc, selenium, cobalt—are affected by the soil. Nutritionists have nothing against pesticide-free food, but there's no guarantee that organic foods are free of pesticides. Pesticides remain in soil for a number of years, so a farm newly converted to an organic method will still produce pesticide-tainted food for a few years. Also, fresh residues from sprays, dusts, and runoff from neighboring farms can contaminate organic farms.

The main difference between organic and regular foods is the price—organic foods are usually twice as expensive. This has on occasion led retailers to slap the label "organic" on foods that are not. The only way to be certain you are eating organically grown food is to know the grower, distributor, and retailer and to check soil and water reports.

Herbs and herbal teas Many herbs carry unfounded claims for curing some fairly serious disorders and some are clearly unsafe to consume. Herbs have been used as drugs for centuries, and they can affect the body. Some are effective for relieving certain disorders, but no more so than current drugs, which have undergone much more extensive testing for safety. Sometimes herbs can affect the body in dangerous ways. Some cause diarrhea, vomiting, paralysis, or can induce abortion. Others are quite simply poisons, such as hemlock, curare, and nightshade, but of the half million known plant species, less than one percent are poisonous. Most herbalists know better than to go around prescribing deadly herbs, but what about the herbs that are commonly found in popular products? Mandrake, a known poison, was added to the Herbalife Slim and Trim formula with the attached claim that the product will "keep the weight off indefinitely." (The company later had to remove it.) Sometimes accepted herbs are dropped from the list of safe products because of new evidence against them. Recently, calamus, sassafras, and the tonka bean were found to be either toxic or cause cancer and were banned from the U.S. food supply.

Herbal teas are easy to spot because they come in brightly colored boxes, often depicting a nature scene and carrying wonderful quotes about the meaning of existence. You do not buy just a tea, you buy an experience.

Most herbs are safe to drink in moderate amounts, including peppermint, chicory, dandelion, catnip, chamomile, hibiscus, linden flowers, passion flower, red clover, rose hips, rosemary, and red bush tea (marketed as Kaffree Tea). These teas are good alternatives to coffee or black tea. But even these herbs carry warnings for large consumption. If you have a heart condition, do not consume linden flower tea in large amounts. If you are allergic to ragweed, asters, chrysanthemums, or other members of this plant family, you may get a severe allergic reaction to chamomile and yarrow. Excessive consumption of any one tea is unwise. Long-term use of ginseng, for instance, has led to a syndrome of high blood pressure, nervousness, insomnia, diarrhea, and skin rashes.

Herb teas already prepared and sold in the store are, on the whole, safe to drink. (If you *do* have any unpleasant side effects, report them to your local Environmental Health Department. Such information helps herb tea companies ensure safe and wholesome products.) But using herbs as medications is less safe. If you do use herbs to make tea for remedies, here are some suggestions:

- Get your problem diagnosed by a doctor. If you won't seek medical advice initially, at least consult with someone who is knowledgeable about herbs, and see a doctor if your condition is serious and does not improve within a few days of using your herbal remedy.
- Let your doctor know if you are taking herbal remedies. Some can interfere with other drugs.
- Use therapeutic herbs only in moderate amounts. Brew a weak tea (one-half to one teaspoon in one or two quarts of warm water). Drink it slowly throughout the day.
- Avoid oils of herbs, most of which are toxic and may be fatal.
- Do not use herbs to make tea for remedies during pregnancy or when you are nursing. The effects to your baby are unknown.
- If you develop a rash, blurred vision, dizziness, diarrhea, or other side effects, see a doctor and stop taking the tea made with herbs.
- If you gather herbs, make sure you know what you are doing. Many herbs look alike, and some can be dangerous.
- Avoid angelica, arnica, belladonna, blue cohosh, calamus, chaparral, comfrey, coltsfoot, Dong Quai, lobelia, mandrake, pennyroyal, poke root, sassafras, tansy, tonka bean, and yohimbe.

Bad advice Health-food stores are often run by people who feel perfectly qualified to dispense nutrition information, though they have no formal training. Much of their advice is at best a good guess and at worst dangerous. In one survey, investigators

In the Kitchen: the Politics of the Pantry

telephoned staff members of various health food stores and described the symptoms of potentially serious medical problems. Over half of the people they spoke with recommended remedies—without ever seeing the "patient"—and failed to suggest that the person see a doctor. None recognized that the medical problem was urgent, and 20 percent actually gave unsound or unsafe advice. Be aware that merely working in a health food store does not qualify a person to diagnose illness or recommend treatment. Get your nutrition information elsewhere.

Supermarkets

To buy nutritious food at a supermarket, take your cart and circumnavigate the inner aisles. Ever notice how the dairy products are farthest away from the entrance? As you run in to get your quart of milk, chances are you will grab something else en route. By staying on the periphery, you will hit the produce, dairy, fish, and meat counters. Make occasional flights into the inner aisles for pasta, beans, grains, cereals, juices, and paper goods. Remember that the prime selling area is eye level. Cheaper items fall somewhere above or below these levels. Not everything that looks as if it is on sale is really a bargain. Watch out for end-of-aisle displays and "economy" buys that are more expensive than a similar product down the aisle. And, of course, steel yourself against the snacks at the checkout line.

BUYING FOOD—PART 2: KNOWING WHAT TO BUY

Estimating your nutrient needs

No one can tell you exactly how much of each nutrient you need. But researchers devise a generous estimate that will cover practically everyone's needs. In Britain, such estimates, established by the Department of Health and Social Security, are called the Recommended Daily Amounts (RDA). Table 16-3 shows the allowances for women. These recommendations are designed to cover the needs of almost all healthy women, and are higher than the average estimated requirements (except for energy).

The exact amounts of nutrients needed are different for each individual, and vary at different stages of life, such as growth,

Table 16–3 Recommended daily amounts of nutrients for girls and women
(Department of Health and Social Security, 1979)

Age ranges		Energy		Protein	Calcium	Iron
		MJ	kcal	g	mg	mg
Girls						
under 1		3.0	720	18	600	6
1		4.5	1,100	27	600	7
2		5.5	1,300	32	600	7
3–4		6.25	1,500	37	600	8
5–6		7.0	1,680	42	600	10
7–8		8.0	1,900	48	600	10
9–11		8.5	2,050	51	700	12[2]
12–14		9.0	2,150	53	700	12[2]
15–17		9.0	2,150	53	600	12[2]
Women						
18–54	Most occupations	9.0	2,150	54	500	12[2]
	Very active	10.5	2,500	62	500	12[2]
55–74		8.0	1,900	47	500	10
75 and over		7.0	1,680	42	500	10
Pregnant		10.0	2,400	60	1,200	13
Lactating		11.5	2,750	69	1,200	15

[1]Most people who go out in the sun need no dietary source of vitam D (p. 51), but children and adolescents in winter, and housebound adults, are recommended to take 10 μg vitamin D daily.
[2]These iron recommendations may not cover heavy menstrual losses.

pregnancy and lactation. Other factors such as stress, infection, height, weight and sex also affect requirements.

Although they are called Recommended Daily Amounts, it is not actually necessary to meet the requirements every day; but the intakes should average out over a week or so.

The DHSS limits its recommendations to energy, protein, two minerals and six vitamins, whereas the US recommendations include a longer list of vitamins and minerals.

Reading food labels—why bother?

Once you have mastered the art of reading food labels, you may find label reading fun, enlightening, and even cause for getting

Vitamin A (retinol equivalent)	Thiamin	Riboflavin	Niacin equivalent	Vitamin C	Vitamin D[1]
µg	mg	mg	mg	mg	µg
450	0.3	0.4	5	20	7.5
300	0.4	0.6	7	20	10
300	0.5	0.7	8	20	10
300	0.6	0.8	9	20	10
300	0.7	0.9	10	20	—
400	0.8	1.0	11	20	—
575	0.8	1.2	14	25	—
725	0.9	1.4	16	25	—
750	0.9	1.7	19	30	—
750	0.9	1.3	15	30	—
750	1.0	1.3	15	30	—
750	0.8	1.3	15	30	—
750	0.7	1.3	15	30	—
750	1.0	1.6	18	60	10
1,200	1.1	1.8	21	60	10

miffed. My favorite label is one for a "natural" yogurt bar with "no preservatives." The ingredients list begins with sucrose (sugar), then follows soon with artificial color and flavor. Just where does the "natural" come in? you might ask. (More on natural foods later.)

Food labels can steer you toward better buys, or they can intimidate you so much that you refuse even to take a peep at them. Here is what to look for and what it all means.

List of ingredients Labels on most prepacked foods must list their ingredients on the label by weight in decreasing order. Though food additives must be listed, specific spices and flavors do not have to appear by name, a potential problem for consumers with allergies.

Many people are suspicious of food additives because they are "chemicals." But everything—including your body and food—is made up of chemicals. Food additives range from the natural to the synthetic and from those intentially added to those that sneak in by themselves. Iron added to bread is intentional; insect legs in flour are not.

About 98 percent of all additives (by weight) are accounted for by sugar, salt, corn syrup, citric acid, baking soda, vegetable colors, mustard, and peppers. The remaining additives (2 percent or so) are there to improve the nutritional value of food, to preserve the ingredients, or to add cosmetic appeal.

Not all additives are bad. Some, such as vitamins and minerals, make up for diet deficiencies. Others, such as preservatives, allow us to eat a wide variety of foods year-round at reasonable prices. The best way to avoid the worst additives is to eat whole foods that are minimally processed, such as dried beans and peas, fresh fruits and vegetables, whole grains, dairy products, and lean meats, poultry, and fish. By doing so, you get a broader range of nutrients, including trace minerals and fiber. But remember that if you buy foods free of preservatives, you will have to refrigerate them or eat them before they go bad. Bread, for example, will mold in a few days.

Nutrition information In the United Kingdom, foods that claim to be especially for diabetics, infants or slimmers must back up their claims with supporting information on the label. For example, slimming foods must state how much energy they provide per 100 grams and per helping, and also that they can aid slimming only as part of a controlled diet. And labels must give details of any foods claiming to contain specific vitamins and minerals, such as "rich in vitamin C".

There are no Government recommendations in Britain for nutritional labelling, but a few manufacturers and supermarket chains already list the energy, protein, carbohydrate, fat, sodium and fibre contents of their food, and include the proportion of sugar and saturated fat.

However, most packaged foods merely show a list of ingredients in order of weight, without specifying the amount of nutritional value.

Product descriptions Food descriptions carry subtle meanings. Take a product that contains "chicken with noodles." This item has to have more chicken than a product called "noodles with chicken."

Product descriptions can explain a lot about flavor additives. In Britain "strawberry yogurt" or "strawberry-flavored yogurt" means its flavor comes mainly from real strawberries. "Strawberry flavor" means the product is flavored either completely by artificial flavorings or by a combination of natural and artificial flavors.

"Fortified" and "enriched" foods contain added nutrients. For instance, iodine is added to table salt and vitamins A and D to some milk products in Britain. Originally, fortification allowed nutrients that were low in the diet to be added to the food supply to avoid deficiency diseases. It is still a good idea, but some manufacturers make a business out of selling the idea of fortification rather than encouraging a good diet. Then they charge more for it. A candy bar fortified with 100 percent of the RDA for several vitamins is still a candy bar loaded with fat and sugar, except now it costs more. A cereal fortified with 100 percent of several vitamins and minerals may be so high in sugar that it can't be considered nutritious. The current Western diet is beset not with vitamin deficiencies, but with excesses of fat, cholesterol, sugar, and calories. Fortification does nothing to get rid of these culprits; it merely dresses them up in vitamins and minerals and calls them wholesome. Your job is to look beyond the fortification claims and check the label for large amounts of unwanted ingredients.

Natural foods have emigrated from their original home in health food stores to special sections in supermarkets. Sometimes they are fully integrated with ordinary foods. These foods are supposed to be safer and more nutritious than processed foods that are teeming with—once again—"chemical" food additives. Originally, the natural foods movement glorified whole, minimally processed food, but in the last few years, the term "natural" has become somewhat slippery. "Natural" is not legally defined, so food manufacturers slap the word on anything they want (it boosts the sales). Highly refined breakfast cereals provide an excellent example of how wholesome food can be ruined through processing and yet still bear a "natural" reputation.

So read labels carefully. Other information that may peer out from labels include recipes, storage and cooking recommendations, place of origin and name and address of manufacturer, packer, or seller.

Getting the most out of your food—taking care of nutrients

Vitamins are fragile. Vitamin C and folacin are the most delicate; niacin, the hardiest. What good does it do to plan a great diet with plenty of fresh food, only to kill off the vitamins or pour them down the drain? To keep vitamins safe from oxygen, heat, light, acid, and alkali, follow the recommendations in table 16-4.

PUTTING IT ALL TOGETHER

A number of my friends have complained that keeping track of all the information they hear about nutrition is impossible. When they sit down to eat, they forget that vitamin C-rich foods help you to absorb iron, for example. They cannot remember what increases the risk of cancer and what does not, or how they are supposed to cook food to lower risk of heart disease. In answer to their dilemma, I offer two aids. The first is a visual guide to food choices (figure 16-1). According to this guide, you choose foods liberally from the highest level, moderately from the second, very moderately from the third, and sparingly from the fourth.

With this plan, meat is no longer the centerpiece on your table but becomes just another face in a crowd of beans, rice, and broccoli. Instead of having a thick slab of steak with a few peas on the side and a baked potato smeared with sour cream, you would have, say, stir-fry broccoli, onions, mushrooms, red pepper, and beef slices, served over rice. You can still enjoy pork, but instead of frying a chop, use small bits to flavor a navy bean soup or a vegetable stew. If you want a meat entree, serve chicken, turkey, fish, or lean cuts of red meat. You can even have your steak dinner, but not too often. According to

In the Kitchen: the Politics of the Pantry

Table 16-4 Protecting the vitamins in food

DAIRY PRODUCTS AND EGGS

Keep milk cold, covered, and out of strong light.
Avoid raw milk. Pasteurization does not destroy many nutrients, and drinking raw milk can increase risk of diphtheria, brucellosis, salmonellosis, and spinal tuberculosis.
Refrigerate according to the following timetable:

Milk	1 week
Natural or processed cheese	4–8 weeks
Cream, ricotta, and cottage cheese	1–2 weeks
Eggs	2–3 weeks

FRUITS AND VEGETABLES

Storing and Preparing

Do not eat old, wilted, or bruised produce.
Sun ripen, then immediately refrigerate.
Store in the refrigerator in plastic bags or put in crisper.
Leave vegetables in pods until ready to use.
Keep potatoes and onions in a cool, well-aired place. Keep potatoes out of light.
Wrap frozen fruits and vegetables tightly in plastic or place in tightly covered, vaporproof containers.
Canning fruits and vegetables destroys some nutrients, but those that remain contribute to the diet.
Canned fruit (opened) may be refrigerated for one week.
Canned vegetables (opened) may be refrigerated for three days.

Preparing and Cooking

Wash quickly without soaking, preferably unpeeled.
Avoid long-term exposure to light or air.
If vegetables must be soaked, do so before paring.
After washing leafy greens, shacke off excess water and blot gently.
When removing peel, do not hack away half the fruit or vegetable. If skin is edible, wash and eat it. When cooking, keep vegetables in whole or large pieces.
Nutrients become more available when some vegetables are cooked rather than eaten raw. These vegetables include dried peas and beans, peanuts, potatoes, spinach, broccoli, cauliflower, and carrots.
To cook, either steam, microwave without water, or use a waterless cooking method.
Save cooking water for soups, casseroles, or preparing grains and beans.
Stir-frying in oil cuts vitamin C losses (but adds calories and fat).
Boil or bake potatoes in their skins.
Cook only enough vegetables for a meal. Storing and reheating destroys nutrients.
Avoid deep-fat frying, adding baking soda to give vegetables a bright green color, cooking in copper pots, thawing frozen vegetables before cooking, running frozen juice under hot water.

GRAINS

Storing

Store whole grains in a cool, dry place. Keep whole-grain flour in refrigerator or freezer.

Cooking

Do not wash enriched rice before cooking (vitamins are added to the outside).

Avoid cooking cereals in too much water and then draining off the excess.

Use only the required amount of baking powder when baking breads (it destroys thiamin).

Compared to unleavened breads, yeasted breads have more B vitamins. Also, the yeast breaks down substances that normally bind iron, calcium, and zinc, so these minerals in yeasted breads are more easily absorbed.

MEAT AND FISH

Storing

Freeze meat by wrapping it tightly and storing at the proper temperature.

Refrigerate according to the following timetable:

Bacon	5–7 days
Beef, lamb, pork, veal (fresh)	2-4 days
Beef, salt	1 week
Minced beef, lamb, pork, veal	1–2 days
Ham slice	3–4 days
Leftover cooked meats	4–5 days
Cold meats	1–2 days

Cooking

Use the nutrient-rich drip from meats for gravies or serve with the meat (refrigerate first and skim off the fat).

Grilling and microwave cooking (because of shorter time) destroy fewer nutrients than roasting and baking. Frying causes few nutrient losses, but adds fat.

Boil leftover chicken and turkey bones and use stock for soups (refrigerate stock first and then skim off fat).

OILS

Store vegetable oils in refrigerator to keep them from going rancid quickly.

William Castelli, present director of the Framingham heart study, Americans eat, night after night, from only ten basic recipes. What you need to do now is find ten new nutritious recipes, so that most of the time you are eating well. Then you

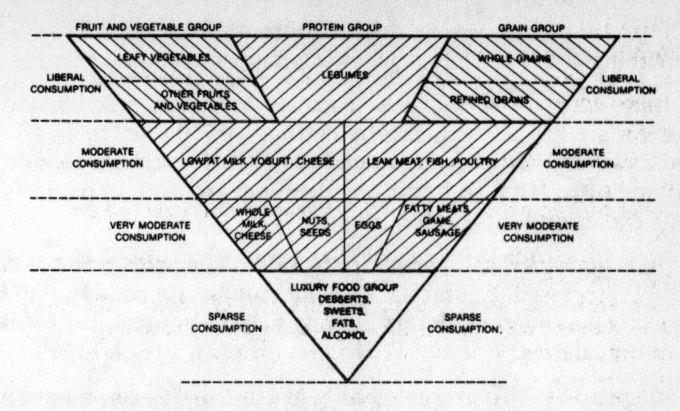

Figure 16-1 The pyramid guide

From Pennington, J. 1981. "Considerations for a new food guide." *Journal of Nutrition Education* 13(53).

can afford to make occasional forays into the land of meat slabs and rich pastries.

The second aid is the guidelines in the Health Education Authority's *Guide to Healthy Eating*:

- Cut down on fat, sugar and salt
- Eat more fiber-rich foods.
- Eat plenty of fresh fruit and vegetables.
- Go easy on alcohol.
- Get plenty of variety in what you eat.

By following these guidelines, you can lower your risk of obesity, heart disease, cancer, gastrointestinal disorders, and Type II diabetes. "Lowering your risk" does not necessarily mean you will avoid these disorders, only that, based on current research, you will be doing your best to lessen your chances of getting them.

If you have trouble remembering them all when you start to prepare or order a meal, ask yourself these three questions:

- Can I cut out any fat from this meal?
- Can I add any fiber?
- Can I add more variety?

Eat Beautiful!

If you answered yes to one or more of these questions, do something about it. Here is what can happen if you take action:

Cutting back on fat Sweets such as breakfast pastries and desserts are loaded with fat; by cutting back on fat, then, you automatically cut back on some sugar. Cholesterol-rich foods, too, are often fatty, so by cutting them out you end up reducing your cholesterol intake, too.

Adding fiber By eating fiber-rich foods, you stop relying on highly processed products, a major source of sodium (and sugar). High-fiber foods are filling, so you automatically cut back on calories.

Adding variety To prevent getting in a nutritional rut, question yourself about variety. Many people eat few fresh fruits and vegetables, so for them adding variety means including some nutrient-rich produce.

Obviously, weaknesses exist in any shortcut method to a complicated subject. But if the alternative is for you to throw up your hands in frustration, stick with these three questions and you will do all right. Consider the following meals:

Breakfast

Original: white toast with butter, sugary cereal, whole milk

Decrease fat? Switch to low-fat milk. Substitute ricotta cheese and fruit for butter.

Add fiber? Switch to whole-wheat toast and less refined cereal like oatmeal (add raisins for sweetness).

Add variety? Add fresh fruit or juice.

Revised: whole-wheat toast with ricotta and fruit spread, oatmeal with raisins, orange juice, low-fat milk

Lunch

Original: luncheon meat on white bread with mayonnaise, orange drink, potato crisps, chocolate-chip cookie

Decrease fat? Switch to lean ham and mustard and forget the potato crisps.

In the Kitchen: the Politics of the Pantry

Add fiber? Switch to whole-wheat bread, add lettuce, have an orange instead of orange drink, and have a date bar instead of a chocolate chip cookie.

Add variety? Have cut-up vegetables instead of crisps.

Revised: ham sandwich on whole wheat with mustard and lettuce, orange, cut-up vegetables, date bar

Dinner

Original: fried chicken, white rolls, peas with butter, mashed potatoes with gravy, wine, ice cream

Decrease fat? Bake chicken, skip butter, and have a baked potato with a little gravy.

Add fiber? Add whole-wheat bread, then have yogurt with fresh fruit for dessert.

Add variety? Substitute a salad for the rolls or potato. Top with a low-fat dressing.

Revised: baked chicken, whole-wheat bread, peas (no butter), salad, wine, yogurt with fresh fruit

Finally, make dietary changes gradually so you do not frighten your tastebuds. Each month make some improvement in your eating habits. Over a year's time, you may not recognize your dinner table:

January	Limit meat to lunch or dinner.
February	Once a week, cook a vegetarian meal or a stir-fry with small bits of meat.
March	Take the salt shaker off the table.
April	Mix your whole milk with one-half low-fat milk, then gradually substitute low-fat or skim milk.
May	Trade in your morning doughnut for a bran muffin.
June	Limit coffee to one cup a day.
July	At every dinner, serve either fresh vegetables (lightly steamed) or a salad with a variety of ingredients (lettuce, spinach, tomatoes, cucumbers, carrots, green peppers, onions, radishes) and a low-fat dressing.

Eat Beautiful!

August	Substitute whole-grain breads (whole wheat, corn, oat, rye) for white breads.
September	Once a week, have fish for dinner.
October	If you regularly eat rich, sugary desserts, limit them to once a week. Instead, try low-fat alternatives, such as fresh fruit, or combine fruit juice with plain gelatin and top with low-fat yogurt.
November	Don't fry any foods. Instead grill, bake, or boil them.
December	Substitute fruit juices and soda water for canned drinks (whether regular or sugarfree). Make your list for next year ...

SHOULD YOU TAKE SUPPLEMENTS?

The woman who ignores her diet and relies on supplements makes the assumption—a wrong one—that supplements provide total nutrition. (Before continuing, you might want to refresh your knowledge of vitamins and minerals from appendix A.)

Some people believe that manufacturers strip foods of their nutrients, then blithely toss in a few token vitamins and minerals. Sure, they reason, these processed foods can support life, but can they support health? So they take supplements. In one sense, they are right: highly processed foods do lose fiber and certain nutrients, particularly trace minerals. But in another sense, they are mistaken: the way to get all the essential nutrients is to eat whole, minimally processed foods, not to take supplements.

Other people take supplements "just to be sure." Perhaps they read that stress depletes certain nutrients or that cigarette smoking lowers levels of vitamin C (even these lowered levels fall within the normal range). So rather than cope with their stress or give up cigarettes, they turn to vitamin-mineral pills. Yet the damage they inflict on body organs and tissues from smoking or being stressed far outweighs any nutritional problems.

Finally, some people admit that they eat poorly—from lack of time or inclination—but prefer to stick with their old habits and rely on supplements to round out their day's eating. Unfortunately, supplements cannot replace a good diet because they

In the Kitchen: the Politics of the Pantry

do not include all the essential nutrients or fiber. Even if they did, substances may exist that we do not yet believe are essential, but really are—perhaps all the elements in the periodic table.

Knowing all this, be aware that there are still certain situations and stages of life when your nutrient requirements increase. Your doctor may recommend the following:

Oral Contraceptive Users	Folacin (0.1–1.0 mg)
	Vitamin B-12 (3–10 µg)
Childbearing Years	Iron (10–30 mg) or one-a-day formula*
	Calcium (400–800 mg)
Pregnancy	Iron (30–60 mg)
	Folacin (300–800 µg)
	Calcium (600–1,200 mg)
Breastfeeding	Iron (10–60 mg)
	Calcium (600–1,200 mg)
Postmenopause	Calcium (500–1,000 mg)

Also, if you are following a reducing diet that provides fewer than 1,500 calories a day, take a multivitamin-mineral supplement. If you are a strict vegetarian, take vitamin B_{12} (3–10 µg).

Vitamin and mineral supplements are of questionable value for the following conditions, but if you decide to take them, here are dosage recommendations:

Heavy alcohol use	One-a-day formula
Cigarette smoking	One-a-day formula
Stress	One-a-day formula
Common cold	Vitamin C (75 mg)

Choosing a supplement

If you have a medical reason for taking supplements, follow your doctor's advice on dosage. However, if you insist on taking vitamins for "insurance," stick with one-a-day formulas that provide close to 100 percent of the RDA (50–150 percent is okay). Avoid supplements of only one or two nutrients because these can throw off the balance of other nutrients in your body

---

*One-a-day formula refers to a multivitamin-mineral supplement that provides nutrients at levels of 50–150% of the U.S. RDA.

(a person is rarely deficient in only one nutrient). You do not need special formulas designed for older women, younger women, athletes, stressed executives, and so on. Besides the higher cost, these pills may not offer the best combination of nutrients. For instance, the label on a multivitamin-mineral pill marketed for your women boasts of its high calcium content. But to be best absorbed, calcium should be taken throughout the day. With this formula you are forced either to take the supplement several times a day (getting too much of the other nutrients) or to pay more for calcium that you cannot absorb. Avoid formulas that claim to be "organic," "therapeutic," "geriatric," and "high potency." No data exist to back up such claims, which in the past have been used by some disreputable firms.

Another claim to avoid is "natural." Your body cannot tell the difference between a synthetic vitamin and a "natural" one. Most laboratory-made vitamins have the same structure as their natural counterparts, and sometimes those that do not (folacin, vitamin E) are actually more effective. Also, natural vitamins may be far from natural. During processing, manufacturers add substances such as ethyl cellulose, polysorbate 80, and gum acadia to glue the tablet together. Because only active ingredients must be listed on the label, you may be unaware of these hidden additives. Some natural products have synthetic vitamins added. Tablets labeled "rose hips vitamin C" have been found to contain natural rose hips with synthetic ascorbic acid. The only difference between the two types of vitamins is the price: "natural" vitamins cost about twice as much. Also, avoid supplements that contain substances (choline, inositol) not required in human nutrition.

Finally, make sure the product has an expiration date. Vitamin supplements become less potent over time, especially in hot, humid places—like the bathroom cabinet.

Megadoses

In large doses, vitamins and minerals no longer act like nutrients but have pharmacological effects like drugs and can pose similar hazards. Megadoses of vitamins and minerals can be toxic. Over four thousand cases of vitamin poisoning happen each year, mostly to children. Of major concern are the fat-soluble vitamins

In the Kitchen: the Politics of the Pantry

because they are easily stored and can accumulate in the body. To some extent water-soluble vitamins can be stored in the body, and recent evidence shows that megadoses of these may not be as harmless as once believed.

Megadoses exert their effects in several ways. Large amounts of one nutrient may interact harmfully with others. Because nutrients work together, megadosing on one may throw off the body's balance of others. Excessive amounts of one vitamin may hide a deficiency of another. Also, your body can sometimes become dependent on large doses; when they are withdrawn, deficiency signs appear.

To avoid toxicity symptoms, never self-medicate with more than ten times the RDA for water-soluble vitamins or more than three times the RDA for fat-soluble supplements (appendix A lists toxicity symptoms for vitamins and minerals).

Future research may find exciting uses for megadoses. Scientists are studying the effects of vitamin A and related retinoids for skin problems. They are looking at vitamin E for treating genetic anemias and preventing a certain eye disorder in newborn babies. And they are trying to determine whether vitamin A, carotene, and folacin may one day be used in cancer prevention. But until then, we have to rely on what past research and experience have revealed: megadosing can be dangerous and life-threatening. If you insist on being a human guinea pig, remember—the average guinea pig lives only seven years.

RESOURCES

Ministry of Agriculture, Fisheries and Food. 1985. *Manual of Nutrition*. HMSO.

Health Education Authority. *Guide to Healthy Eating*. Order from your local health education unit.

Cookbooks for Vegetarians:
Spencer, Colin, and Sanders, Tom. 1986. *The Vegetarians' Health Diet Book*. Positive Health Guide.

Elliot, Rose. 1976. *Not Just a Load of Lentils*. Fontana.

17
In the Workplace: Earning and Eating your Daily Bread

> After working for three years on a morning
> newspaper she had an allusion of maturity and
> experience; but it was fatigue merely. . . .
> Katherine Anne Porter, *Pale Horse, Pale Rider*

The alarm goes off at 7:00 A.M. You ignore it. You got to bed late last night, and your head seeks the peace of the pillow. Around 7:30, a wave of guilt sweeps over you, and you begin to think about getting to work. By 7:45, panic sets in. You succumb, drag yourself out of bed, turn on the water for coffee, and fall into the shower. You manage to gulp down half a cup of coffee before you race out the door to catch your bus. As you rush toward your office, you grab a Danish pastry and eat it at your desk while you plan your schedule. It is only nine o'clock, and you have already made four big mistakes.

Fatigue is one of the main causes of poor work performance. You know the feeling—you have no energy, you cannot think clearly, people talk to you and you hear only a distant buzz (or roar, depending on the state of your head). Fatigue occurs when you are either emotionally or physically drained. Nutritional factors may also be at fault. Here is how diet can affect your work.

Breakfast

Breakfast is not critical to health. If you lived in a society of foragers, you could nibble on berries, roots, and nuts over the course of the morning and be none the worse for it. But you live in a technological society where skipping breakfast usually means grazing on bizarre combinations of vending machine snacks or fasting until noon (or later). And by that time you may be tired, depressed, and grouchy.

No single way of eating is best for everyone, but eating your

In the Workplace: Earning and Eating your Daily Bread

heaviest meals at breakfast and lunch will keep your energy up during the workday. People who skip breakfast tend to snack more later, and for some women this may lead to unwanted weight. Laura, for instance, is a woman who carried meal skipping to extremes. She would avoid both breakfast and lunch, then devour a 2,800-calorie dinner about an hour before bedtime. She was not only exhausted during her workday, she was also overweight. Once she started dividing up her food into three meals, she had energy to be active during the day and got rid of both her fatigue and her fat.

Just eating breakfast is not enough, of course. You have to eat the *right* kind of breakfast. This means about 300–400 calories from a mix of carbohydrate, protein, and some fat. Sugary meals can leave you more fatigued than if you skipped breakfast altogether.

No matter how many minutes you can spare in the morning, it is always possible to eat something:

The forty-five-minutes-or-more breakfast

Basics: Fresh fruit or juice
Low-fat or skim milk or coffee mixed with ½ cup milk

- Homemade biscuits with ricotta cheese and bits of peaches or apricots
- Fresh muffins (bran, corn, fruit)
  Add a spread of ricotta cheese, low-fat cream cheese, and grated orange peel
- Omelet stuffed with fresh vegetables (limit eggs to three per week)
- Crepes stuffed with meat or cheese filling
- Any dinner entrees (with a microwave oven, some entrees will take fewer than forty-five minutes)

The twenty-to-thirty-minute breakfast

Basics: Fresh fruit or juice
Low-fat or skim milk or coffee mixed with ½ cup milk

- Hot cereal (combine different cereals for a taste change)
  Add to water: raisins, nonfat powdered milk
  Top with applesauce, fresh fruit, cinnamon, nuts, yogurt, cottage cheese

- French toast
  Top with ricotta cheese, low-fat cottage cheese, or fresh fruit
- Concoct a blender meal with a base of
  low-fat milk
  yogurt
  buttermilk
  evaporated milk (mixed 1:1 with water)
  Add:
  peanut butter
  wheat germ
  dry cottage cheese
  nonfat powdered milk
  Flavor with:
  fruit
  vanilla
  almond extract
  carob
- Whole-wheat bread or English muffin with ricotta cheese or low-fat cream cheese or cottage cheese
  Add: small amounts of jam or poppy seeds
- Whole or pita bread with cheese (melt under broiler)
  Add: tomato, pizza sauce

Be more daring and try a nontraditional breakfast (remember, all your body cares about is getting 300–400 calories from carbohydrates, protein, and fat; it doesn't care what it looks like!)

- Sandwiches: tuna, grilled cheese, peanut butter (for fewer calories, mix in ricotta cheese)
- Bean burrito
- Homemade soup, made earlier and frozen (split pea is great in wintertime)
- Dinner leftovers: casseroles, spaghetti, chicken, and so on

The ten-minute breakfast

Basics: Fresh fruit or juice
Low-fat or skim milk
(Save your coffee for later; use your time to eat)

In the Workplace: Earning and Eating your Daily Bread

- Put ¾ cup of dry oatmeal in a preheated pint-sized thermos, fill it with hot water, and let it sit overnight; in the morning, add more hot water if the cereal is too thick
- Cold cereal—watch out for sugary ones; avoid those that list sugar as one of the first ingredients
- Rice pudding (make the night before)
- Peanut butter crackers
- Make a sandwich the night before and eat it now.

The 0-minute breakfast

- Toss in your handbag: Bran or corn muffin (baked and frozen on the weekend and thawed out the night before); see recipe 10 in appendix D.
  Yogurt (low-fat)
  Hard-boiled eggs (limit eggs to three per week)
  Fresh or dried fruit
  Raisins and peanuts
  Bagel with low fat cream cheese
  Cartons of fruit or vegetable juice
  Homemade hot-chocolate mix (⅔ cup cocoa, 2 cups nonfat dry milk, and ¼ cup sugar; put 2 heaping teaspoons in cup and add hot water)
  Peanut butter crackers

If possible, schedule some time in the morning for an unhurried breakfast. You can use the nutrients, and starting off with a calm meal can help keep your entire day under control.

The coffee break

Exercise If your energy slumps halfway through the morning, go for a ten- or fifteen-minute walk. Psychologist Robert Thayer of the California State University in Long Beach compared the effects of brisk walking and candy-bar munching on energy levels and tension. Walking outdoors, he found, boosted energy levels for up to two hours and lowered tension. Eating a candy bar elevated energy levels for a brief period, but half an hour later, tension mounted. So if possible, walk.

Caffeine "This little bean is the source of happiness and wit," said British physician William Harvey in 1657. By the 1800s, a

German chemist discovered the reason behind that little bean's appeal—caffeine.

Caffeine is a member of the chemical family called methylxanthines. A natural ingredient of coffee, tea, chocolate, and cola nuts, it is also an added ingredient in some soft drinks and coffee-flavored foods, in certain medications such as "wake up" pills, and in menstrual, painkilling, and cold compounds (table 17-1). Chemical relatives of caffeine are theophylline and theobromine, present mostly in tea, which can exert similar effects.

Within fifteen to forty-five minutes after drinking a cup of coffee, almost all the caffeine penetrates your tissues. Within one hour, caffeine's peak stimulating effect hits, diminishing to half within three hours. Certain factors affect how long you take to metabolize caffeine:

- The average adult—five to six hours
- A woman on the Pill—ten to thirteen hours
- A woman in the latter stages of pregnancy—eighteen to twenty hours
- A woman with liver failure—several days

Cigarette smoking zips the caffeine through at a rate of three to four hours. Here is what goes on during that time.

After one or two cups of coffee, you become more alert and less drowsy and fatigued. You have fewer lapses of attention, and your performance on tasks related to speed improves. Caffeine shrinks the blood vessels in the brain while expanding those in the abdomen. Drinking three to five cups of brewed coffee can speed up your metabolism. You may experience headaches, trembling, nervousness, and irritability. You produce more urine, and your stomach pumps out more acid. Sleep may elude you, and if you succeed in dozing off, you may thrash around all night. At high levels, caffeine has druglike effects and, as with all drugs, some side effects are harmful. Caffeinism, or "coffee nerves," is a state of sleeplessness, nervousness, irritability, and anxiety, sometimes accompanied by upset stomach, diarrhea, and heart palpitations. After consuming eight to fifteen cups of coffee a day, individuals have sought both medical and psychiatric help for dizziness, agitation, headaches, "ringing" ears, and even hearing loss.

In the Workplace: Earning and Eating your Daily Bread

Table 17-1 Caffeine content of beverages and foods

Item	MILLIGRAMS CAFFEINE	
	Average	Range
Coffee (5-oz. cup)		
Brewed, drip method	115	60–180
Brewed, percolator	80	40–170
Instant	65	30–120
Decaffeinated, brewed	3	2–5
Decaffeinated, instant	2	1–5
Tea (5-oz. cup)		
Brewed	60	25–110
Instant	30	25–50
Iced (12-oz. glass)	70	67–76
Cocoa beverage (5-oz. cup)	4	2–20
Chocolate milk beverage (8 oz.)	5	2–7
Milk chocolate (1 oz.)	6	1–15
Dark chocolate, semi-sweet (1 oz.)	20	5–35
Baker's chocolate (1 oz.)	26	26
Chocolate-flavored syrup (1 oz.)	4	4

Caffeine content of soft drinks

Brand	MILLIGRAMS CAFFEINE (12 oz. serving)
Coca-Cola	45.6
Diet Coke	45.6
Dr. Pepper	39.6
Sugar-Free Dr. Pepper	39.6
Pepsi-Cola	38.4
Diet Pepsi	36.0
Pepsi Light	36.0

Adapted from Lecos, C. "The latest caffeine scoreboard." *FDA Consumer*, March 1984.

Caffeine is mildly addictive, but even after long-term use, you continue to feel alert and active. (Your kidneys and circulatory system, however, may develop some tolerance to its effects.)

Your reaction to caffeine may differ from the reactions of those around you. Some people become jittery after one cup of coffee; others can sleep peacefully after two. Ten grams is considered lethal. But what about lesser amounts? Are there health risks to drinking a cup or two of coffee?

Heart disease No one has the final word on caffeine and heart disease. In two studies from the 1970s, researchers found that the more coffee you drink, the higher your risk of heart attack. Later research, however, found no link between coffee drinking and heart disease, angina, or heart attacks. Then, in 1983, researchers studying Norwegians, who are estimated to drink twice as much coffee as Americans, found coffee drinking was associated with higher levels of total cholesterol, higher levels of blood fats, and, in women, lower levels of high-density lipoproteins (HDLs)—all risk factors for heart disease. The study was highly criticized for its weaknesses in design.

Yet a Stanford group recently found that drinking more than three cups of coffee a day was linked to higher levels of low-density lipoproteins (LDLs), total cholesterol, and a particular protein associated with heart disease. (Drinking tea showed no similar rises and the effect of decaffeinated coffee was not studied.)

While we wait for this issue to be resolved, one thing is known: Caffeine may trigger irregular heartbeats, so patients with existing heart problems should cut back or avoid it.

Cancer Caffeine (in coffee) was first linked to bladder cancer in the 1960s, but later studies failed to confirm a direct relationship. What they did find was the not-so-surprising fact that many coffee drinkers smoke cigarettes (and cigarette smoking greatly increases the risk of bladder cancer).

A more recent and highly controversial suggestion is that drinking coffee causes cancer of the pancreas. In 1981, Dr. MacMahon and colleagues at the Harvard School of Public Health found that patients with pancreatic cancer habitually drink more coffee than persons without this cancer. Some drank as little as one or two cups a day. However, the study was highly criticized, and other researchers could not duplicate these findings.

In a 1983 Norwegian study, researchers found no association between coffee drinking and pancreatic cancer. They did find a link with smoking cigarettes—and an even stronger one with drinking alcohol.

On the positive side, caffeine appears to intensify the effectiveness of radiation therapy and cancer drugs, possibly by preventing cancer cells from repairing themselves.

Decaffeinated coffee is not free of problems, either. Until recently, decaffeinated coffee was processed with trichloroethylene (TCC), a chemical known to cause cancer in animals. General Foods, which used TCC for Sanka and Brim coffees, claimed that a person would have to drink 50 million cups of decaffeinated coffee daily to match the amount used in the animal study but voluntarily switched to a different chemical, methylene chloride. Today, the question of the safety of this solvent is unanswered.

Fibrocystic breast disease Fibrocystic breast disease usually refers to any breast lump that is not cancerous. Such benign cysts can make breasts feel lumpy, nodular, and painful.

Caffeine has never been shown to cause fibrocystic breast disease, but many women with lumpy, painful breasts improve once they eliminate coffee, tea, colas, and chocolate from their diet, according to a 1979 study by Dr. John Minton of Ohio State University. Later studies have repeatedly failed to confirm this result, but if you want to try it, go ahead. It cannot hurt to cut back on caffeine. An added bonus for some women is that by giving up caffeine (and other methylxanthines), they feel less premenstrual breast tenderness.

Other nutritional approaches to fibrocystic breast disease may be recommended:

- Prescribed vitamin E supplements of 600 I.U. daily to eliminate the pain (not the lumps); if no improvement is noted after eight weeks, the supplementation should be discontinued
- Weight-reducing diet for overweight women
- A low-sodium diet, or some restriction of salty foods

Birth defects In 1981, Harvard researchers released the results of a three-year study involving twelve thousand women interviewed after delivery. They found no correlation between birth defects and caffeine consumption but noted a suspicious link between heavy coffee drinking and heavy cigarette smoking. Because babies might experience other problems from caffeine, research continues.

Other effects Coffee, both regular and decaffeinated, stimulates the production of stomach acid, a clue that caffeine is probably not the ingredient to blame. Though coffee will not *produce* ulcers, it can make an already existing one act up. In some people, it may trigger heartburn.

Besides caffeine, other components of tea and coffee can block the absorption of certain minerals. Tea contains flavorful tannins that inhibit absorption of calcium, iron, and B vitamins. The darker the tea, the more tannins. Tea drunk with a meal can reduce absorbed iron by as much as 87 percent. Coffee does this, too, but less so: drinking coffee an hour before a meal will not interfere with iron, but drinking it with or after a meal can reduce absorbed iron by more than one-third, regardless of whether your coffee is black, creamed, sweetened, decaffeinated, or instant. To get a much iron as possible:

- Drink your tea or coffee between meals, preferably at least an hour before eating.
- Drink orange juice or grapefruit juice with meals. Vitamin C will boost the iron absorption.

If you habitually drink coffee and then stop, you may experience withdrawal symptoms, such as headaches, depression, nausea, constipation, nervousness, and inability to concentrate. These symptoms usually disappear within a week. (Do not treat a withdrawal headache with medications such as Anacin and Excedrin: they contain caffeine, so you will just be setting yourself up for recurring headaches.)

Drinking coffee and tea may not be as bad as the habits that accompany it: skipping breakfast, adding lots of cream and sugar, staying awake instead of sleeping, and lighting up a cigarette whenever you pause for a coffee break.

Soft drinks When you sip that Coke or Pepsi, you are refreshing yourself with a beverage whose history is studded with Civil

In the Workplace: Earning and Eating your Daily Bread

War casualties, religious fundamentalism, and the temperance movement. When the Civil War ended, the North treated its wounded with alcohol-based nostrums. The South, spurred by religious convictions, reached instead for cocaine, opium, and heroin—all licit drugs. Cocaine laced such popular concoctions as Ryna's Hay-Fever Remedy, Dr. Tucker's Specific, and Dr. Mitchell's Coco-Bola.

Once the federal government moved to restrict the sale of hard drugs, the cocaine extracts were finally removed. Today, sodas have lost their status as medicinal tonics and are now peddled as "fun, now generation" drinks.

Just how do these fun drinks rate nutritionally? The only two nutrients present in any significant amount are water and sugar. Unlike milk or juice, soft drinks provide few vitamin and minerals. The sugar can cause dental caries (cavities) and adds unnecessary calories. If you drink sodas occasionally, you should have no problem. However, if, like the average American teenager, you drink about twenty-two ounces of the stuff a day, soft drinks will edge out nutritious foods, and your diet will suffer. In 1985 soft drinks comprised a £15 billion industry, so *somebody* out there is drinking a lot of "fun."

When the svelte look became popular, the soft drink industry, ever ready to accommodate the diet-conscious American, began to artificially sweeten beverages. Now many soft drinks are sweetened with aspartame (NutraSweet), and though the long-term risks of using aspartame are still being studied, this sweetener is expected to double the sale of soft drinks.

Most, but not all, colas contain caffeine. Besides sweeteners and caffeine, soft drinks may contain orange, red, and green dyes; caramel color; phosphoric acid to trap metal atoms that could discolor or spoil the drink; sodium citrate (or citric acid) to preserve the drink and give it a tart taste; and brominated vegetable oil, which is currently under study for its possible negative effects on health.

Today's promotional war is not over what sodas have, but what they don't have. Riding the wave of public concern over caffeine, Coke and Pepsi introduced a line of caffeine-free colas, while 7-Up created its "Caffeine: Never Had It, Never Will' campaign. Next, 7-Up moved into food colorings, which it avowed never to have had, either. RC Cola joined the fray by getting rid of most of the sodium in its sodas. Then, "natural" sodas appeared, boasting no caffeine, no preservatives, no artificial flavors, no sodium. Some even contain over half fruit juice. Soon, with soft drink companies battling to strip their products of offending ingredients, we may finally end up with a nutritious beverage—plain water or juice.

Water—tap and bottled When thirsty, many people's knee-jerk reaction is to drink soda, milk, tea, or coffee. They forget about one of the least expensive and most available beverages—water.

Water from the ground, lakes, rivers, or reservoirs is naturally flavored with carbon dioxide, calcium, iron, sodium, fluoride, and other minerals. The only "pure" water is distilled, and it tastes horrible. Some minerals may be removed from water and others added to improve flavor. Hard water, high in magnesium and calcium, is difficult to make sudsy and usually leaves a residual scum on dishes, clothes, and skin, so sodium is often added to "soften" it. However, some evidence shows that in areas where water is soft, rates of heart disease are higher. Still highly controversial, this research has offered several explanations for such a link: soft water may dissolve toxic minerals like cadmium, cobalt, and lead from pipes or may contain excessive sodium or too few minerals, such as magnesium. Also, hard water contains calcium, which may protect against heart disease. To reduce levels of possible toxic minerals in soft water, let the water run a few minutes before using it. Also, if you must use a softener, soften only the hot water.

A few people are afraid of fluoridated water. They claim that fluoridation is the cause of cancer. In fact, fluoridation is a public health measure to adjust an essential nutrient, naturally present in water and foods, to a level favorable to health. Fluoride prevents cavities in teeth and possibly protects against bone loss from osteoporosis. In high doses, fluoride can cause brown spots on the teeth in children, but this happens only in areas where fluoride is naturally high. To get a toxic dose, a person would have to consume 20–80 mg of fluoride a day for years (fluoridated water provides only about 1 mg a day).

Some people choose to pay extra for bottled water because they believe it is a safer alternative to tap water. A few people

In the Workplace: Earning and Eating your Daily Bread

drink these waters believing they are therapeutic. However, no benefits have even been shown. But just what are these people getting for their money?

Like tap water, bottled water may have minerals added or removed to improve the taste. Types of bottled waters that you can buy include mineral water drawn from a natural spring and left unaltered by the manufacturer (outside of California no standard exists for how many minerals the water has to contain, so the term is meaningless); mineral-free water, in which most of the minerals have been removed; and natural water from a protected well or spring that contains only those minerals from the ground.

Bottled water is usually cleansed of impurities and treated with ozone to kill bacteria. If present, chlorine is removed. Bottlers must meet standards for permissible levels of arsenic, barium, cadmium, chloride, chromium, copper, cyanide, fluoride, and other minerals as well as for levels of pesticides, mercury, and radioactive substances.

In short, not all tap water is bad, and not all bottled varieties are better. And both types are refreshing alternatives to colas, coffee, and tea, which are usually sweetened, colored, lightened, and caffeinated.

Snacks If you get light-headed and weak during the five to six hours between breakfast and lunch, snack during your morning break. Here are some suggestions:

- Low-fat or skim milk
- Low-fat yogurt
- Raisins and nuts
- Unsalted whole-wheat crackers with cheese or peanut butter
- Sunflower seeds
- Popcorn
- Unsalted pretzels
- Fresh fruit
- Cut-up vegetables (carrots, green peppers, celery, raw mushrooms, radishes, broccoli, cauliflower, cherry tomatoes)
- Bran muffin
- Rusk

Eat Beautiful!

- Melba toast
- Bagel

Avoid eating from vending machines unless you can choose any of the above.

Cigarette smoking For smokers, the "coffee break" translates into a "cigarette break." The hazards of smoking are well publicized, but what is less well known are the effects of cigarette smoking on nutrition.

Over a long period of time, smokers—regardless of the number of cigarettes they smoke—show a lower level of vitamin C in their blood, though this level is still within normal range. No one is sure what this lower level means, but smokers should eat plenty of vitamin C-rich foods, including citrus fruits, strawberries, red and green peppers, tomatoes, broccoli, and potatoes. Avoid vitamin and mineral supplements "for smokers."

If you smoke cigarettes, you may reduce your lung cancer risk by eating carotene-rich foods, such as leafy greens, carrots, pumpkin, tomatoes, and broccoli. However, your risk will never reach that of a nonsmoker unless you quit.

Many smokers fear that if they quit smoking, they will gain weight. Part of this fear results from advertising. Beginning in the 1920s, the tobacco industry turned its eye to the potentially large market of women, and ads began to associate smoking with slimness and attractiveness—"Have a Lucky Instead of a Sweet." But this fear also results from knowing that smoking speeds up the metabolism, slows food from emptying out of your stomach so you stay full longer, and, for some people, cuts the desire for sweets. Though all this can help keep your weight under control, weight gain is not inevitable when you stop smoking. When you quit, find some way to deal with the stress. Have a carrot instead of a Lucky. Better yet, find ways to handle stress besides grabbing for cigarettes or food.

Lunchtime

For most workers, lunchtime falls somewhere between ten and four. Meals are rare, particularly for people under age thirty-five. With their real or perceived shortages of time, women are turning into grazers, noshers, and snackers. While on the run,

In the Workplace: Earning and Eating your Daily Bread

a woman is likely to grab a hotdog, a yogurt, some Chinese food, or just some plastic-wrapped raisins and nuts. Half the time, you probably eat lunch at your desk or skip it for a cup of coffee and a cookie. The other half, you schedule a meeting and try to eat while working out details on your latest project. (If possible, avoid using your lunch hour for work sessions. You not only need the break, but you may start associating working with eating.)

Nothing is wrong with replacing three meals a day with five or six minimeals, as long as those minimeals offer variety. By not planning your nibbles, you may end up with some strange results—like nothing fresh having touched your lips in a week. Following are some suggestions.

Brown bagging Bringing your own food to work not only cuts costs but lets you prepare food the way you like it. Take turns bringing lunch with a friend. You get more variety and only have to prepare the meal every other day. Eat it outside on warm days, then go for a walk. Try these ideas:

Sandwiches:
Chicken salad
Turkey
Tuna (water-packed)
Lean beef
Cheese (mix hard cheese with low-fat cottage cheese for a spread)
Peanut butter (mix with ricotta)

The "unsandwich":
Sesame crackers and cheese
Celery/cucumber stuffed with cottage cheese, peanut butter, tuna, or chicken salad
Low-fat yogurt with fresh fruit
Hard-boiled egg, mustard, capers
Hummus on pita bread
Aubergine dip with pita bread
Tofu marinaded and baked in wine
Vinegar, garlic, ginger, and soy sauce (a little), and water

Eat Beautiful!

Hot lunches:
Soups
Dinner leftovers
Stews
Baked beans

"Nibbles":
Popcorn Sunflower or pumpkin seeds
Digestive biscuits
Chunks of fresh fruits and vegetables
Dried fruit (raisins, pears, apricots, peaches, figs)
Nuts
Fig bars
Oatmeal cookies

Tips
- To keep food cold (a must for chicken, turkey, fish, and eggs), buy a freezer gel or fill an old margarine tub with water and freeze it, making sure the lid stays on tight. Or wrap a small can of frozen juice or yogurt in foil or plastic and put it in with your lunch.
- Make and freeze a week's worth of sandwiches (frozen, these will be good for up to three weeks). Do not freeze eggs, mayonnaise, tomatoes, lettuce, jelly, or raw vegetables. Instead of mayonnaise, use yogurt or cottage-cheese spreads.
- To keep foods hot, invest in a wide-mouth Thermos.
- Some evidence shows that eating high-carbohydrate lunches will leave you listless and tired a few hours later, while high-protein foods will keep your energy up. So save the pasta for dinner and have a tuna salad or baked chicken for lunch.

Eating at home If you work at home, whether caring for children, tending the house, or free-lancing, you may find your weight ballooning upward. The refrigerator is always beckoning, and frequent breaks are refreshing. To avoid this, use your breaks to take a walk, pick up a different assignment, or do a few exercises.

Plan your snacks ahead of time, and eat in dining areas. Keep

In the Workplace: Earning and Eating your Daily Bread

food out of your office or you will begin to think of your desk as a cafe counter. Schedule a regular lunch hour. Half is for lunch and half for a walk. Occasionally arrange to meet a friend for lunch, or invite someone over.

If you use your lunch hour to exercise, be sure and have something to eat, even if it is just yogurt, a bagel, and fruit. For details on restaurant eating, see chapter 18.

After work

When you spend all day sitting, you do not burn off many calories. Some women compensate by eating very little food, and though they may not gain weight, they are constantly tired and hungry. A better solution is to eat normal amounts of food and work off the calories with exercise. Cultivate the Daisy Duck look. Put your sneakers on and commute to work on foot or take short walks during the day. The extra food keeps your energy levels up; the exercise keeps your weight down.

Stress

A stressor is a situation that forces your body to readjust in some way. Stressors can be physical, such as injury, burns, exercise, surgery, pregnancy, cold or hot temperatures, high altitudes, noise, or pollution. They can also be psychological, such as fear, boredom, love, embarrassment, or rage.

The body response In the face of stress, your body readies itself to fight or flee. First, it shoots "alarm" hormones into your bloodstream, pumping the heart faster and raising blood pressure. Glucose and fats surge into the blood, which desert your stomach and intestines and head for your head, arms, and legs, engorging the muscles with quick energy. Metabolism speeds up. The electrical patterns in the brain shift, clearing your head for fast thinking. Your skin gets clammy. Hearing sharpens. Vision sharpens. Breathing becomes rapid. Your body is set to react. If these symptoms continue, the result can be illness, disease, even death.

Stress and diet Stress can disrupt your nutritional status by causing you to binge, skip meals, or take in too few calories. Being well nourished helps you withstand more severe pressures with less damage. If you are malnourished, being under pressure will only worsen your condition. Drastic weight gains and losses are signs that you are overeating or overdrinking—or not eating at all.

We know that emotional alarms bring on certain biochemical changes. Stores of fat and protein are broken down to release energy, and some loss of zinc, copper, magnesium, calcium, and especially potassium may occur. The adrenal glands are intimately tied into the stress reaction (they speed up heart rate, dilate eyes, and so on). These glands have the highest concentration of vitamin C of any body organ, and under stress may excrete extra amounts. You may also lose vitamin A and B vitamins. Absolutely *no* evidence exists to show that these losses are too high to be replaced by eating a good diet. Stress-formula vitamins that provide ten times the recommended amount of vitamin C and thiamin and twice the amount of other B vitamins are no better than one-a-day formulas and are usually priced much higher. Because they are relatively harmless, however, no concerted effort is being made to get them off the market. Also, by relying on supplements—*any* supplements—instead of your diet, you assume that researchers know exactly which nutrients are depleted when you are under stress. But they do not.

Instead, when under stress, do the following:

- Eat moderate, balanced meals at regular times. Try not to let stress make you overeat or undereat.
- Take time to prepare meals so you give yourself a sense of independence and control.
- Choose mostly low-fat, low-sugar, nutrient-rich foods.
- Despite the previous suggestion, it is okay to eat "comfort foods" that give you emotional security. Often these are high in fat and sugar, like chocolate or cookies. Accept the fact that you are emotionally vulnerable at this time and that these foods give you some comfort. Do not feel guilty about eating them. But keep to moderate amounts: do not binge.
- Eat foods rich in vitamin C, such as citrus fruits, green and red peppers, broccoli, tomatoes, and potatoes.
- Drink fruit juices, which are rich in potassium.

In the Workplace: Earning and Eating your Daily Bread

- If you habitually drink coffee, try to cut back. Giving it up completely will only add more stress to your situation. If you normally do not drink coffee, do not start when you are stressed.
- Exercise regularly.
- If you decide to take a supplement, choose a one-a-day variety, not special, high-priced "stress formulas."
- Do not take drugs, drink alcohol, or smoke cigarettes as a means of coping with your stress.

Headaches

When you get a headache, you might as well forget about concentrating on anything. Headaches can result from tension, but sometimes the culprit is something you ate. Certain foods are vasoactive, meaning they dilate or constrict the blood vessels. When this happens to vessels in your brain, your head may start throbbing. Foods affect people differently, but ones to look out for include:

- Histamines—in some alcoholic beverages, especially red wine
- Fusel oils—in wine, brandy, liqueurs
- Tyramine—in peanuts, cashews, coconut, aged cheese, processed cheese, other dairy products
- Phenylethylanine—in chocolate
- Nitrites—in hotdogs, luncheon meat
- Salt and monosodium glutamate—in Accent, Chinese food
- Too much caffeine—in coffee, tea, colas, chocolate, medications
- Caffeine withdrawal

Other diet-related causes are hunger, low blood sugar, hangovers, or eating ice cream (when cold ice cream touches a warm mouth, two nerves transmit "pain" to the brain).

Diet is even beginning to be linked to migraine headaches. Some intractable migraine sufferers experience headaches after consuming wheat, corn, chocolate, and sometimes cinnamon and Coca-Cola—all possible food allergens. No nutritional treatment exists, but if you have been vomiting, replace fluids with soups, water, juices, or low-fat or skim milk.

Special considerations

The woman with no time When you get home from work, are you so rushed and exhausted that dinner becomes a plate of crackers and cheese, a glass of wine, and a bowl of maple-walnut ice cream? If so, learn how to schedule your time so that dinner—though quick—does more than just kill hunger pangs. Following are some suggestions created with the help of Teri Reifer, a behavioral therapist and licensed clinical social worker in the San Francisco Bay area.

- Keep a notepad handy for writing down items that need restocking.
- Buy in bulk, then divide larger packages (meat, fish) into meal-sized portions and freeze. Each morning, take out the number of servings you want for that evening and place in refrigerator.
- Always have available ingredients for "fast food":

In the cupboard
nuts
popcorn
tuna (water-packed)
nonfat dry milk
dried fruits
canned beans
tomato sauce and paste
pasta
grains (rice, bulgur, couscous)
breadsticks
sesame crackers

In the refrigerator
fruit
milk
juices
tortillas
eggs
raw vegetables
yogurt
cooked chicken
cheese

In the Workplace: Earning and Eating your Daily Bread

In the freezer
cooked beans
spaghetti sauce
cooked turkey
homemade soups
stews
casseroles
meat or vegetable pies
lasagna
cheese sauces
enchiladas

To save cooking time:
- Cook enough staples for two to three days. Warm portions by steaming. Add fresh vegetables to leftover rice or pasta to make great salads. (When you cook beans, make enough for freezing.)
- Occasionally buying frozen dinners is okay, but these foods can be high in sodium. (The ones billed as "dieter's dinners" are often lower in fat.) Avoid relying on them all the time.
- Cook in batches, then freeze meal-sized portions for later use. Table 17-2 shows how such a system can work. All the recipes are in appendix D.
- Find recipes that require little preparation time, such as grilled fish, burritos and beans, salads, and couscous (faster than rice).
- In the morning throw some chicken and vegetables into a slow cooker; by the time you return home, dinner is ready.
- Consider investing in a microwave oven to heat up frozen foods or a pressure cooker for cooking beans and grains.
- Find a local deli or restaurant that serves nutritious food and occasionally buy a take-out dinner.

Enlist the aid of others:

- Arrange with a friend to cook three times as much of an entree. One-third goes to your friend (she is probably just as busy as you), one-third to your freezer, and one-third to your dining room table for dinner. Sometime that week

Eat Beautiful!

Table 17-2 Batch cooking

	Mexican casserole (9)	Chicken Korma (4)	Lentil soup (8)	Stir-fry sauce (7) and salad dressing (3)
(—)1:30	Beans to soak and boil Or soak overnight			
0:00	Bring beans to boil	Prepare chicken marinade		
0:15				
0:3	Prepare and assemble Mexican casserole	(Chicken marinates 2½ hrs.)		
0:45				
1 hour				
1:15	Clean up: wrap casseroles; wash pot			
1:30			Prepare soup	
1:45				
2 hours			Clean up (Soup cooks)	
2:15				
	BREAK			
2:30		Chop onions for chicken		
2:45			Wash soup pot; portion soup	
3 hours		Cook onions and add chicken		
3:15		(chicken cooks)		
3:30				Prepare stir-fry sauce and salad dressing
3:45				
	Clean up, portion, and store remaining foods			
4:15				

In the Workplace: Earning and Eating your Daily Bread

Meal plans
(A) Mexican casserole, salad with yogurt-herb dressing
(B) Vegetable stir-fry, brown rice
(C) Chicken Korma, bulgur pilaf with raisin-peanut garnish, steamed vegetables
(D) Lentil soup, salad with yogurt-herb dressing, cheese with whole grain crackers or bread

Serve each of these meals in order, then start over again. You will have enough food to last two weeks (13 dinners) with one night off to eat out.

SHOPPING LIST
Meat and dairy

- 12 serving pieces of chicken (any combination of legs, thighs, breasts) or two whole chickens cut in parts
- 1 pound mild cheddar cheese (for Mexican casserole and cheese sandwiches)
- 1 package (12) corn tortillas
- 1 quart plain, low-fat yogurt (32 ounces)

Bulk or Dry Goods

- safflower or corn oil
- 1 pound bulgur wheat (more for larger servings)
- 1 pound dry pinto beans (or two 15-ounce cans of pinto or kidney beans. Sugar and salt are added to canned beans and should be avoided when possible.)
- 12 ounces dried lentils
- 1 pound brown rice (more for larger servings)
- peanuts, raisins, sesame seeds for garnish (optional)

Canned Goods

- Two 28-ounce cans tomatoes
- 1 can (4 ounces) chopped green chillies
- 1 can (6 ounces) low-sodium V-8 juice or salt-free tomato juice

Produce

- (#) 2 pounds firm tofu (only one additional half pound needed the second week)
- 1 head garlic
- 6 medium onions
- 1 bunch parsley
- 4 lemons
- small piece fresh ginger root (2 to 3 ounces) or use dried powdered ginger if fresh is not available
- 1 bunch celery
- 2 carrots
- salad makings of your choice. Buy in large enough quantities to accompany soup and two casserole meals for two persons.
- (#) fresh vegetables such as broccoli, carrots, Brussels sprouts, green beans, or other vegetables of your choice to steam and serve with two chicken Korma meals for two persons.
- (#) assorted vegetables for stir-fry in quantities large enough for two stir-fry meals for two persons.

Eat Beautiful!

For instance: ¼ pound mushrooms, 1 bunch spring onions, small bunch broccoli, 2 courgettes, 2 green peppers, ¼ pound mung bean sprouts. (Note: Frozen vegetables can be used for the stir-fry and chicken Korma recipes, if fresh are expensive or look wilted. Fresh vegetables add a crisp texture desired in stir-frying.)

Herbs, spices and condiments

- Mild (salt-reduced) soy sauce
- red wine vinegar
- oriental sesame oil (optional)
- basil
- bay leaves
- black pepper or cayenne
- caraway seed (optional)
- chili powder (no salt added)
- coriander seed, ground (optional)
- cumin seed (optional)
- curry powder (no salt added)
- dill weed
- dry mustard
- ginger, dried powdered (if not using fresh ginger root)
- oregano

COOKING UTENSILS

Four eight-inch (or smaller) cake pans, pie tins or baking dishes; a heavy four-quart soup pot; plastic wrap, foil *or* freezer wrap; and labels *or* masking tape.

STORAGE CONTAINERS

Chicken Korma: Three one-quart (or larger) plastic containers or jars with tight-fitting lids. (Or six smaller containers if portioning full recipe for one.)

Lentil soup: Four three-cup (or larger) containers with tight lids. (Or eight smaller containers if portioning for one.)

Stir-fry and salad dressing: Two two-cup containers.

Extra pinto beans: If you are cooking beans for Mexican casserole from scratch, you will need two two-cup containers or four one-cup containers.

Source: Turner, S. "If this is Tuesday, it must be Chicken Korma." *Nutrition Action*, May 1983, pp. 10–14.

(or month), have your friend bring over a third of her batch. Prepare foods that freeze well.
- Send your children off with a friend or babysitter one day a week. Then use that time for a marathon of cooking and

In the Workplace: Earning and Eating your Daily Bread

prepare your meals for the week (see batch cooking ideas, table 17-2). As thanks, your friend may even enjoy a portion of your food. By swapping children and meals, you both get more variety—and more time.
- Strike a bargain with your partner. One of you cooks, and the other does the cleaning up.

The woman who travels Good eating does not come easy to the woman whose job requires extensive traveling. First, there are the airlines. If you order twenty-four hours in advance, you can get special foods served to you on the flight. These include kosher foods, fresh-fruit or seafood plates, and diabetic, vegetarian, or low-calorie meals. In case of delays, carry a sandwich, fruit, and seeds or nuts in your purse. Airport food is usually expensive and often revolves around hotdogs and hamburgers. During the flight, pass up the alcohol for soda water, fruit juice, tomato juice, or V-8.

When you arrive at your destination, avoid drinking alcohol or taking tranquilizers to fall asleep. Try a warm bath or go for a brisk walk. If you are staying at a hotel, check to see if they offer any fitness facilities or if there is a nearby leisure centre. Keep up your exercise routine. For business lunches, follow the guidelines in chapter 18 for ordering at restaurants. Have a big salad at least every other day to ensure your supply of vitamins, minerals, and fiber. If you have time at conferences or conventions, search out a local grocery and bring back fresh fruits to your hotel room for nibbles. Watch out for the cocktail hour, where unwinding means drinks and salty nuts. Skip the predinner festivities and go for a run or swim. If your banquet dinner is horribly high in fat, salvage what you can by removing visible fat, including poultry skin, butter, and salad dressing. Skip dessert unless it is fruit.

18
On the Town: the Good, the Bad, and the Bubbly

> Dost thou think, because thou art virtuous, there shall be no more cakes and ale?
>
> Sir Toby Belch asked of the Clown. *Twelfth Night*, William Shakespeare

Crouching behind each of your food choices is some need or desire of your body, your mind, or your heart. Your body wants foods stuffed with vitamins and minerals, entwined with fiber, and low in fat. It clamors for meals to descend on the stomach at regular intervals so it has an unwavering source of energy. Your body is a no-frills consumer.

Your mind seeks out foods that it thinks it needs (coffee), that it thinks your body needs (seaweed, bran, and brewer's yeast), and that are popular to eat (barbequed anything). Your mind has an uncanny knack for being wrong and, ever capricious, is inclined to grab at fads.

Meanwhile, your heart remembers the sugar cookies your mom used to bake. Your heart searches for security and love in food. It wants birthday cakes and bottles of champagne.

Somehow you must satisfy your body, your mind, and your heart and keep the bickering to a minimum. After writing seventeen chapters for the body and the mind, I dedicate this one to the heart.

The "cakes"

When a drop of sweetened solution is placed on a newborn's tongue, the baby's face lights up with surprise and joy. But for sugar, as for many of life's little pleasures, killjoys lurk around every corner. Sugar, we are told, rots teeth, packs on unwanted pounds, and has been accused of causing everything from heart disease to juvenile delinquency to temporary insanity. Should

On the Town: the Good, the Bad, and the Bubbly

sugar be banned as some have suggested? Is it really imperiling our health and lives? Could that baby be so deceived?

At the heart of the sugar controversy is this bitter fact: Sugar contains virtually no vitamins or minerals, only empty calories. Considering that sugar is the most popular food additive and that it is often a "hidden" ingredient in food, it is clear why nutritionists and the public are worried. The British consume an average of 84 pounds of refined sugar per person per year, of which half is found in sweets, sweet foods and soft drinks. About 10 ounces per person is added to foods and drinks at home, every week.

The consumer is no longer the one who adds sugar to food. It is the food manufacturer. But in processed foods, sugar is more than a flavoring. It provides a medium for the growth of yeasts and fermenting agents in the manufacture of pickles, bread, and alcoholic beverages. It preserves jams, jellies, syrups, and candies. (If you buy low-sugar jams, you usually have to refrigerate them.) Sugar is also part of the curing process for meats. When you look on labels to see how much sugar there is, remember that any one of the following is a "nickname" for sweetener: brown sugar, honey, molasses, malto dextrin, maltose, glucose, mannitol, sorbitol, dextrose, corn syrup, and high-fructose corn syrup.

"Sugar" is sucrose and can take the form of white table sugar, brown sugar, and powdered (icing) sugar. Honey provides a few nutrients, but in very small amounts; tablespoon for tablespoon, it contains eighteen more calories than sugar. Of all the sweeteners, blackstrap molasses contains the most nutrients, particularly potassium, calcium, magnesium, thiamin, riboflavin, and iron. The darker the molasses, the more nutrients, but also the stronger the flavor.

Fructose is slightly sweeter than sucrose (although its sweetness depends on how it is used in cooking) and provides the same number of calories. It does not require insulin to be metabolized, so diabetics can use it in limited amounts.

Sorbitol occurs naturally in fruits and is half as sweet as sucrose, contains the same number of calories, but is absorbed from the gastrointestinal tract much more slowly so it causes less drastic rises in blood sugar. It is also less likely to promote tooth decay. However, if consumed in large amounts (twenty-

Eat Beautiful!

five sticks of chewing gum daily), sorbital can cause severe diarrhea.

The quantity of nutrients in any sweetener is so small as to be inconsequential. Choose your sweetener for its taste, not its nutrients.

If sugar is sugar, does this mean that all these sweeteners are bad for us? The only solid link between any sugar and health problems is with tooth decay. And even here, you can minimize tooth damage if you limit the number of times you eat (regardless of the amount). Eat sweets right after a meal, and brush and floss your teeth regularly. Sugar does not cause obesity unless you take in more calories than you use, as is true with any food. Though sugar does not cause diabetes or hypoglycemia, people with these disorders must often restrict their intake to avoid wide swings in blood sugar. Finally, despite the warnings in the popular book *Pure, White and Deadly* (Viking, 1986) by Dr. John Yudkin, little research supports the view that sugar causes heart disease, except in individuals who are genetically predisposed to develop high blood fats on sugary diets.

Though sugar may not be killing us, it is not helping us get any healthier. Here are ways to cut your sugar consumption, while still enjoying your celebrations:

- For snacks and desserts, buy fresh fruits or fruits frozen in water.
- Bake your own cakes, pies, cookies, and other goodies and cut the sugar content by one-third to one-half what the recipe recommends.
- When baking sweet desserts, find recipes that contain nutritious ingredients, such as pumpkin pie, apple crisp, date bars, or biscuits made with oatmeal, raisins, apple chunks, nuts, and seeds.
- To get a sweet effect without using sugar, add "sweet" spices and herbs, such as cinnamon, nutmeg, coriander, cardamom, basil, ginger, or mace. Place grapefruit, bananas, or tomatoes under a broiler for a few minutes. Small amounts of shredded coconut also impart a sweet taste.
- Avoid soft drinks. These account for a high proportion of all refined sugar consumed. Even those with artificial sweeteners serve only to perpetuate your desire for sweets.

Instead, create your own soft drinks with fruit juice and soda water.
- For sweet treats, try these:
  Fresh (or frozen) fruit topped with yogurt
  Cinnamon toast
  Ice milk, sorbet, or frozen yogurt
  Hot low-fat milk with cinnamon, vanilla, or almond extract
  Biscuits—fig bars, arrowroot cookies, ginger snaps, vanilla wafers
  Digestive biscuits
  Gingerbread
  Plain gelatin mixed with fruit juice and cut-up fruit. Top with plain yogurt.

The "ales"

Alcohol lives a Jekyll and Hyde existence. As Jekyll, it is a social lubricant, smoothing the tensions of everyday troubles. As Hyde, it is the most abused substance in the West and has destroyed more lives than any other social drug.

Alcohol (or ethanol) is the fermented wastes of yeast growing on grains, fruit, and molasses. Alcoholic beverages differ in strength according to their alcohol content. Table 18-1 compares common alcoholic beverages.

A minute or two after you sip a drink, most of the alcohol zips past your stomach into the small intestine, where you absorb it into your bloodstream. Your liver breaks down about 95 percent of the alcohol into carbon dioxide and water. If alcohol is absorbed faster than your liver can detoxify it, it accumulates in your blood. Tissues with the highest blood flow (liver, brain, lungs, kidneys) will be affected before tissues with less blood flow (muscles).

Given the same amount of alcohol per pound of body weight, women will have higher blood levels than men. The menstrual cycle can even affect a woman's response. Just before her period, a woman will show higher blood levels of alcohol after drinking. Premenstrual bloating probably accounts for this, since alcohol levels parallel those of body water. Lowest levels occur on the first day of menstrual bleeding.

The uncertain benefits of alcohol Whether you benefit from or

Table 18-1 Energy Constituents of some Alcoholic Drinks, Average Values per 100 ml

	Alcohol g	Carbohydrate g	Energy kcal	kJ
Beer, bitter	4.1	2.3	37	156
Lager	3.9	<0.1	29	122
Cider, sweet	3.7	4.3	95	176
Sherry, medium	16.8	5.9	140	582
Red wine	12.1	0.1	85	353
White wine, dry	9.1	0.6	66	275
White wine, sweet	10.2	5.9	94	390
Spirits	31.7	0	222	919
Liqueurs, medium strength	25.1	32.8	299	1,253

1 ml of pure alcohol weighs 0.79 g.

Source: *Manual of Nutrition*–MAFF.

are harmed by alcohol depends on your drinking habits and your body's reaction.

Heavy drinking has no benefits, but moderate inbibing of alcohol—about four to fourteen drinks a week—may relax you after a frantic day. Of course, turning to alcohol whenever you are tense is flirting with alcohol abuse. In high amounts, alcohol destroys your taste for food and impairs your ability to absorb and use nutrients.

The most tantalizing possible benefit of alcohol is that moderate drinking may reduce the risk of heart disease. Yet scratching below the surface of this presumed benefit reveals some conflicting evidence and inconsistencies in the studies. Some data show that drinkers have higher levels of high-density lipoproteins (HDLs) than do nondrinkers (HDLs lower risk of heart disease). Moderate drinkers do have higher levels of HDLs, but not necessarily the right kind. Though both HDL-2 and HDL-3 are found in humans, HDL-2 is the one that protects against heart disease. As luck would have it, moderate drinking increases HDL-3.

In short, if alcohol does reduce risk of death from heart disease, it is no monumental drop. Drinking, of course, can work against you. Heavy drinking is associated with hypertension, possibly because these drinkers are more likely to be obese (obesity is linked to high blood pressure).

So what does all this mean? If you enjoy a drink in the evening, fine—have one. However, if you normally do not drink, do not start now just to lower your risk of heart disease. Though all the data are not in on this possible benefit of alcohol, we have reams of information on its dangers.

Alcohol and nutrition Alcohol comes on with a broad smile, hand extended, but you soon learn how unfriendly it can be. Besides irritating the stomach lining, alcohol interferes with the digestion and absorption of nutrients, increases nutrient loss, and to be detoxified requires precious vitamins, minerals, and protein.

Alcohol is a nutritional lightweight. Wine contains insignificant amounts of vitamins and minerals (though some red wines are high in iron); beer, small amounts of B vitamins; and liquor, none. At seven calories per gram, alcohol is loaded with empty calories. Because the body wastes about one-fourth of alcohol's calories, figure on getting five to six calories per gram. And though your body burns up alcohol calories (none are stored as fat), it will fuel itself on alcohol and instead convert your food calories into fat.

Ironically, the heavy drinker may suffer from obesity or under weight, vitamin deficiency or toxicity. The woman who is exposed to social occasions where food and drink are both served may end up chronically overeating. Sheer volume of drinking can add on pounds.

The woman who eats irregularly and abstains from food during drinking sprees may lose weight. If she smokes cigarettes or suffers from depression or liver disease, her appetite is further eroded. Some heavy drinkers purposely avoid eating, knowing that without food they get drunk faster. Heavy daily drinkers may miss at least one meal a day, and binge drinkers may miss a few meals a week. The more a person drinks, the worse her diet is likely to be. And though not all alcoholics are malnourished, those with liver disease usually are.

Besides consuming too few nutrients, heavy drinkers may poorly absorb and metabolize thiamin, niacin, B_{12}, folacin, calcium, protein, and sugar. Damage to the liver, the storage site for vitamins A and B_{12}, can lower body levels of these two nutrients. Because alcohol is a diuretic, it pulls water from the body along with water-soluble vitamins, sodium, potassium, chloride, magnesium, and zinc. Alcohol can cause a thiamin-deficiency disease called Wernicke-Korsakoff syndrome, which produces stumbling, amnesia, impaired ability to think or focus eyes, and inability to function independently. Alcohol damages the bone marrow cells that are destined to become blood cells, so alcoholics are often anemic.

To avoid these problems, heavy drinkers may megadose on vitamin and mineral supplements. Overdoses of vitamin A and niacin are common. Though supplements or a good diet can offset deficiencies, they cannot prevent damage to body organs. A better strategy for the heavy drinker (besides finding ways to cut down on alcohol) is to eat plenty of leafy greens, whole grains, lean meats, and fish and take a daily multivitamin-mineral supplement.

How to drink sensibly When drinking, pace yourself so that you absorb alcohol at a rate similar to your liver's ability to detoxify it. Here is how to coordinate the two:

- Keep track of how much you are drinking.
- At parties, delay your first drink for as long as possible.
- Eat some food first, preferably something with protein or fat in it. When your stomach is empty, the alcohol makes a clean break for your stomach and bloodstream. When you drink during or after eating, the alcohol has to slog through all the food before it comes in contact with the intestinal wall.
- Choose watery drinks like beer over concentrated beverages (liquors), or dilute a liquor in fruit juice and lots of ice.
- Be aware that bubbly sodas or champagne speed alcohol into your blood. If you consume mixed drinks with carbonated beverages or sweet mixers on an empty stomach, you can end up with sudden hypoglycemia, including headache, dizziness, and nausea.
- Avoid two-liquor drinks like manhattans or martinis.
- Whatever you decide to drink, sip, do not gulp, and limit yourself to two or three drinks in an evening.

On the Town: the Good, the Bad, and the Bubbly

When you host a party, serve nonalcoholic alternatives such as juices, tea, coffee, sparkling cider, or club soda with lemon or lime. Offer nutritious snacks such as pita bread with aubergine or chickpea spread, yogurt dips, cut-up vegetables and fruits, chicken wings, marinated tuna, slices of turkey and lean ham, cocktail sauce, sesame crackers, and pretzels. (Forget the frankfurters and sour cream dips.)

The pleasures and perils of eating out

If you eat out only a couple of times a year, perhaps for a birthday or anniversary, order what you want, have a good time, and skip the rest of this section. But if you eat away from home often, the effects on your diet and health can be enormous. Well-paid professionals are often comfortable in every corner of the city except their own kitchens. Instead, they eat breakfast in a coffee shop, lunch in a diner, and dinner in a restaurant. If, like these professionals, you eat most of your meals out, be selective about what you order. Following are some suggestions for eating out and eating well.

Choosing the restaurant Foods naturally low in fat are specialties of certain restaurants—seafood, Italian, French, Chinese, Japanese, Thai, Indonesian, Vietnamese, Korean, Indian, Polynesian, Spanish, Mexican, Cuban, and vegetarian. Other restaurants offer fattier fare, such as steaks, burgers, and pizza. Yet in almost any restaurant you can order menu items cooked in a manner to cut the fat.

Ordering from the menu Even if you are not dieting, think like a dieter. Cut out unnecessary calories from fat, alcohol, and sweets, and you automatically improve your diet. Study the menu and ask your waiter or waitress how foods are prepared when you are uncertain. Table 18-2 lists menu terms and phrases that carry subtle meanings about the fat and sodium content of your meals.

Drinks and appetizers For beverages, try skim or low-fat milk, fruit or tomato juice, or sparkling water with lemon or lime. If you want an alcoholic beverage, dilute the calories with water, juice, or club soda.

Table 18-2 What restaurant terms really mean

Low in fat

"Steamed;" "In its own juice;" "Garden fresh;" "Broiled;" "Roasted;" "Poached;" "Tomato juice;" "Dry broiled" (in lemon juice or wine)

High in sodium

"Pickled;" "In cocktail sauce;" "Smoked;" "In broth;" "In a tomato base"

High in saturated fat, cholesterol, and sodium

"Buttery," "buttered," "in butter sauce"
"Sautéed," "fried," "pan-fried," "crispy," "braised"
"Creamed," "in cream sauce," "in its own gravy," "hollandaise"
"Au gratin," "parmesan," "in cheese sauce," "escalloped"
"Marinated" (in oil), "stewed," "basted"
"Casserole," "prime," "hash," "pot pie"

From *Dining Out: A Guide to Restaurant Dining*. 1984. American Heart Association.

For appetizers, try steamed seafood, raw vegetables, or fresh fruit. Avoid pâtés, quiches, and cream soups. Clear soups are fine unless you are watching your sodium. Enjoy the bread or breadsticks, but skip the butter or margarine.

Salads The term "salad" is commonly applied to everything from a plate of anemic-looking lettuce to a mound of lettuce, spinach, cucumbers, radishes, tomatoes, carrots, onions, beans, cauliflower, and other garden delights. Salad bars can enrich a meal, but go lightly on the cheese, eggs, meat, bacon bits, potato and pasta salads, olives, pickles, and croutons—all high in fat. Order your dressing on the side and then dab, don't drench, your salad with it. For a fat-free alternative, use lemon juice.

Sandwiches Good choices are chicken, turkey, ham, or roast beef sandwiches on whole-wheat bread.

Entrees When you are barely hungry, choose an appetizer or two for your main course, or order à la carte. When with a companion, you may each want to order salads, then split an entree. Ask for any sauces, dressings, and butter or margarine served on the side, so you can decide how much of these fat-laden accouterments to add. Order your meat, fish, or poultry grilled, baked, steamed, or poached—not sautéed or fried. Request that broiled items be basted with lemon juice or wine, not fat. Trim visible fat off meat before eating. Avoid casseroles or foods dripping with sauces. If vegetables come with your entree, ask that they be prepared and served without fat. Forget about smothering your baked potato under butter or sour cream. Instead, add yogurt, when available, or trace amounts of butter, or eat it plain. Coleslaw and potato salad are both high in fat, so eat them only occasionally.

Desserts If you desire dessert, try sorbets, gelatin, fruit ices, or fruit, even if this last one is listed as an appetizer. If you go for a pastry, split it with your dinner partner. Avoid nondairy creamers and whipped toppings, which are often made from coconut oil, a highly saturated fat.

Table 18-3 gives tips on eating at specific types of restaurants. (For information on fast-food restaurants, see chapter 1.)

Special considerations

Two additives commonly used in restaurants can cause some unpleasant and serious side effects. The first, monosodium glutamate (MSG), brings out the flavor of vegetables and is often sprinkled on Chinese dishes. (It is sold commercially under the brand name Accent.) People sensitive to MSG may experience tightening of the face and neck muscles, headaches, nausea, and giddiness, a group of symptoms known as "the Chinese restaurant syndrome." When you eat at Chinese restaurants, ask that the cook omits the MSG.

Second, a class of additives called sulfiting agents or sulfites are often used to keep salad bar ingredients looking fresh and to keep potatoes and fish looking attractive. Processed foods such as fruit drinks, beer, wine, baked goods, vegetables, and dried fruit may also contain sulfites. Look on the label for potassium metabisulfite, sodium metabisulfite, sodium sulfite, sodium bisulfite, and sulfur dioxide. Some people, especially those with asthmas or allergies, are hypersensitive to these agents and experience faintness, hives, nausea, diarrhea, shortness of

Table 18-3 Tips for ordering in restaurants

Preferred choices	Have less often (high in fat, cholesterol, or sodium)
CHINESE	
Boiled, steamed, lightly stir-fried dishes	Sautéed and deep-fried dishes
Ask for sauces, like soy, served on side	Szechuan-style meat fried in hot oil
Ask that no MSG be added	Soups
	Fried noodles
FRENCH	
Steamed mussels	Onion soup
Wine sauces, such as bordelaise	Butter sauces, such as hollandaise, béchamel, and béarnaise
GREEK	
Tzatziki (yogurt and cucumbers)	Dishes made with phyllo dough
Pita bread	Caviar
Greek salads (avoid the anchovies and olives to reduce sodium)	Babaganoosh (aubergine appetizer)
Plaki (fish dish)	
Shish kebob	
INDIAN	
Lentil Soup	Vegetables prepared with ghee (clarified butter)
Tandoori chicken and fish	
Breads like pulkas or naan	
Salads	
Dishes prepared with yogurt-based curry sauce	
ITALIAN	
White or red clam sauces	Scallopine or parmagiana dishes
Marsala or marinara sauces	
Baked chicken or fish	
Italian ices	
JAPANESE	
Sashimi	Tempura (deep-fried)
Nabemono	Salty soups or sauces
Chicken teriyaki	
Menrui	
Yakimono (grilled) dishes	
Tofu dishes	

MEXICAN

Salads with tomato, onion, and avocado
Seviche (marinated fish)
Chicken tostados

Fried tortillas
Refried beans (cooked in lard)
Sour cream

MIDDLE EASTERN

All the appetizers (can include dolma, mussels, pine nuts, aubergine)
Shish kebob
Couscous and steamed bulgur

Entrees basted with butter

STEAKHOUSES

Grilled
Mixed grill, filet mignon, round and flank steaks (no fat or salt added)
Salads with a small amount of dressing

Butter or sour cream on potatoes
Fatty cuts of meat
Rich desserts

VEGETARIAN

Yogurt-based dishes
Salads
Whole-grain breads

Dishes made with lots of cheeses, eggs, nuts, or oils

From *Dining Out: A Guide to Restaurant Dining*. 1984. American Heart Association.

---

breath, and fatal shock. If you are sensitive, before you order, ask if any foods have been treated with a commercial sulfiting agent.

A final word

Given our social nature, our inclination is to celebrate with food and drink. Eating out is a time to meet with people, share a meal, and, as one philosopher said, to "gossip about the Universe." With some restraint you can have your cakes and ale, retain your "virtue," and long enjoy the company of friends.

APPENDIX A
The Basics of Nutrition

Food is the divine packaging for nutrients. It lures the eye and charms the taste buds. Food makes nutrients desirable, but nutrients give the real life-and-death meaning to food.

Nutrients fall into six classes. Each class either provides energy, regulates biochemical reactions, or serves as raw materials for tissues. Essential nutrients are those you must get from your diet because the human body cannot manufacture them at all or not in amounts sufficient for health. A substance can be essential for one species and not for another. If you were a gerbil, you would need myoinositol; if you were a cat, taurine. But you are human, so you can ignore both.

The six nutrient classes are carbohydrates, fats, proteins, water, vitamins, and minerals. Because your body must have carbohydrates, fats, proteins, and water in relatively large amounts (grams), these are called macronutrients. Vitamins and minerals are micronutrients, which your body requires in smaller amounts (milligrams and micrograms). No matter how much or how little of each essential nutrient you need, a deficiency of any one will lead to severe abnormalities, and possibly death.

Carbohydrates

Of the six classes of nutrients, you get energy only from carbohydrates, fats, and proteins, but carbohydrates are your main source. Based on size, carbohydrates fall into three categories: monosaccharides (one sugar), disaccharides (two sugars), and polysaccharides (many sugars). The first two groups are known as simple sugars:

Monosaccharides
Glucose

Appendix A

Fructose
Galactose

Disaccharides
Sucrose (glucose + fructose)
Lactose (glucose + galactose)
Maltose (glucose + glucose)

The last group, formed from long chains of glucose units, are dubbed complex carbohydrates:

Starch
Glycogen
Cellulose

Your body breaks down all carbohydrates and extra protein into glucose, which your cells ultimately use for energy. So glucose is often referred to as "blood sugar." Fructose, the sweetest of sugars, is present with glucose in fruits, vegetables, and honey. Galactose does not exist in nature as a single sugar but is only attached to other sugars.

Sucrose is common table sugar, brown sugar, and molasses. Lactose is the sugar in milk, while maltose is the sugar in malt and germinating grains. It is partly the removal of maltose units that makes "light beer." Starches are the storage form of carbohydrates in plants like wheat, rice, corn, tubers, and peas, while glycogen is the storage form in your body. Cellulose (or fiber) is the part of plants that cannot be digested and hurries food through your digestive tract.

Try to get your carbohydrates from foods that contain vitamins and minerals, too. In general, choose from the following:

Fruits and juices
Vegetables
Dried beans, peas, lentils
Whole or enriched grains (flours, breads, cereals, pasta, noodles, brown rice)

Eat less of these:

Sugar, honey, syrup
Pastries, cookies, cakes, pies
White flour, not enriched

White rice, not enriched
Highly processed cereals

Fat (lipids)

Fats and fatlike substances are classified as lipids, meaning they cannot dissolve in water but can dissolve in solvents like fingernail polish. Fats are composed of carbon, hydrogen, and oxygen, fashioned together into fatty acids. If every bond in the fatty acid chain is filled to its limit with hydrogen, the fatty acid is "saturated." If a part of the chain is missing a hydrogen atom, the fatty acid is "unsaturated." If two or more parts are missing hydrogen atoms, the fatty acid is "polyunsaturated," sometimes abbreviated PUFA. The parts of the chain that are missing hydrogen atoms are structurally weak and open to attack by oxygen. For this reason, refrigerate polyunsaturated fats (vegetable oils, margarines) and keep them only for short periods of time, or they will go rancid. Sometimes antioxidants such as BHA, BHT, vitamin C, or vitamin E are added to foods to prevent oxygen damage.

Polyunsaturated fats tend to be liquid at room temperature, and saturated fats tend to be solid. To make polyunsaturated margarines look more like butter, manufacturers bombard the polyunsaturated chains with hydrogen, a process called hydrogenation. The margarine becomes more saturated—and harder. (If you are trying to cut down on saturated fats, hardened margarines are not much better than butter.)

Your body can make all the fat it needs from carbohydrates and proteins, except for one polyunsaturated fat called linoleic acid. You must get this from your diet, and the best sources are vegetable oils (corn, peanut, soybean, safflower).

Fats from food either become part of your body (like cell membranes), are burnt for quick energy, or are stashed in fat cells, where they pad vital organs, insulate the body, and provide energy. While carbohydrates are short-term energy sources for your body, fats are available for the long run. Compared to carbohydrates, fats are much more compressed forms of energy because they are stored with very little water. Your fat cells can stretch like elastic bags to accommodate quite a lot of fat. Though you can pull the fat out of these cells when you need

Proteins

Your entire genetic machinery is designed to direct the creation of proteins. Proteins are chains of smaller units called amino acids, twenty-two in all. Each amino acid has a side chain with a distinctive shape, size, composition, and electrical charge. Given the proper diet, your body can concoct all but eight of the amino acids, which it must get from food. These are isoleucine, leucine, lysine, methionine, phenylalinine, valine, threonine, and tryptophan. (To make these other nonessential amino acids, your body also needs a certain amount of nitrogen.)

Once consumed, proteins are broken down into their nitrogen-containing amino acids, which then move through the blood. When your body needs to create tissues, enzymes, antibodies, and hormones, it recruits and reassembles these amino acids. Your genes determine how the amino acids line up to form a specific protein. Deoxyribonucleic acid (DNA) tells your cells what proteins to produce. Ribonucleic acid (RNA) carries out the instructions. Depending on their amino acids, proteins may construct long, stiff, hardy bones, tendons, ligaments, and hair. Other softer, more maleable proteins form hemoglobin, enzymes, and milk curd.

If a mistake is made and the wrong amino acid is inserted into a sequence, serious problems can result. The blood disorder sicklecell anemia occurs when an incorrect amino acid is incorporated into the protein chain of hemoglobin. Also, when building protein chains, cells must have all the essential amino acids available at that time. If one is missing, the entire production comes to a halt, and whatever function that protein was destined for remains unfilled. (This is why strict vegetarians must combine plant proteins to get all essential amino acids at once.)

Proteins attract water, so cells keep a constant store of proteins within and outside their membranes to maintain water balance. Also, because of their electrically charged side chains, proteins can prevent the blood from getting too acidic or too alkaline.

Once the nitrogen is removed from proteins, your body can break down amino acids to release energy or may convert them to fat. The nitrogen is released first as poisonous ammonia, then soon forms the less toxic urea, which your kidneys flush out of your body with water.

Water

Water comprises a little over half of your weight. (Men have more body water than women because they have more lean tissue, which is more watery than fat.) Often forgotten as a nutrient, water is part of the blood and lymph that transport nutrients to cells and carry away wastes. Water can dissolve glucose, amino acids, and minerals. Those fat-soluble substances that do not dissolve in water are carried wrapped in water-soluble protein coats. Water makes a perfect medium for biochemical reactions.

Because water resists being compressed, it can lubricate and cushion joints and other vital body parts. Also, water pushes on the inside and outside of cells, helping them to hold their shape. Finally, water keeps body temperature within a survivable range, cooling you through evaporation.

You can survive without food for weeks, but without water you could die in two to four days. Losing 15–20 percent of body water is fatal. To replace daily water losses, drink six to eight glasses (eight-ounce) of fluid a day. Watch out for too much coffee or tea, which as diuretics can actually pull water from the body.

Vitamins

Vitamins are less like a family than they are workers in a common trade—carpenters, for instance. Unrelated to each other, they are bunched together as a class of nutrients because they are all organic (contain carbon) and perform similar functions, like members of a vitamin guild. In your body they assist enzymes to speed the rate of biological reactions from weeks or months to seconds. During these reactions, the vitamins are not used up, which is why you need them in only small amounts. Without enzymes or their vitamin assistants, the nutrients in a chicken enchilada might not ever reach your cells. Unlike the fuel nutrients (proteins, carbohydrates, and fats), vitamins cannot be broken down to supply energy; they contain no calories. But like these other essential nutrients, vitamins must come from the

Appendix A

diet. (Because vitamin D can be made in skin exposed to sunlight, some consider it a hormone, not a vitamin.)

Vitamins are measured in micrograms (μg) and milligrams (mg). Vitamin A is often measured in International Units (IU). Table A-1 lists essential vitamins, their sources, functions, and deficiency and toxicity signs.

Minerals

Minerals are inorganic, derived from rock or soil rather than living things. Like vitamins, minerals do not provide calories and cannot be broken down to release energy. Their functions fall loosely into the categories of regulating and building. What they regulate are heartbeat, blood clotting, body fluids, acid-base balance, nerve transmission, muscle contraction, and oxygen transport. What they build are bones, teeth, and soft tissues. Unlike vitamins, minerals can be built into body tissues. Iron colors hemoglobin red. Cobalt affixes itself to vitamin B_{12}. Sulfur is enmeshed in the vitamins thiamin and biotin.

Minerals are divided into two general categories: those you need in relatively large amounts (macrominerals) and those you need in much smaller amounts (trace minerals). Some of the macrominerals appear as single, electrically charged particles, called electrolytes. In this form, they attract water and can regulate how much water stays inside and outside cells, which prevents cells from shrinking or swelling. Electrolytes also keep the acid-base balance of your body within an acceptable range. Table A-2 lists essential minerals, their sources, functions, and deficiency and toxicity signs.

Other substances in food

Whenever a substance appears in food, you wonder why it is there. Some of these things are essential for other animals but have not been shown to be necessary for humans. These include cobalt, nickel, vanadium, silicon, arsenic, tin, and cadmium. Researchers continue to explore whether these may actually be essential for humans, too.

Also, certain growth factors in food that are essential for lower forms of life (such as bacteria and insects) do not seem to be necessary for higher animals, including humans. These factors include asparagine, Bifidus factor, cholesterol, lecithin, lipoic acid, nucleic acids, and para-aminobenzoic acid. Finally, substances appear in food that have no known function for any animal. Among these are amygdalin (laetrile), chlorophyll, orotic acid, "pangamic acid," and "vitamin U."

Table A-1 Vitamins*

Food sources	To conserve	Functions in body	Deficiency signs	Toxicity signs
VITAMIN A, RETINOL (RDA = 750 mg)				
Beef liver Eggs Fortified milk and dairy products Carotene (converted to vitamin A in the body): spinach cantaloupe leafy greens kale carrots broccoli apricots	Cook in covered pots Avoid frying at high temperatures Avoid overexposing food to air	Smooth, healthy-looking skin Resistance to infections and other diseases Normal vision Healthy mucous membranes Strengthens tooth enamel and favors growth of strong bones	Night blindness and eye disease Failure of tear secretions Susceptibility to respiratory and intestinal infections Dry, rough skin Changes in mucous membranes Poor growth	Loss of appetite and weight Nausea and vomiting Dry, cracked skin; hair loss Severe headache; blurred vision, mimics brain tumor Fatigue, lethargy, irritability Damage to liver, spleen and nervous system Swelling of feet and ankles; joint pain Eye hemorrhages Poor growth; possible death Too much carotene: yellowing of skin; menstrual irregularities

Food sources	To conserve	Functions in body	Deficiency signs	Toxicity signs
—————————————————————————— VITAMIN D ——————————————————————————				
Fish oils Beef Butter Eggs Fortified milk Salmon Tuna Made by skin when exposed to sun	Avoid overexposing food to air	Needed for strong bones and teeth	Bowleg, knock knee, curvature of spine, pelvic and chest deformities Softening of bones Excessive tooth decay Listlessness	Nausea, vomiting, loss of weight Excessive thirst Headache, weakness, muscle stiffness Kidney stones Calcium deposits in kidney and heart; high blood pressure Growth and mental retardation Kidney failure; death
————————————————————————— VITAMIN E, TOCOPHEROL —————————————————————————				
Vegetable oils Whole grains Wheat germ Almonds Sunflower seeds Peanuts Hazel nuts Yellow and green vegetables	Avoid deep-fat frying Avoid freezing	Formation of red blood cells and other tissues Antioxidant: protects cells from air pollutants Healthy heart and skeletal muscles	Premature and low-birth-weight infants: breakdown of red blood cells	Uncertain. Some reports of nausea, fatigue, blurred vision. May interfere with vitamin K made in intestine.

Food sources	To conserve	Functions in body	Deficiency signs	Toxicity signs
VITAMIN K				
Leafy greens Peas Potatoes Liver Cabbage Cereals Made by intestinal bacteria (except in new-borns)		Needed for blood clotting Needed for healthy bones	Rare in adults except in those with impaired fat absorption, cancer, kidney disease, or those on prolonged antibiotic therapy Bruising, poor blood clotting In newborns, hemorrhage	None reported in adults. In babies, jaundice Synthetic vitamin K (menadione) has produced irritation of skin and respiratory tract; no known toxicity for natural vitamin K
Water-soluble vitamins				
VITAMIN B₁, THIAMIN (RDA = 0.7–1.0 µg)				
Pork Liver Oysters Whole grains Soybeans Rolled oats Green peas	Cook with a minimum of water or steam Avoid cooking at high temperatures or cooking for a prolonged time Avoid using baking soda to color vegetables green	Release of energy from carbohydrates Healthy heart and nerves	Beriberi (muscle weakness, heart and nerve damage) Mental confusion Depression Constipation Loss of appetite and weight Fatigue Painful calf muscles Numbness in toes and feet Occurs mainly among alcoholics	None reported, but excess of any B vitamin can cause deficiency of others; headache, insomnia, rapid pulse, weakness

Food sources	To conserve	Functions in body	Deficiency signs	Toxicity signs
VITAMIN B$_2$, RIBOFLAVIN (RDA = 1.3 mg)				
Beef liver Milk Eggs Meat Broccoli Whole and enriched grains Dried peas and beans	Avoid cooking in large amounts of water Cut vegetables into large, not small, pieces Avoid overexposure to light Cover pots when cooking	Release of energy from proteins, carbohydrates, fats Maintains healthy skin and mucous membranes	Visual fatigue and light sensitivity Cracks around the mouth Burning and itchy eyes Reduced strength Swollen, magenta tongue; swollen, reddened lips; sore throat Greasy skin around face and ears Retarded growth; anemia	None reported, but excess of any B vitamin can cause deficiency of others; causes yellow discoloration of urine
VITAMIN B$_3$, NIACIN, NICOTINAMIDE, NICOTINIC ACID (RDA = 15 mg)				
Liver Tuna Poultry Meat Peanuts Whole and enriched grains Dried beans and peas Can be synthesized in body from the essential amino acid	Niacin is very stable Avoid throwing out cooking water from vegetables	Aids metabolism of carbohydrates, fats, and proteins Mental and emotional health Needed for oxygen use by cells	Pellagra (skin scaling, diarrhea) Mental confusion Loss of appetite and weight Anemia; weakness Loss of balance Irritability, sleeplessness, headaches Sore mouth and	Flushing and itching of skin Ulcers Abnormal liver function Irritability, headache Nausea Rapid heartbeat Stomach pain

Food sources	To conserve	Functions in body	Deficiency signs	Toxicity signs
		VITAMIN B6, PYRIDOXINE, PYRIDOXOL, PYRIDOXAMINE		
Whole grains Liver Meat Spinach Bananas Nuts Potatoes Tomatoes Wheat germ	Avoid cooking in large amounts of water Freezing vegetables destroys 30–56% Canning vegetables destroys 57–77%	Needed for protein metabolism Formation of red blood cells Helps the body use fats Healthy nervous system Healthy skin	Skin disorders; greasy scaliness around eyes, nose, and mouth Mental depression Anemia, weight loss, stomach pains, vomiting Convulsions Kidney stones Deficiencies are rare except for borderline cases among oral contraceptive users	High doses produce dependency May produce liver disease, unsteady gait, numb feet, numbness and clumsiness of hands At risk: women taking high doses for pre-menstrual water retention

Food sources	To conserve	Functions in body	Deficiency signs	Toxicity signs
—————————— VITAMIN B_{12}, CYANOCOBALAMIN, COBALAMIN ——————————				
Clams Beef liver Oysters Mackerel Sardines Meat Eggs Milk Brewer's yeast	Avoid extreme heating of meat products	Formation of red blood cells Helps build genetic material Healthy nervous system Normal growth	Pernicious anemia (severe reduction in number of red blood cells; muscle weakness) Irritability, apathy, drowsiness, depression, hallucinations Weight loss Nervous system damage Raw scarlet tongue with a smooth surface At risk: strict vegetarians who do not eat reliable sources of B_{12}; Persons with part of stomach removed; Persons who inherited defect in ability to absorb B_{12}	None reported, but excess of any B vitamin can cause deficiencies of others

Food sources	To conserve	Functions in body	Deficiency signs	Toxicity signs
—————————————————————— FOLACIN, FOLATE, FOLIC ACID ——————————————————————				
Spinach Broccoli Asparagus Wheat germ Liver Orange juice Dried beans Brewer's yeast	Avoid high temperatures Avoid cooking in large amounts of water Avoid overexposure to light Avoid storing at room temperature	Needed for production of RNA and DNA Formation of red blood cells	Megaloblastic anemia (enlarged blood cells; smooth, red tongue; diarrhea) Fatigue During pregnancy, deficiency may cause fetal abnormalities or loss	None reported, but body stores vitamin so it is potentially hazardous Large amounts can mask a deficiency of vitamin B_{12} Malaise, irritability
——————————————————————————— PANTOTHENIC ACID ———————————————————————————				
All foods, especially Liver Kidney Milk Whole grains Green vegetables Nuts Eggs Soybeans Made by intestinal bacteria	Avoid extreme heat Avoid heavily processed foods	Metabolism of carbohydrates, proteins, and fats Formation of some adrenal hormones	None reported except in experiments: abdominal pain, vomiting, nausea, fatigue, insomnia, tingling in hands and feet	May cause thiamin deficiency; diarrhea, water retention

Food sources	To conserve	Functions in body	Deficiency signs	Toxicity signs
—BIOTIN—				
Egg yolk
Liver
Kidneys
Leafy greens
Made by bacteria in intestines		Formation of fatty acids
Metabolism of carbohydrates
Use of B_{12} and folacin	None reported under natural conditions
Large amounts of raw egg white contain avidin, which can bind biotin	None reported, but excess amounts of any B vitamin can cause deficiencies of others
—VITAMIN C, ASCORBIC ACID (RDA = 30 mg)—				
Green peppers
Citrus fruits
Melon
Broccoli
Brussels sprouts
Strawberries
Potatoes
Tomatoes
Dark green vegetables	Eat foods raw or minimally cooked
Boil water before adding vegetables
Steam or cook vegetables in very little water
Cut foods in large, not small, pieces
Do not keep foods at room temperature for long periods
Avoid overexposing food to air and light
Do not soak vegetables	Formation of collagen; helps maintain bones, teeth, and blood vessels
Antioxidant: may block cancer-causing nitrosamines from forming
Wound healing
Resistance to infection	Scurvy: bleeding gums, poor healing, muscle loss; brown tough skin; loose teeth
Dry, itchy skin
Hair loss
Fatigue
Loss of appetite and weight	High doses can cause dependency, leading to deficiency when doses reduced in amount (particularly for newborns whose mothers took large doses during pregnancy)
Diarrhea, kidney stones, urinary tract discomfort
Blood tends to clot
Can trigger B_{12} deficiency
Interferes with copper absorption, leading to anemia

Table A-2 Minerals*

Food sources	Functions in body	Deficiency signs	Toxicity signs
Macrominerals			
CALCIUM (RDA = 500 mg)			
Milk and dairy products Canned fish eaten with bones Dark leafy greens Citrus fruits Dried beans	Strong bones and teeth Heart and nerve action Blood clotting Muscle contraction Vitamin B_{12} absorption Activates certain enzymes	In children: rickets (bowed legs, stunted growth) In adults: osteoporosis (loss of bone) Weak bones and teeth	Calcium deposits in tissues Severe fatigue, drowsiness Poor absorption of iron, zinc, and manganese
CHLORIDE			
Table salt Other naturally occurring salts	Regulation of body fluids Part of stomach acid Activates starch-splitting enzyme in saliva	Uncommon, but upsets acid-base balance in body fluids	Upsets acid-base balance in body fluids
MAGNESIUM			
Raw leafy greens Nuts Seeds Whole grains Soybeans	Strong bones Release of energy from muscle glycogen Nerve action Manufacture of proteins	Muscle weakness, irregular heartbeat Convulsions Anorexia, nausea, vomiting Shaky hands At risk: persons with diabetes, epilepsy, or alcoholism; or those with prolonged use of diuretics	Disorders in nervous system Paralysis Dangerous for persons with poor kidney function

Food sources	Functions in body	Deficiency signs	Toxicity signs
— PHOSPHORUS —			
Meat Poultry Fish Eggs Dried peas and beans Dairy products Whole grains Phosphates in processed foods such as soft drinks	Strong bones and teeth Energy release from proteins, fats, and carbohydrates Needed for genetic material, cell membranes, and some enzymes Acts as buffer for proper acid-base balance in blood	Loss of appetite Fatigue, weakness Pain in bones At risk: persons with prolonged use of antacids	Imbalanced ratio of calcium to phosphorus; mimics calcium deficiency
— POTASSIUM —			
Oranges Bananas Meat Milk Bran Dried beans Potatoes Peanut butter Coffee, tea, cocoa	Fluid balance in cells Transmission of nerve impulses Muscle contractions Energy release from carbohydrates, fats, and proteins	Abnormal heart action Fatigue, muscle weakness At risk: persons who work hard in hot weather; those taking diuretics; those with prolonged diarrhea	Muscle paralysis Abnormal heartbeats
— SODIUM —			
Table salt Naturally present in most foods and water, especially cheese, milk, shellfish	Internal water balance Transmission of nerve impulses	Muscle cramps and weakness Nausea Diarrhea	High blood pressure in some people

Food sources	To conserve	Functions in body	Deficiency signs	Toxicity signs
SULFUR				
Beef Wheat germ Dried beans and peas Peanuts Clams		Formation of body cells Component of insulin and sulfur amino acids Builds hair, nails, skin	None reported in humans	Unknown
Trace minerals				
CHROMIUM				
Brewer's yeast Meat Cheese Whole grains Dried beans Peanuts		Needed for insulin activity	Uncertain, but possibly adult-onset diabetes and abnormal glucose metabolism	Unknown
COPPER				
Oysters Nuts Liver Cocoa Kidneys Dried beans Corn oil margarine		Formation of red blood cells Part of several enzymes	Unknown in adults In children: anemia, bone disease	Violent vomiting and diarrhea Nausea Low levels of vitamin A in blood

Food sources	Functions in body	Deficiency signs	Toxicity signs
—FLUORINE, FLUORIDE—			
Fish Animal foods Fluoridated water Tea	Strong teeth that are resistant to decay Strong bones	Excess dental decay Stunted growth Possibly osteoporosis	Mottling of teeth Toxic in large doses
—IODINE—			
Seafood Saltwater fish Iodized salt Sea salt	Component of thyroid hormone Normal reproduction	Adults: goiter (enlarged thyroid) Newborns: cretinism (poor growth, protruding abdomen, enlarged tongue)	None reported, but possible sensitivity or poisoning
—IRON (RDA = 18–54 years: 12 mg, 55+ years: 10 mg)—			
Red meats Egg yolk Leafy greens Dried beans Enriched and whole grains Blackstrap molasses	Formation of red blood cells Part of enzymes and proteins	Anemia, fatigue Loss of appetite Susceptibility to infection Pale skin Shortness of breath	Toxic buildup in liver, pancreas, heart Diarrhea, constipation
—MANGANESE—			
Whole grains Nuts Vegetables Fruit Tea Instant coffee	Healthy nervous system and bones Reproduction Part of enzymes needed for metabolism of carbohydrates, protein,	None reported in humans	None reported from diet Overexposure to manganese dust in air: slurred speech, muscle spasms

Food sources	Functions in body	Deficiency signs	Toxicity signs
MOLYBDENUM			
Meats Cereal grains Legumes Liver Kidney	Part of an enzyme	None reported in humans	Goutlike syndrome Loss of copper
SELENIUM			
Seafood Whole grains Meat Eggs Milk Garlic	Antioxidant: prevents breakdown of body substances, including fat	None reported in humans	None reported in humans, but has led to death in animals
ZINC			
Meat Liver Eggs Poultry Seafood (oysters) Milk Whole grains (less available form)	Formation of enzyme	Delayed wound healing Loss of taste Stunted growth Reproductive failures Infants with low birth weights and birth defects Loss of appetite Skin changes	Nausea, vomiting, stomach bleeding Fever, diarrhea, abdominal pain Anemia Premature birth, still birth May aggravate atherosclerosis Interferes with copper

Some evidence exists that other trace minerals, including cobalt, nickel, vanadium, silicon, arsenic, tin, and cadmium, may be essential to humans.

APPENDIX B
Where to Find Nutrition Information

Your local health education unit, listed in the telephone book under the district health authority, will have a resources centre.

The Health Education Authority, 78 New Oxford Street, London WC1A 1AH, is the central body. It has a resources centre and publishes booklets on nutrition. Their publications address is PO Box 877 London SE99 6YE.

The Ministry of Agriculture, Fisheries and Food is responsible for the safety of food. Their publications on labelling and additives can be obtained from the Publications Unit, Lion House, Willowburn Trading Estate, Alnwick, Northumberland NE66 2PF. (In Scotland, from the Scottish Home and Health Department, Foods Branch, Room 40, St Andrew's House, Edinburgh EH1 3DE. In Northern Ireland, from the Department of Health and Social Services, Medicines and Food Control Branch, Annex A, Dundonald House, Upper Newtownards Road, Belfast BT4 3SF.)

For nutritional information about various food products, contact the manufacturer. For own brand goods and general information, write to the community relations department of leading supermarket chains. Some of those who already put nutritional information on products also produce free booklets and other publications on diet, nutrition and health.

The Food and Drink Federation, 6 Catherine Street, London WC2B 5JJ, provide literature and information on nutrition.

Your local community dietician and hospital dietician can also provide advice on nutrition.

For special needs such as diabetes, heart and cancer, write to the appropriate voluntary body. A large, stamped address envelope is appreciated (and a donation is always welcome).

Appendix B

Many provide free diet and other fact sheets, booklets and, in some cases, resources centres.

There is a growing concern for healthy eating in the United Kingdom, and information and guidance is becoming more widely available.

Evaluating Nutrition Claims

While waiting for the dentist, you pick up a magazine and start reading an article about diets. Sandwiched between pages of the article are advertisements claiming their products can give you thin ankles in 30 days or can dissolve your fat without your lifting a finger (after you write a check for the product, of course). As the messages of both the article and ads reach your brain, what should you be thinking? How can you scrutinize these claims?

First, is more attention paid to the packaging than the contents? Is an unrealistic aura being given to the product? (The model with the thin ankles, for instance, was no doubt *born* with thin ankles.) Does the promoter ask you to diagnose yourself or try to convince you that you are unhealthy? What about intimidating tactics? Does the person suggest that if you truly loved your child/partner/self you would buy this product?

Next, examine the logic. Does the claim run counter to the laws of nature? For instance, are cures promised for diseases such as arthritis for which science has yet to find a cure? Are quick results promised? ("Twenty pounds in seven days!") Because of such miracle cures, does the person claim to be persecuted by the Food and Drug Administration?

Also, watch the language. A statement that reads "Sugar, fat, cholesterol, and salt cause diabetes, cancer, hypertension and heart disease" does not tell you which disease correlates with which diet factor. Do all these things cause all these diseases?

Another gimmick is to place together two sentences that imply an association where none exists. Consider this: "High intakes of saturated fats contribute to heart attacks. This product is low in saturated fat." The mind naturally concludes that this product can prevent heart attacks—quite a mental leap.

Word choices can distort a product's worth. For instance, a food that is promised to "give 'em quick energy" is relying on the public's positive view of the word "energy." If the ad were

Eat Beautiful!

to read "gives 'em quick calories," the reader might hesitate before buying and wonder what else she is getting besides calories. Any vitamins or minerals?

Beware of dangling comparisons such as "Sugar intake is higher in the United Kingdom." Higher than what? Closely related to this is the practice of spurious comparison. For instance, an ad that claims a product has more iron than an 8-ounce glass of milk is misleading because milk is a recognized poor source of iron. It is like saying a product has more vitamin C than a bonbon. So what? All these techniques can indicate possible bias or inaccurate claims.

Ask yourself how the research was conducted. Was it on humans or animals? Is the evidence purely anecdotal? ("I took product X and immediately lost ten pounds.") Testimonials are the worst sort of evidence because not all possible intervening factors are controlled. Let's say you have a cold. You take 4 grams of vitamin C for two days and you feel better. Plus your symptoms seem less severe than usual. This type of account is anecdotal because you have no way of knowing if the vitamin C was responsible or if you caught a less vigorous strain of virus this time. Also, if you expect to feel better, you usually do, a situation known as the placebo effect.

APPENDIX C
The Food Exchange

1¼ US teaspoons	= 1 UK teaspoon
1¼ US tablespoons	= 1 UK tablespoon
1 cup.	= 8 fluid ounces
1 cup flour	= 4 ounces
1 cup sugar	= 8 ounces

Eating plans at five calorie levels
Number of portions at each calorie level

	Calories				
Exchanges	1,000	1,200	1,500	1,800	2,100
1. Free foods	Unlimited	Unlimited	Unlimited	Unlimited	Unlimited
2. Vegetables	3	2	3	3	4
3. Fruits	3	3	4	4	5
4. Starches	3	5	7	9	11
5. Proteins	6	7	7	8	10
6. Milk	2	2	2	3	2
7. Fats	3	3	5	6	7

Food exchange lists

1. *Free Foods*

Coffee (black), tea
Clear broth (salt-free)
Cranberries (unsweetened)
Gelatin (unsweetened)
Garlic
Horseradish
Lemon, lime
Low-calorie soft drinks
Mustard
Onion flakes
Pickle, dill
Spices
Vinegar

Chicory
Chinese cabbage
Endive
Lettuce
Parsley
Radishes
Watercress

The following are unlimited if eaten raw:
Broccoli
Mushrooms
Peppers (red or green)

Eat Beautiful!

2. Vegetables *(1 exchange equals ½ cup, cooked)*

- Asparagus
- Aubergine
- Bean Sprouts
- Beets
- Broccoli
- Brussels sprouts
- Cabbage
- Carrots
- Catsup (2 Tbsp.)
- Cauliflower
- Celery
- Courgettes
- Cucumber
- Greens (beet, kale, spinach, etc.)
- Mushrooms
- Okra
- Onions
- Pepper (green or red)
- Rhubarb
- Sauerkraut
- String beans (yellow, green)
- Swede
- Tomatoes or Tomato juice
- Turnips
- Vegetable juice

3. Fruit *(amount equals one exchange)*

Fruits:
- Apple—½ med.
- Applesauce—½ cup
- Apricots, fresh—2 med.
- Apricots, dried—4 halves
- Bananas—½ small
- Blueberries—½ cup
- Cantaloupe—¼ med. (6″ dia.)
- Cherries—10 large
- Dates—2
- Figs, dried—1 small
- Fruit cocktail, canned—½ cup
- Grapefruit—½ small
- Grapes—12
- Honeydew Melon—⅓ (7″ dia.)
- Mango—½ small
- Nectarine—1 small
- Orange—1 small
- Papaya—⅓ med.
- Peach—1 med.
- Pear—1 small
- Pineapple—½ cup
- Prunes, dried—2
- Raisins—2 Tbsp.
- Strawberries—¾ cup
- Tangerine—1 large
- Watermelon—1 cup cubed

Juices:
- Apple, Pineapple—⅓ cup
- Grapefruit, Orange—½ cup
- Grape, Prune—¼ cup

4. Starch Exchanges *(cooked servings)*

Breads:
- Any loaf—1 slice
- Bagel—½
- Danish pastry, 1¼ oz.—omit 2 fat exchanges
- Doughnut, plain, 1—omit 1 fat exchange
- Dinner roll—1 (2″ dia.)
- English muffin—½
- Bun, hamburger or hotdog—½
- Tortilla—1 (6″ dia.)

Cereals:
- Hot cereal—½ cup
- Dry flakes—⅔ cup
- Dry puffed—1½ cups
- Bran—5 Tbsp.
- Wheatgerm—2 Tbsp.
- Pastas—½ cup
- Rice—½ cup

Appendix C

Crackers:
Digestive—2 (2½" sq.)
Matzoh—½ (4"×6")
Melba Toast—4
Oysters—20 (½ cup)
Pretzels—8 rings
Rye Krisps—3
Potato crips or cornchips, 15—omit 2 fat exchanges

Desserts:
Brownie, 2" square—omit 2 fat exchanges
Chocolate cake, 1 oz.—omit ½ fat exchange
Angel cake—1½" square
Fruit pie, 1/14—omit 2 fat exchanges and ½ fruit exchange
Hard candy—½ oz.
Chocolate chip cookies, 2—omit 1 fat exchange
Ginger snaps—5 small
Ice cream, ½ cup—omit 2 fat exchanges
Ice milk, ½ cup—omit 1 fat exchange
Sorbet—4 oz.

Vegetables:
Beans or Peas, (plain) cooked—½ cup
Corn—1/3 cup or ½ med. ear
Parsnips—2/3 cup
Potatoes, white—1 small or ½ cup
Potatoes, sweet or yams—¼ cup
Pumpkin—¾ cup

Alcohol:
Beer—5 oz.
Whiskey—1 oz.
Wine, dry—2½ oz.
Wine, sweet—1½ oz.

5. Protein, cooked weight (amount equals one exchange)

Beef, dried, chipped—1 oz.
Beef, Lamb, Pork, Veal (lean only)—1 oz.
Cottage cheese, uncreamed—¼ cup
Poultry without skin—1 oz.
Fish—1 oz.
Lobster—1 small tail
Oysters, Clams, Shrimp—5 med.
Tuna, packed in water—¼ cup
Salmon, pink, canned—¼ cup
Egg—1 med.
Hard cheese—½ oz.
Peanut butter—2 tsp.

6. Milk Exchanges

Buttermilk, fat free—1 cup
Yogurt, plain, made with nonfat milk—¾ cup
Skim milk—1 cup
1% fat milk—7 oz.

7. Fat (amount equals one exchange)

Avocado—1/8
Bacon (crisp)—1 slice
Butter, margarine—1 tsp.
Cream, light or sour—2 Tbsp.
Cream, heavy—1 Tbsp.
Cream cheese—1 Tbsp.
Gravy (meat)—1 Tbsp
French dressing—1 Tbsp.
Mayonnaise—1 tsp.
Roquefort dressing—2 tsp.
Oil—1 tsp.
Olives—5 small
Almonds, Peanuts—10
Walnuts—6 small

Eat Beautiful!

Tips for Success with the Exchange System

1. Be accurate with amounts. A 3-ounce serving of cooked meat counts as 3 exchanges and is equal to approximately 4 ounces of raw lean meat.
2. Note that some foods require you to omit certain exchanges from other categories. For example, you would need to omit ½ fat exchange for *each* ounce of chocolate cake. If you ate a 3-ounce piece of cake, you would omit 1½ fat exchanges.

Source: The Exchange Lists are based on material in the "Exchange Lists for Meal Planning," prepared by committees of the American Diabetes Association and the American Dietetic Association, in cooperation with the National Institute of Arthritis, Metabolism and Digestive Diseases and the National Heart and Lung Institute of Health, PHS, U.S. DHHS.

Appendix C

Your plan: 1,500 calorie level

Food (portions)	1. Free _1_	2. Vegs. _3_	3. Fruits _4_	4. Starches _7_	5. Prots. _7_	6. Milk _2_	7. Fats _5_
Breakfast 1/2 c. orange juice 1 c. hot cereal 1 tsp. butter 2 Tbs. raisins 1 c. skim milk			1 1	2		1	1
Lunch lettuce, pickle 3/4 c. tuna 2 sl. whole wheat bread 2 tsp. mayo 3 sl. tomato 1 apple 1 c. low-fat milk 1 carrot	2	1 1	1	2	3	1	2 1 (for low-fat milk)
Dinner 1/2 c. green beans 4 oz. chicken (no skin) sm. can on cob 1/2 c. mashed potato 1 tsp. butter 3 oz. white wine 1/4 cantaloupe lettuce	1	1	1	1 1	4		1
Other times							
Totals for Day:	3	3	4	7	7	2	5
Goals for Day:	3	3	4	7	7	2	5

345

APPENDIX D
Recipes

Recipe 1
APRICOT-COTTAGE CHEESE MUFFINS
serves 4

4 English muffins, split
1 cup low-fat cottage cheese
¼ teaspoon cinnamon
16 canned apricot halves (2½-pound can of water or juice-packed, only)

In toaster, oven or grill, toast muffin halves. Combine cottage cheese and cinnamon. Mash 8 apricot halves; stir into cheese. Place apricot-cheese mixture on each of the muffin halves; heat under broiler.

Top each muffin with 1 each of remaining apricot halves. Serve immediately.

Each serving provides:
Calories: 235
Fat: 2 g
Cholesterol: 8 mg
Sodium: 153 mg
Vitamin A: 2,440 IU

From the California Apricot Advisory Board

Appendix D

Recipe 2
GINGERBREAD SQUARES
serves 12

1½ cup plain flour, sifted
½ cup whole-wheat flour
1½ teaspoons baking soda
1½ teaspoons ginger
½ teaspoon salt
1 cup molasses, blackstrap
⅓ cup (2½ ounces) margarine
½ cup buttermilk
1 egg
½ cup raisins
½ cup chopped walnuts

Sift all dry ingredients together. Bring molasses and shortening just to a boil and cool.

In large bowl, combine dry ingredients, molasses mixture, buttermilk, egg, raisins, and nuts. Mix until blended well. Bake at 350 degrees in a greased and slightly floured 9-inch square or 8-inch rectangular pan.

Each serving provides:
Calories: 240
Fat: 10 g
Cholesterol: 23 mg
Sodium: 49 mg
Iron: 5.5 mg

From the Columbia University *Nutrition and Health* newsletter.

Recipe 3
YOGURT-HERB DRESSING
makes about 1¾ cups

1 cup fresh parsley sprigs (chopped if not using blender)
⅔ cup plain low-fat yogurt
⅓ to ½ cup lemon juice
⅓ cup safflower or corn oil
1¼ tsp. dill weed
1 tsp. dry mustard

1 tsp. oriental sesame oil (optional)
¼ tsp. black pepper (or to taste)

Put all the ingredients in a blender or two-cup jar with a tight-fitting lid.

Blend or shake until all ingredients are well-mixed. Store in a refrigerator.

Each serving (2 tablespoons) provides:
Calories: 60
Fat: 6 g
Cholesterol: 15 mg
Sodium: 8 mg

From Turner, S. "If this is Tuesday, it must be Chicken Korma." *Nutrition Action*, May 1983, pp. 10–14.

Recipe 4
CHICKEN KORMA
serves 6

12 pieces chicken (any combination of legs, thighs, breasts) or 2 whole fryers cut into pieces
3 cups plain low-fat yogurt
4 tsp. curry powder
2 tsp. ground coriander (optional)
2 tsp. peeled grated ginger root or 1 tsp. powdered ginger
6 cloves garlic, minced
⅛ tsp. cayenne or black pepper (or to taste)
1 tbsp. lemon juice
2 tbsp. oil
2 medium onions, chopped
2 bay leaves

Cut chicken into serving pieces if purchased whole. Remove skin.

In a large, deep bowl combine the yogurt, curry powder, coriander (optional), ginger, garlic, pepper, and lemon juice.

Add the chicken pieces and stir to coat with marinade. Cover and refrigerate for at least 30 minutes.

Heat oil in a large, heavy soup pot.

Appendix D

Add the onion and cook until soft (5 to 8 minutes).
Add the bay leaves and cook 5 more minutes.
Add the chicken and yogurt marinade to the pot. Mix well.
Bring to a boil, then simmer over medium heat for 40 minutes.
Stir often.

Each serving provides:
Calories: 306
Fat: 11g
Cholesterol: 117 mg
Sodium: 176 mg

From Turner, S. "If this is Tuesday, it must be Chicken Korma." *Nutrition Action*, May 1983, pp. 10–14.

Recipe 5
HERB BLENDS TO REPLACE SALT
these can be placed in shakers and used instead of salt

Saltless surprise:
2 teaspoons garlic powder
1 teaspoon each of basil, oregano, and powdered lemon rind (or dehydrated lemon juice)

Put ingredients into a blender and mix well. Store in glass container, label well, and add rice to prevent caking.

Pungent salt substitute:
3 teaspoons basil
2 teaspoons each of savory (summer savory is best), celery seed, ground cumin seed, sage and marjoram
1 teaspoon lemon thyme

Mix well, then powder with a mortar and pestle.

Spicy saltless seasoning:
1 teaspoon each of cloves, pepper, and coriander seed (crushed)
2 teaspoons paprika
1 tablespoon rosemary

Mix ingredients in a blender. Store in airtight container.

From Shimizu, H. "Do yourself a flavor," *FDA Consumer*, April 1984, p. 19.

Eat Beautiful!

Recipe 6
A PRECOMPETITION LIQUID MEAL
one cup equals 200 calories

Nonfat dry milk (¼ cup)
Skim milk (3 cups)
Water (½ cup)
Sugar (¼ cup)
Flavoring, vanilla (1 teaspoon)

From American Alliance for Health, Physical Education, Recreation and Dance, 1900 Association Dr., Reston, VA 22091.

Recipe 7
STIR-FRY SAUCE
serves 6 (makes 1¼ cups)

1 can (6 oz.) low-sodium V-8 or low-sodium tomato juice
3 tbsp. red wine vinegar
1 tbsp. mild (salt-reduced) soy sauce
1 tbsp water
4 to 6 cloves garlic, minced, or coarsely chopped (if using blender)
¾-inch cube of fresh ginger, peeled and grated, or coarsely chopped (if using blender). You may substitute 1 tsp. dry powdered ginger
1½ tsp. oriental sesame oil (optional: if not using oil, add one tsp. dried mustard)
⅛ tsp. cayenne (or to taste)

Put all the ingredients into the blender or two-cup jar with a tight-fitting lid.

Blend or shake until all ingredients are well-mixed. Store in refrigerator.

Each serving (2 tablespoons) provides:
Calories: 12
Fat: 1.4 g
Cholesterol: 0 mg
Sodium: 66 mg

From Turner, S. "If this is Tuesday, it must be Chicken Korma." *Nutrition Action*, May 1983, pp. 10–14.

Appendix D

Recipe 8
LENTIL SOUP
serves 10

2 cups (12 oz.) dried lentils
2 tbsp. oil
2 medium onions, chopped
2 medium carrots, diced
2 celery ribs with leaves, diced
3 cloves garlic, minced
2 tsp. dried basil
1 tsp. dried oregano
1 bay leaf
¼ tsp. cayenne or black pepper (or to taste)
1 lb. 12 oz. canned tomatoes
8 to 9 cups water
red wine vinegar
chopped fresh parsley

Rinse and drain lentils.

In a large soup pot, heat oil and cook onions until soft (5 to 8 minutes).

Add chopped celery and carrots. Cook 5 minutes more.

Add garlic, basil, oregano, bay leaf, tomatoes and juice. Crush tomatoes with a spoon.

Add the water and lentils, bring to a boil, and simmer 45 minutes.

Serve with chopped parsley and a dash of red wine vinegar.

Each serving provides:
Calories: 213
Fat: 4 g
Cholesterol: 0 mg
Sodium: 160 mg

From Turner, S. "If this is Tuesday, it must be Chicken Korma." *Nutrition Action*, May 1983, pp. 10–14.

Eat Beautiful!

Recipe 9
MEXICAN CASSEROLE
serves 8

4 cups cooked pinto beans
2 tbsp. oil
2 medium onions, chopped
4 cloves garlic, minced
1 lb. 12 oz. canned tomatoes
2 tsp. chili powder (or to taste)
1½ tsp. oregano
½ tsp. caraway (optional)
½ tsp. cumin (optinal)
⅛ tsp. cayenne or black pepper (or to taste)
1 can (4 oz.) chopped green chilies
1 lb. firm tofu, drained and crumbled
12 corn tortillas
4 oz. (1½ cups) mild cheddar cheese, grated

Preheat oven to 375 degrees.
Mash beans with a fork and set aside. (Mashing one cup at a time on a dinner plate works well.)
In a medium saucepan, heat oil, add chopped onions and cook about 5 minutes or until soft.
Add garlic and cook on low heat for 3 minutes.
Add tomatoes and juice, chili powder, oregano, caraway and cumin (optional), and pepper. Crush tomatoes with back of spoon.
Bring to a boil, reduce heat, and simmer for 15 minutes, stirring often.
Toast tortillas on oven rack in single layers until golden (about 10 minutes).
When sauce is done, add beans, crumbled tofu, and chopped chillies.
Spread a small amount of the sauce-bean mixture (just to cover) on the bottom of four eight-inch cake or pie pans.
Layer 1½ broken tortillas in each pan.
Divide half of the sauce-bean mixture among four pans and spread over tortillas.

Appendix D

Repeat with another layer of tortillas and the remainder of sauce-bean mixture. Top with grated cheese.

Wrap well and freeze. If you are planning to serve the casserole for tonight's dinner, bake at 375 degrees for 20 to 30 minutes. If baked frozen, add 10 to 15 minutes additional baking time.

Each serving provides:
Calories: 419
Fat: 12 g
Cholesterol: 14 mg
Sodium: 262 mg

From Turner, S. "If this is Tuesday, it must be Chicken Korma." *Nutrition Action*, May 1983, pp. 10-14

Recipe 10
BANANA BRAN MUFFINS
makes 12 muffins

1¼ cups whole wheat flour
¼ cup sugar
3 tsp. baking powder
1½ cups whole bran cereal or bran
¾ cup skim milk
1 cup mashed ripe banana (2 medium-size)
1 egg
¼ cup oil

Preheat oven to hot (400°). Grease 12 muffin-pan cups or use paper muffin cups to avoid more fat. Sift flour, sugar and baking powder into a bowl; stir in any particles of bran remaining in sifter.

Combine bran, milk and banana in a medium-size bowl; let stand a few minutes for bran to soften. Beat in egg and oil. Stir in flour mixture just until flour is moistened. Divide mixture among prepared muffin cups.

Bake for 25 minutes or until muffins are golden brown. Remove from pan to wire rack; cool slightly.

Each muffin contains:
Calories: 156

Eat Beautiful!

Fat: 6 g
Cholesterol: 23 mg
Sodium: 208 mg

From *Menus and Recipes to Lower Cancer Risk*. 1984. Washington, D.C.: American Institute for Cancer Research, p. 23.

APPENDIX E
Food Sources of Nutrients

Table E1 Vitamin A (carotene) in Foods
Recommended daily amount = 2,500 I.U. Lactating women = 2,000 I.U.

Food	Serving size	Vitamin A (I.U.)
Vegetables		
Broccoli, cooked	⅔ cup	2,500
Carrots, raw	1 large	11,000
Corn, yellow, cooked	1 ear (4″)	400
Greens	¾ cup cooked	7,400
Spinach, cooked	½ cup	7,300
Fruits		
Apricots	2 to 3 medium	2,700
Cantaloupe	¼ melon	3,400
Peaches	1 medium	1,330

Table E-2 Iron in foods
Recommended daily amount for women: 12 mg

Food	Serving size	Iron (mg)
Meat, poulty, fish*		
Beef, lean (all cuts)	3 ounces	4–5
Calves' liver	3 ounces	12
Chicken livers	3 ounces	7
Clams and oysters	3 ounces	5
Lamb, lean (all cuts)	4 ounces	4–5
Liver sausage	3 ounces	4.5
Poultry	3 ounces	1.5
Shrimp	3 ounces	2.5
Beans and lentils		
Baked beans	½ cup	3
Beans, kidney	1 cup	4.5

Eat Beautiful!

Food	Serving size	Iron (mg)
Black-eyed peas, cooked	1 cup	3.5
Black beans, cooked	1 cup	7.9
Chickpeas, cooked	1 cup	6.9
Green split peas, cooked	1 cup	3.4
Lentils, cooked	1 cup	4.2
Peanut butter	2 tablespoons	0.6
Peanuts, roasted	½ cup	2.7
Soy milk	1 cup	1.8
Tofu	4 ounces	2.3
Grains		
Bread, whole wheat/white	1 slice	0.7
Oatmeal, cooked	1 cup	1.7
Pasta, enriched	½ cup	1
Rice, enriched, cooked	1 cup	1.8
Rice, brown, cooked	1 cup	1
Wheat germ	1 tablespoon	0.5
Vegetables		
Bean sprouts, raw	1 cup	1.4
Beet greens, cooked	1 cup	2.8
Broccoli	1 cup	2
Kale, cooked	1 cup	1.3
Spinach, cooked	1 cup	4.8
Fruits		
Apricots, dried	12	6
Dates	9	5
Figs, large	1	0.6
Peaches, raw	1	0.5
Prune juice	½ cup	5
Raisins	½ cup	2.7
Miscellaneous		
Almonds	½ cup	3.5
Blackstrap molasses	1 tablespoon	3.2
Brewer's yeast	1 tablespoon	1.4
Cashews	6–8	0.6
Pecans	½ cup	1.2

*The iron in animal products is more easily absorbed than the iron in plant foods.

Appendix E

Table E-3 Vitamin C in foods
Recommended daily amount = 30 mg. Pregnant women = 60 mg.

Food	Serving size	Vitamin C (mg)
Vegetables		
Broccoli, cooked	2/3 cup	90
Brussels sprouts, cooked	6–7	87
Cabbage, raw	1 cup	47
Cauliflower, raw	1 cup flower pieces	78
Green peppers, cooked	3½ ounces	96
Parsley, chopped, raw	1 tablespoon	17
Peas, boiled	2/3 cup	20
Potatoes, baked	1	20
Spinach, cooked	½ cup	25
Tomatoes, raw	1 small	23
Turnip greens, boiled	½ cup	139
Fruits		
Cantaloupe	¼ melon	33
Guava	1 medium	242
Lemon	1 medium	53
Orange	1 medium	80
Pineapple, raw	¾ cup	17
Strawberries	10 large	59

Table E-4 Folacin in foods

Food	Serving size	Folacin (µg)
Meat, poultry, fish		
Beef, veal, pork (lean)	6 ounces	5–20
Kidney	3 ounces	20–50
Liver	3 ounces	100–150
Shellfish	6 ounces	20–50
Dairy products and eggs		
Egg	1 large	20–50
Cheese, hard	1 ounce	5–20
Milk	8 ounces	5–20
Yogurt	8 ounces	20–50
Vegetables		
Broccoli	2 stalks	100–150
Green beans	1 cup	20–50
Cucumber	1 small	20–50
Spinach	4 ounces	200–300

Eat Beautiful!

Food	Serving size	Folacin (µg)
Fruit		
Grapefruit	½ medium	5–20
Orange juice	6 ounces	100–150
Strawberries	1 cup	20–50
Miscellaneous		
Brewer's yeast	1 tablespoon	200–300
Sesame seeds	1 tablespoon	5–20

Source: *Nutrition and Health* 4(1), 1982, M. Winick, ed.

Table E-5 Calcium in foods

Recommended daily amount for women: 500 mg. Pregnant and lactating: 1200 mg.

Food	Serving size	Calcium (mg)
Meat, poultry, fish		
Chicken	3 ounces	10
Haddock	1 fillet	23
Hamburger	3 ounces	10
Oysters	1 cup	226
Salmon (canned, with bones)	3 ounces	165
Sardines (with bones)	3 ounces	370
Shrimp (canned)	3 ounces	100
Tuna	3 ounces	5
Beans and lentils		
Baked beans	½ cup	70
Chili with beans	1 cup	90
Lentils, cooked	1 cup	75
Navy beans, cooked	½ cup	48
Tofu (processed with calcium sulfate)	4 ounces	145
Dairy products and eggs		
Buttermilk	1 cup	285
Cheese:		
Cheddar	1 ounce	210
Cottage, lowfat	½ cup	75
Cream	2 tablespoons	20
Ricotta	½ cup	335
Swiss	1 ounce	270
Egg	1 large	30
Ice cream, vanilla	½ cup	100

Appendix E

Food	Serving size	Calcium (mg)
Ice milk, vanilla	½ cup	275
Milk, lowfat	1 cup	300
Milk, whole	1 cup	290
Pudding, chocolate	½ cup	187
Soybean milk	1 cup	60
Yogurt, lowfat, plain	1 cup	415
Grains		
Bread, whole-wheat	1 slice	20
Oatmeal, cooked	1 cup	22
Pancakes, buttermilk	3 (4-inch)	174
Spaghetti, cooked	1 cup	15
Tortilla, corn	1 (6-inch diameter)	60
Vegetables		
Beans, green	½ cup	30
Bok choy	1 cup	116
Broccoli	½ cup	70
Kale, cooked	½ cup	74
Okra, cooked	½ cup	74
Swede, cooked	½ cup	71
Spinach*	½ cup	85
Turnip greens	1 cup	267
Watercress, chopped	1 cup	189
Fruits		
Apple	1 medium	10
Apricots, dried, cooked	½ cup	25
Figs, dried	1 large	26
Orange	1 medium	55
Prunes, uncooked	4	14
Miscellaneous		
Almonds	12–15	40
Blackstrap molasses	1 tablespoon	135
Brewer's yeast	1 ounce	60
Peanut butter	1 tablespoon	20
Pizza, cheese	¼ of 14-inch pie	330
Sesame seeds, whole	¼ cup	348

*Calcium in spinach is not easily absorbed.

Eat Beautiful!

Table E-6 Cholesterol in foods

Food	Serving size	Cholesterol (mg)
Meat and poultry		
Beef, lean	3 ounces	77
Hotdog, all-beef	1	27
Beef liver	3 ounces	372
Pork and ham, lean	3 ounces	80
Bacon	2 slices	11
Chicken, (no skin)		
light meat	3 ounces	76
dark meat	3 ounces	82
Fish, lean	3 ounces	43
fat	3 ounces	40
Shellfish		
lobster	½ cup	90
shrimp	11 large	96
Tuna (in water)	3 ounces	55
Dairy products and eggs		
Milk, whole	1 cup	33
skim	1 cup	4
Cheese, hard	1 ounce	30
Cottage cheese,		
creamed	1 cup	31
uncreamed	1 cup	10
Mozzarella (part skim)	1 ounce	16
Egg	1 medium	274
Fats		
Butter	1 tablespoon	31
Margarine	1 tablespoon	0
Peanut butter	2 tablespoons	0

Table E-7 Dietary fiber in foods
Daily fiber goal: 30 grams

Food	Serving size	Fiber (grams)
Breads and crackers		
Rye crackers	3 wafers	2.3
Rye bread	1 slice	2.0
Whole-wheat bread	1 slice	2.4

Appendix E

Food	Serving size	Fiber (grams)
Cereals		
All-Bran or 100% Bran	1 cup	23.0
Cracked wheat (bulgur), dry	1/3 cup	5.6
Grape-Nuts	1/3 cup	5.0
Rolled oats, dry	1/2 cup	4.5
Shredded wheat	2 biscuits	6.1
Fruits		
Apple	1 small	3.1
Applesauce	1/2 cup	1.7
Banana	1 medium	1.8
Cantaloupe, cubes	3/4 cup	1.4
Cherries, raw	10	0.8
Grapefruit	1/2	2.6
Grapes, raw	16	0.4
Orange	1 small	1.8
Peach, raw	1 medium	1.3
Peaches, canned slices	1/2 cup	1.3
Pear, raw	1 medium	2.8
Pears, canned	1/2 cup	1.4
Plum, raw	2 small	1.6
Strawberries	1/2 cup	2.6
Tangerine	1 medium	2.1
Vegetables		
Beans, green	1/2 cup	1.2
Beets, cooked	2/3 cup	2.1
Broccoli, cooked	3/4 cup	1.6
Cabbage, cooked	3/4 cup	2.2
Cabbage, raw	1 cup	2.1
Carrots, raw	1 medium	3.7
Cauliflower, cooked	1/2 cup	1.2
Cauliflower, raw	1 cup	1.8
Celery, cooked	2/3 cup	2.4
Celery, raw	2½ stalks	3.0
Corn kernels	2/3 cup	4.2
Cucumber	1/2 of 7-inch cucumber	1.5
Kale, cooked	1/2 cup	2.0
Kidney beans, cooked	1 cup	3.6
Lentils, cooked	1/2 cup	4.0
Lettuce	1 cup	0.8
Parsnips, cooked	3/4 cup	5.9

Eat Beautiful!

Food	Serving size	Fiber (grams)
Peas, cooked	½ cup	3.8
Potatoes, cooked	⅔ cup	3.1
Rice, brown, cooked	1 cup	1.1
Rice, white, cooked	1 cup	0.4
Spinach	2 large leaves	1.8
Summer squash, cooked	½ cup	2.2
Summer squash, raw	1 5-inch squash	3.0
Turnips, raw	1 cup	2.2

From fiber analyses prepared by Dr. James W. Anderson, professor of medicine and clinical nutrition at the University of Kentucky Medical Center in Lexington, Kentucky.

Selected References

ADOLESCENCE

Frisch, R. E., and J. W. McArthur. "Menstrual cycles: Fatness as determinant of minimum weight for height necessary for their maintenance or onset." *Science* 185:949–51, 1974.

Garn, S. M., and M. LaVelle. "Reproductive histories of low weight girls and women." *American Journal of Clinical Nutrition* 37:862–66, 1983.

Hallberg, L., A. M. Hogdahl, L. Nilsson, and G. Rybo. "Menstrual blood loss: A population study." *Acta Obstetricia et Gynecologica Scandinavica* 45:320, 1966.

Hamill, P., T. Drizd, C. L. Johnson, R. B. Reed, A. F. Roche, and W. M. Moore. "Physical growth: National Center for Health Statistics percentiles." *American Journal of Clinical Nutrition* 32:607–29, 1979.

Hill, P., L. Garbaczewski, J. Huskisson, E. Sporangisa, and E. L. Wynder. "Diet, lifestyle, and menstrual activity." *American Journal of Clinical Nutrition* 33:1192–98, 1980.

Katchadourian, H. *The Biology of Adolescence*. San Francisco: W. H. Freeman and Company, 1977.

Marynick, S. P., Z. H. Chakmakjian, D. L. McCaffree, and J. H. Herndon, Jr. "Androgen excess in cystic acne." *New England Journal of Medicine* 308:981–86, 1983.

Matsuoka, L. Y. "Acne." *Journal of Pediatrics* 103:849–53, 1983.

Pugliese, M., F. Lifshitz, G. Grad, P. Fort, and M. Marks-Katz. "Fear of obesity: A cause of short stature and delayed puberty." *New England Journal of Medicine* 309:513–17, 1983.

U.S. Department of Health, Education, and Welfare. *Ten-State Nutrition Survey, 1968–1970: V. Dietary*. DHEW Publication no. (HSM) 72-8133, 1972.

Vincent, L. M. *Competing with the Sylph: Dancers and the Pursuit of the Ideal Body Form*. New York: Andrews & McMeel, Inc., 1979.

YOUNG ADULTHOOD

Abraham, G., and M. Lubran. "Serum and red cell magnesium levels in patients with premenstrual tension." *American Journal of Clinical Nutrition* 34:2364–66, 1981.

Adams, P. W., D. Rose, J. Folkard, V. Wynn, M. Seed, and R. Strong. "Effect of pyridoxine hydrochloride (vitamin B_6) upon depression associated with oral contraception." *Lancet* 1:897–904, 1973.

Bothwell, T.H., and R. W. Charlton. *Iron Deficiency in Women: A Report of the International Nutritional Anemia Consultative Group.* Washington, D.C.: The Nutrition Foundation, 1981.

Dalvit, S. "The effect of the menstrual cycle on patterns of food intake." *American Journal of Clinical Nutrition* 34:1811–15, 1981.

Foss, S., and R. Keith. "Food habits and dietary adequacy of single, professional women." *Nutritional Reports International* 26:613–29, 1982.

Pliner, P., and A. S. Fleming. "Food intake, body weight, and sweetness preferences over the menstrual cycle in humans." *Physiology and Behavior* 30:663–66, 1983

Prasad, A., D. Oberleas, K. Y. Lei, K. Moghassi, and J. Stryker. "Effect of oral contraceptive agents on nutrients: I. Minerals." *American Journal of Clinical Nutrition* 28:377–84, 1975.

Prasad, A., K. Y. Lei, D. Oberleas, K. Moghassi, and J. Stryker. "Effect of oral contraceptive agents on nutrients: II. Vitamins." *American Journal of Clinical Nutrition* 28:385–91, 1975.

Reid, R., and S. Yen. "Premenstrual syndrome." *American Journal of Obstetrics and Gynecology* 139:85–104, 1981.

Schaumburg, H., J. Kaplan, A. Windebank, N. Vick, S. Rasmus, D. Pleasure, and M. J. Brown. "Sensory neuropathy from pyridoxine abuse: A new megavitamin syndrome." *New England Journal of Medicine* 309:445–48, 1983.

Solomon, S., M. Kurzer, and D. Calloway. "Menstrual cycle and basal metabolic rate in women." *American Journal of Clinical Nutrition* 36:611–16, 1982.

PREGNANCY

Bates, G. W., S. R. Bates, and N. S. Whitworth. "Reproductive failure in women who practice weight control." *Fertility and Sterility* 37(3):373–78, 1982.

Clarke, H., ed. "Physical activity during menstruation and pregnancy." President's Council on Physical Fitness and Sports. *Physical Fitness Research Digest*, ser. 8(3), July, 1978.

Frisancho, A., J. Matos, and P. Flegel. "Maternal nutritional status and adolescent pregnancy outcome." *American Journal of Clinical Nutrition* 38:739–46, 1983.

Higginbottom, M. C., L. Sweetman, and W. L. Nyhan. "A syndrome of methylmalonic aciduria, homocystinuria, megaloblastic anemia and neurologic abnormalities in a vitamin B_{12}-deficient breast-fed infant of a strict vegetarian." *New England Journal of Medicine* 299:317–23, 1978.

Linn, S., S. C. Schoenbaum, R. Monson, B. Rosner, P. Stubblefield, and K. Ryan. "No association between coffee consumption and adverse outcomes of pregnancy." *New England Journal of Medicine* 306:141–45, 1982.

Metzger, B. E., V. Ravnikar, R. A. Vileisis, and N. Freinkel. "'Accelerated starvation' and the skipped breakfast in late normal pregnancy." *Lancet*: 588–92, March 13, 1982.

National Research Council. Food and Nutrition Board. Committee on Nutrition of the Mother and Preschool Child. *Alternative Dietary Practices and Nutritional Abuses in Pregnancy*. Washington, D.C.: National Academy Press, 1982.

Roepke, J., and A. Kirksey. "Vitamin B_6 nutriture during pregnancy and lactation: II. The effect of long-term use of oral contraceptives." *American Journal of Clinical Nutrition* 32:2257–64, 1979.

Rosenberg, L., A. A. Mitchell, S. Shapiro, and D. Slone. "Selected birth defects in relation to caffeine-containing beverages." *Journal of the American Medical Association* 247:1429–32, 1982.

Ulleland, C. N. "The offspring of alcoholic mothers." *Annals of the New York Academy of Sciences* 197:167, 1972.

Zaharieva, E. "Olympic participation by women: Effects on pregnancy and childbirth." *Journal of the American Medical Association* 221:992–95, 1972.

BREASTFEEDING

Berlin, C. M., H. M. Denson, C. H. Daniel, and R. M. Ward. "Disposition of dietary caffeine in milk, saliva, and plasma of lactating women." *Pediatrics* 73:59–63, 1984.

Chopra, J. "Effect of steroid contraceptives on lactation." *American Journal of Clinical Nutrition* 25:1202–14, 1972.

Committee on Drugs. "The transfer of drugs and other chemicals into human breast milk." *Pediatrics* 72:375–83, 1983.

Perez-Reyes, M., and M. E. Wall. "Presence of 9-tetrahydrocannabinol in human milk" (correspondence). *New England Journal of Medicine* 307:819–20, 1982.

Rogan, W., A. Bagniewska, and T. Damstra. "Pollutants in breast milk." *New England Journal of Medicine* 302:1450–53, 1980.

MIDDLE ADULTHOOD

Anon. "Smoking and the age of menopause." *Research in Reproduction* 9(4):2, 1977.

Heaney, R., J. Gallagher, C. Johnston, R. Neer, A. Parfitt, B. Chir, and G. Whedon. "Calcium nutrition and bone health in the elderly." *American Journal of Clinical Nutrition* 36:986–1013, 1982.

Heaney, R., and R. R. Recker. "Effects of nitrogen balance, phosphorus, and caffeine on calcium balance in women." *Journal of Laboratory and Clinical Medicine* 99:46–55, 1982.

Parfitt, A., B. Chir, J. Gallagher, R. Heaney, C. Johnston, R. Neer, and G. Whedon. "Vitamin D and bone health in the elderly." *American Journal of Clinical Nutrition* 36:1014–31, 1982.

Raisz, L. "Osteoporosis." *Journal of the American Geriatrics Society* 30:127–38, 1982.

Roberts, H. J. "Potential toxicity due to dolomite and bonemeal." *Southern Medical Journal* 76:556–59, 1983.

Spencer, H., L. Kramer, and D. Osis. "Factors contributing to calcium loss in aging." *American Journal of Clinical Nutrition* 36 (supplement):776–87, 1982.

THE LATER YEARS

Abraham, S., M. D. Carroll, C. M. Dresser, and C. L. Johnson. *Dietary Intake Findings, United States 1971–74*. DHEW Publication no. HRA 77-1647, 1977.

Andres, R. "Effect of obesity on total mortality." *International Journal of Obesity* 4:381–86, 1980.

Harper, A. "Nutrition, aging, and longevity." *American Journal of Clinical Nutrition* 36 (supplement):737–49, 1982.

Insogna, K. L., D. R. Bordley, J. F. Caro, and D. H. Lockwood. "Osteomalacia and weakness from excessive antacid ingestion." *Journal of the American Medical Association* 244:2544–46, 1980.

Jeffay, H. "Obesity and aging." *American Journal of Clinical Nutrition* 36 (supplement):809–11, 1982.

Kohrs, M. B. "A rational diet for the elderly." *American Journal of Clinical Nutrition* 36 (supplement):796–802, 1982.

Kohrs, M. B., and S. K. Kamath, eds. "Symposium on nutrition and aging." *American Journal of Clinical Nutrition* 35 (supplement):1–96, 1982.

McCay, C. M., M. F. Crowell, and L. A. Maynard. "The effect of retarded growth upon the length of life span and upon the ultimate body size." *Journal of Nutrition* 10:63–79, 1935.

Mishara, B. L., and R. Kastenbaum. *Alcohol and Old Age*. New York: Grune & Stratton, 1980.

Selected References

Morrison, S. D. "Nutrition and longevity." *Nutrition Reviews* 41:133–42, 1983.

Rivlin, R., and E. Young, eds. "Symposium on evidence relating selected vitamins and minerals to health and disease in the elderly population in the United States." *American Journal of Clinical Nutrition* 36 (supplement):977–1086, 1982.

Ross, M. H. "Length of life and caloric intake." *American Journal of Clinical Nutrition* 25:834–38, 1972.

Watkin, D. "The physiology of aging." *American Journal of Clinical Nutrition* 36 (supplement):750–58, 1982.

WEIGHT CONTROL

A. C. Nielsen Company. *Who's Dieting and Why* (a survey), 1978.

Bjorntorp, R., and L. Sjostrom. "Number and size of adipose tissue fat cells in relation to metabolism in human obesity." *Metabolism* 20:703–713, 1971.

Bray, G. A., ed. *Obesity in America*. Public Health Service, National Institutes of Health. NIH Publication no. 79–359, 1979.

Coates, T. J. "Eating—A psychological dilemma." *Journal of Nutrition Education* 13 (supplement):S34–S48, 1981.

Dwyer, J., J. Feldman, and J. Mayer. "The social psychology of dieting." *Journal of Health and Social Behavior* 11:269–87, 1970.

"Exercising within several hours of eating can burn more kilo-calories." *Journal of the American Dietetic Association* 83:290, 1983.

Garrison, R. J., M. Feinleib, W. P. Castelli, and P. M. McNamara. "Cigarette smoking as a confounder of the relationship between relative weight and long-term mortality." *Journal of the American Medical Association* 249—2199–2203, 1983.

Goldblatt, P. B., M. E. Moore, and A. J. Stunkard. "Social factors in obesity." *Journal of the American Medical Association* 192:1039–44, 1965.

HEW News, December 20, 1979, p. 40 (results of saccharin and bladder cancer study).

Hirsch, J., and J. L. Knittle. "Cellularity of obese and nonobese human adipose tissue." *Federation Proceedings* 29:1516, 1970.

Keesey, R. "Set-points and body weight regulation." In *The Psychiatric Clinics of North America*. Vol. 1, *Obesity: Basic Mechanisms and Treatment*, edited by A. J. Stunkard, pp. 523–43. Philadelphia: W. B. Saunders, 1978.

Keys, A. "Overweight, obesity, coronary heart disease and mortality." *Nutrition Reviews* 38:297–307, 1980.

Knapp, T. R. "A methodological critique of the 'ideal weight' concept." *Journal of the American Medical Association* 250:506–10, 1983.

Mancini, M., G. DiBiase, F. Contaldo, A. Fischetti, L. Grasso, and P. Mattioli. "Medical complications of severe obesity: Importance of treatment by very-low-calorie diets. Intermediate and long term effects." *International Journal of Obesity* 5:341, 1981.

Morrison, A. S., and J. E. Buring. "Artificial sweeteners and cancer of the lower urinary tract." *New England Journal of Medicine* 302:537–41, 1980.

Rolls, B. J., E. A. Rowe, and E. T. Rolls. "How sensory properties of food affect human feeding behavior." *Physiology and Behavior* 29:409, 1982.

Sclafani, A., and D. Springer. "Dietary obesity in adult rats: Similarities to hypothalamic and human obesity syndromes." *Physiology and Behavior* 17:461, 1976.

Sorlie, P., T. Gordon, and W. B. Kannel. "Body build and mortality: The Framingham Study." *Journal of the American Medical Association* 243:1828–31, 1980.

Stunkard, A. J., W. J. Grace, and H. G. Wolff. "The night-eating syndrome: A pattern of food intake among certain obese patients." *American Journal of Medicine* 19:78, 1955.

Stunkard, A. J., ed. *Obesity*. Philadelphia: W. B. Saunders, 1980.

Van Itallie, T. "Obesity: Adverse effects on health and longevity." *American Journal of Clinical Nutrition* 32:2723–33, 1979.

Wurtman, R. J. "Neurochemical changes following high-dose aspartame with dietary carbohydrates" (letter). *New England Journal of Medicine* 309:429–30, 1983.

SHAPE-UP PROGRAM

Craighead, L. W., A. J. Stunkard, and R. O'Brien. "Behavior therapy and pharmacotherapy of obesity. *Archives of General Psychiatry* 38:763–68, 1981.

Mahoney, M. J., and K. Mahoney. *Permanent Weight Control*. New York: Norton, 1976.

Stuart, R. B. "Behavioral control of overeating: A status report." In *Obesity in America*, edited by G. A. Bray. DHEW Publication no. NIH 75–708, 1976.

Stuart, R., and B. Davis. *Slim Chance in a Fat World: Behavioral Control of Obesity*. Champaign, Ill.: Research Press, 1972.

Stunkard, A. J. "Obesity." In *International Handbook of Behavior Modification and Therapy*, edited by A. S. Bellack, M. Hersen, and A. E. Kazdin, pp. 535–73. New York: Plenum Press, 1982.

Selected References

EATING DISORDERS

Bruch, H. *Eating Disorders: Obesity, Anorexia Nervosa, and the Person Within.* New York: Basic Books, 1973.

Bruch, H. *The Golden Cage: The Enigma of Anorexia Nervosa.* Open Books, 1980.

Neuman, P., and P. Halvorson. *Anorexia Nervosa and Bulimia: A Handbook for Counselors and Therapists.* New York: Van Nostrand Reinhold, 1983.

ATHLETES

Barnett, S. W., and R. K. Conlee. "The effects of a commercial dietary supplement on human performance." *American Journal of Clinical Nutrition* 40:586–90, 1984.

Bonen, A., and H. Keizer. "Athletic menstrual cycle irregularity: Endocrine response to exercise and training." *The Physician and Sportsmedicine* 12(8):78–94, 1984.

Bullen, B. A., et al. "Induction of menstrual disorders by strenuous exercise in untrained women." *New England Journal of Medicine* 312:1349–53, 1985.

Carlberg, K. A., M. T. Buckman, G. T. Peake, and M. L. Riedesel. "Body composition of oligo/amenorrheic athletes." *Medicine and Science in Sports and Exercise* 15(3):215–17, 1983.

Costil, D. L., and J. M. Miller. "Nutrition for endurance sports: Carbohydrate and fluid balance." *International Journal of Sports Medicine* 1:2, 1980.

Drinkwater, B., K. Nilson, C. Chesnut, III, W. Bremner, S. Shainholtz, and M. Southworth. "Bone mineral content of amenorrheic and eumenorrheic athletes." *New England Journal of Medicine* 311:277–81, 1984.

Frisch, R. E., G. Wysak, and L. Vincent. "Delayed menarche and amenorrhea in ballet dancers." *New England Journal of Medicine* 303:17–19, 1980.

Grandjean, A. "Vitamins, diet, and the athlete." *Clinics in Sports Medicine* 2:105–14, 1983.

Gray, M., and L. Titlow. "B_{15}: Myth or miracle." *The Physician and Sportsmedicine* 10(1):107–12, 1982.

Keller, K., and R. Schwarzkopf. "Preexercise snacks may decrease exercise performance." *The Physician and Sportsmedicine* 12(4):89–91, 1984.

Parr, R. B., L. A. Bachman, and R. A. Moss. "Iron deficiency in female athletes." *The Physician and Sportsmedicine* 12(4):81–86, 1984.

Stein, T. P., M. D. Schluter, and C. E. Diamond. "Nutrition, protein turnover, and physical activity in young women." *American Journal of Clinical Nutrition* 38:223–28, 1983.

Williams, M., ed. *Ergogenic Aids in Sport*. Champaign, Ill.: Human Kinetics Publishers, 1983.

BEAUTY

Barrett, S. "Commercial hair analysis: Science or scam?" *Journal of the American Medical Association* 254:1041–45, 1985.

Hambridge, K. M. "Hair analyses: Worthless for vitamins, limited for minerals." *American Journal of Clinical Nutrition* 36:943–49, 1982.

Rivlin, R. S. "Misuse of hair analysis for nutritional assessment." *American Journal of Medicine* 75:489–93, 1983.

ATHEROSCLEROSIS

Gruchiow, H., K. Sobocinski, and J. Barboriak. "Alcohol, nutrient intake, and hypertension in U.S. adults." *Journal of the American Medical Association* 253:1567–70, 1985.

Havlik, R. J., and M. Feinleib, eds. *"Proceedings of the conference on the decline in coronary heart disease mortality."* USDHEW, PHS, NIH Publication no. 79–1610, May, 1979.

Hayes, S., and M. Feinlieb. "Women, work, and coronary heart disease: Prospective findings from Framingham." *American Journal of Public Health* 70(2):133–41, 1980.

Kromhout, D., E. B. Bosschieter, and C. de Lezenne Coulander. "The inverse relation between fish consumption and 20-year mortality from coronary heart disease." *New England Journal of Medicine* 312:1205–9, 1985.

Marx, J. "The HDL: The good cholesterol carriers?" *Science* 205:677–79, 1979.

McCarron, D., C. Morris, H. Henry, and J. Stanton. "Blood pressure and nutrient intake in the United States." *Science* 224:1392–98, 1984.

Wood, P. D., W. Haskell, H. Klein, S. Lewis, M. P. Stern, and J. W. Farquhar. "The distribution of plasma lipoproteins in middle-aged male runners." *Metabolism* 25:1249–57, 1976.

CANCER

Ames, B. "Dietary carcinogens and anticarcinogens: Oxygen radical and degenerative diseases." *Science* 221:1256–64, 1983.

Brown, R. R. "The role of diet in cancer causation." *Food Technology*: 49–79, March 1983.

Kromhout, D., E. Bosschieter, and C. de Lezenne Coulander. "Dietary fibre and 10-year mortality from coronary heart disease, cancer, and

Selected References

all causes: The Zutphen Study." *Lancet*: 518–521, September 4, 1982.

Moertel, C. G., et al. "A clinical trial of amygdalin (laetrile) in the treatment of human cancer." *New England Journal of Medicine* 306:201–6, 1982.

National Research Council. Assembly of Life Sciences. Committee on Diet, Nutrition, and Cancer. *Diet, Nutrition, and Cancer*. Washington, D.C.: National Academy Press, 1982.

Pollack, E. S., A. Nomura, L. Heilbrun, G. Stemmermann, and S. B. Green. "Prospective study of alcohol consumption and cancer." *New England Journal of Medicine* 310:617–21, 1984.

Sandler, R. S. "Diet and cancer: Food additives, coffee, and alcohol." *Nutrition and Cancer* 4:385–92, 1983.

Willett, W. C., and B. MacMahon. "Diet and cancer: An overview" (first of two parts). *New England Journal of Medicine* 310:697–703, 1984.

Wynder, E. L. "The dietary environment and cancer." *Journal of the American Dietetic Association* 71:385–92, 1977.

DIABETES

Anderson, J. W. "Dietary fiber and diabetes." In *Dietary Fiber in Health and Disease*, edited by G. V. Vahouny and D. Kritchevsky, pp. 151–67. New York: Plenum Press, 1982.

Crapo, P. A., J. Insel, M. Sperling, and O. G. Kolterman. "Comparison of serum glucose, insulin, and glucagon response to different types of complex carbohydrates in noninsulin-dependent diabetic patients." *American Journal of Clinical Nutrition* 34:184–90, 1981.

Evans, D. J., R. G. Hoffman, R. K. Kalkhoff, and A. H. Kissebah. "Relationship of body fat topography to insulin sensitivity and metabolic profiles in premenopausal women." *Metabolism* 33:68–75, 1984.

Horwitz, D. "Diabetes and aging." *American Journal of Clinical Nutrition* 36 (supplement):803–8, 1982.

Jenkins, D. J. A., et al. "Glycemic index of foods: A physiological basis for carbohydrate exchange." *American Journal of Clinical Nutrition* 34:362–66, 1981.

Kalkhoff, R. K., A. H. Hartz, D. Rupley, A. H. Kissebah, and S. Kelber. "Relationship of body fat distribution to blood pressure, carbohydrate tolerance, and plasma lipids in healthy obese women." *Journal of Laboratory and Clinical Medicine* 102:621–27, 1983.

Yager, J., and R. T. Young. "Non-hypoglycemia is an epidemic condition." *New England Journal of Medicine* 291:907–8, 1974.

GASTROINTESTINAL DISORDERS

Eastwood, M. A., and R. M. Kay. "An hypothesis for the action of dietary fiber along the gastrointestinal tract." *American Journal of Clinical Nutrition* 32:364–67, 1979.

Eisele, J. W., and D. T. Reay. "Deaths related to coffee enemas." *Journal of the American Medical Association* 244:1608–9, 1980.

Fontana, V. J., and F. Moreno-Pagan. "Allergy and diet." In *Modern Nutrition in Health and Disease*, 6th ed., edited by R. S. Goodhart and M. E. Shils, pp. 1071–81. Philadelphia: Lea & Febiger, 1980.

Kelsay, J. L. "A review of research on effects of fiber intake on man." *American Journal of Clinical Nutrition* 31:142–59, 1978.

Parker, C. "Food allergies." *American Journal of Nursing* 80:262–65, 1980.

Slavin, J. "Dietary fiber." *Ross Dietetic Currents* 10(6):27–32, 1983.

Spiller, G., and H. Freeman. "Recent advances in dietary fiber and colorectal diseases." *American Journal of Clinical Nutrition* 34:1145–52, 1981.

IN THE KITCHEN

American Dietetic Association. Position paper on the vegetarian approach to eating. *Journal of the American Dietetic Association* 77:61–69, 1980.

Bergan, J. G., and P. T. Brown. "Nutritional status of 'new' vegetarians." *Journal of the American Dietetic Association* 76:151–55, 1980.

Dubick, M. "Dietary supplements and health aids—A critical evaluation. Part 3: Natural and miscellaneous products." *Journal of Nutrition Education* 15:123–28, 1983.

Ellis, F. R., and V. M. E. Montegriffo. "Veganism, clinical findings and investigations." *American Journal of Clinical Nutrition* 23:249–55, 1970.

Frader, J., B. Reibman, and D. Turkewitz. "Vitamin B_{12} deficiency in strict vegetarians" (letter). *New England Journal of Medicine* 299:1319, 1978.

Gourdine, S. P., W. W. Traiger, and D. S. Cohen. "Health food stores investigation." *Journal of the American Dietetic Association* 83:285–90, 1983.

Hergenrather, J., G. Hlady, B. Wallace, and E. Savage. "Pollutants in breast milk of vegetarians" (letter). *New England Journal of Medicine* 304:792, 1981.

Hogan, R. "Hemorrhagic diathesis caused by drinking an herbal tea." *Journal of the American Medical Association* 249:2679–80, 1983.

Selected References

Jukes, T. H. "Pesticides reported used in growing 'health foods.'" *AIN Nutrition Notes*: 6, June 1979.

Marsh, A., T. Sanchez, F. Chaffee, G. Mayor, and O. Mickelsen. "Bone mineral mass in adult lacto-ovo-vegetarian and omnivorous males." *American Journal of Clinical Nutrition* 37:453–56, 1983.

Mertz, W. "Mineral elements: New perspectives." *Journal of the American Journal of Clinical Nutrition* 37:453–56, 1983.

Mertz, W. "Mineral elements: New perspectives." *Journal of the American Dietetic Association* 77:258–63, 1980.

Sacks, F. M., et al. "Effect of ingestion of meat on plasma cholesterol of vegetarians." *Journal of the American Medical Association* 246:640–44, 1981.

Sacks, F. M., W. P. Castelli, A. Donner, and E. H. Kass. "Plasma lipids and lipoproteins in vegetarians and controls." *New England Journal of Medicine* 292:1148–51, 1975.

Stookey, H. E., B. Miller, and K. A. Meister. ACSH Survey: "Do health food stores give sound nutrition advice?" *ACSH News and Views* 4(3):1, 8–9, 13–14, 1983.

Svec, L. V., C. A. Thoroughgood, and H. C. S. Mok. "Chemical evaluation of vegetables grown with conventional or organic soil amendments." *Communications in Soil Science and Plant Analysis* 7(2):213–28, 1976.

IN THE WORKPLACE

Criqui, M. H., et al. "Cigarrete smoking and high density lipoprotein cholesterol—the lipid research clinics prevalence study" (abstract). *CVD Epidemiology Newsletter* 28:26, 1980.

Curatolo, P. N., and D. Robertson. "Health consequences of caffeine." *Annals of Internal Medicine* 98:641–53, 1984.

Dawber, T. R., W. B. Kannel, and T. Gordon. "Coffee and cardiovascular disease: Observations from the Framingham Study." *New England Journal of Medicine* 291—871–74, 1974.

Dickie, N. H., and A. E. Bender. "Breakfast and performance." *Human Nutrition: Applied Nutrition* 36A:46–56, 1982.

Ernster, V. L., et al. "Effects of caffeine-free diet on benign breast disease: A randomized trial." *Surgery* 91:263–67, 1982.

Feinstein, A. R., R. I. Horwitz, W. O. Spitzer, and R. N. Battista. "Coffee and pancreatic cancer, the problems of etiologic science and epidemiologic case-control research" (commentary). *Journal of the American Medical Association* 246:957–61, 1981.

Gillespie, A. H., and M. M. Devine. "Nutrition and the management of stress." *Cornell Human Ecology Forum* 13(1):14–17, 1982.

Heyden, S., H. Tyroler, G. Heiss, C. Hames, and A. Barte. "Coffee consumption and mortality: Total mortality, stroke mortality, and coronary heart disease mortality." *Archives of Internal Medicine* 138:1472–1475, 1978.

IFT's Expert Panel on Food Safety and Nutrition. "Caffeine: A scientific status summary." *Food Technology*: 87–91, April 1983.

MacMahon, B., S. Yen, D. Trichopoulos, K. Warren, and G. Nardi. "Coffee and cancer of the pancreas." *New England Journal of Medicine* 304:630–33, 1981.

Marshall, J., S. Graham, and M. Swanson. "Caffeine consumption and benign breast disease: A case-control comparison." *American Journal of Public Health* 72:610–13, 1982.

Minton, J. P., M. K. Foecking, D. J. T. Webster, and R. H. Matthews. "Response of fibrocystic disease to caffeine withdrawal and correlation of cyclic nucleotides with breast disease." *American Journal of Obstetrics and Gynecology* 135:157–58, 1979.

Monro, J., C. Carini, and J. Brostoff. "Migraine is a food-allergic disease." *Lancet*: 719–21, Sept. 29, 1985.

"The selling of H_2O." *Consumer Reports* 45:531–38, September 1980.

Thelle, D. S., E. Arnesen, and O. H. Forde. "The Tromso Heart Study: Does coffee raise serum cholesterol?" *New England Journal of Medicine* 308:1454–57, 1983.

Williams, P. T., P. Wood, K. Vranizan, J. J. Albers, S. C. Garay, and C. B. Taylor. "Coffee intake and elevated cholesterol and apolipoprotein B levels in men." *Journal of the American Medical Association* 253:1407–11, 1985.

ON THE TOWN

Klatsky, A., G. D. Friedman, and A. Siegelaub. "Alcohol and mortality: A ten-year Kaiser-Permanente Experience." *Annals of Internal Medicine* 95:139–45, 1981.

Marshall, A. W., D. Kingstone, M. Bass, and M. Y. Morgan. "Ethanol elimination in males and females: Relationship to menstrual cycle and body composition." *Hepatology* 3:701–6, 1983.

Roe, D. "Nutritional concerns in the alcoholic." *Journal of the American Dietetic Association* 78:17–21, 1981.

Yano, K., G. G. Rhoads, and A. Kagan. "Coffee, alcohol and risk of coronary heart disease among Japanese men living in Hawaii." *New England Journal of Medicine* 297:405–9, 1977.

APPENDIX A

Alhadeff, L., C. Gualtieri, and M. Lipton. "Toxic effects of water-soluble vitamins." *Nutrition Reviews* 42:33–40, 1984.

Index

abortion, 72
acid-base balance, 323
acne, 22–25
additives, 227
  allergies to, 249
  listed on food labels, 269–70
  restaurant use of, 315, 317
adolescence, 13–33
  eating strategy in, 30–33
  health concerns of, 15–33
  physical changes in, 13–15
  pregnancy in, 73
  psychological changes in, 15
aerobic exercise, 147–48
aflatoxin, 228
aging:
  diabetes and, 237–38
  first signs of, 34–35
  of skin, 203
  see also elderly
alcohol, 309–13
  breastfeeding and, 18
  cancer and, 226
  content in beverages, 310
  heart disease and, 219, 310–11
  nutrition and, 311–12
  during pregnancy, 63–64
allergies, 249–51
  headaches and, 299
amenorrhea, 41–42
  among athletes, 197–98
American College of Obstetrics and Gynecology, 73
American Dietetic Association, 191
Ames, Bruce, 228
amino acid supplements, 262–63
amphetamines, 140–41
  anorexia nervosa and, 173

Anderson, James, 238
androgens, 16, 23
anemia, 26–27
  in alcoholics, 312
  iron-deficiency, *see* iron-deficiency anemia
  in IUD users, 45
  pernicious, 49, 61
  during pregnancy, 60–61
  sickle-cell, 321
anorexia nervosa, 145, 171–77
  dry skin and, 203
  osteoporosis and, 94–95
Anorexia and Bulimia Nervosa Association, 181
Anorexic Aid, 181
Anorexic Family Aid, National Information Centre, 181
antacids, 105
antiaging theories, 111–12
anticellulite therapy, 143
antioxidants, 112
anxiety, breastfeeding problems caused by, 79
appendicitis, 247
appetite, menstrual cycle and, 37–38
appetite suppressants, 20, 140–41
  anorexia nervosa and, 173
apricot-cottage cheese muffins, 346
Aristotle, 38
Arnaz, Desi, 54
arthritis, 106–07
arthritis care, 95
artificial sweeteners, 139–40
aspartame, 64, 139–40, 228
  in soft drinks, 291
aspirin:
  for arthritis, 106

Index

intestinal bleeding caused by, 47
atherosclerosis:
   cholesterol and, 212–13
   development of, 210–11
athletes, 182–98
   anorexia nervosa among, 172, 196–97
   body composition of, 194–96
   diet for, 189–94
   energy needs of, 182–86
   ergogenic aids for, 186–189
   menstrual cycle of, 42, 197–98
   precompetition liquid meal for, 190, 350
Atwood, Margaret, 153

BACUP, 198
balanced diet, 164–65
Balanchine, George, 172
Ball, Lucille, 54
banana bran muffins, 353–54
basal metabolic rate (BMR), 136–37
batch cooking, 302
bee pollen, 263
Bennett, William, 111
Benoit, Jean, 182
benzopyrene, 227
Beverly Hills diet, 181
bifidus factor, 76–77
bingeing, 131
   in adolescence, 31–32
   see also bulimia
bioflavonoids, 189
biotin, 332
birth control, 43–45
   see also oral contraceptives
birth defects, caffeine and, 289–90
birth weight, 56–58
bloating, premenstrual, 38–39
blood pressure readings, 214
body fat:
   in adolescence, 13–14, 16–20
   of athletes, 194–97
   body weight versus, 125–27
   in elderly, 104
   during pregnancy, 57, 71
   surgical removal of, 153
body image, 121–22
   acceptance of, 153–55
   in anorexia nervosa, 171–75
   changes in, after weight loss, 153–4

bonding, 79
bone disease, *see* osteoporosis
bone loss in athletes, 197–98
bonking, 183
bottlefeeding, 82
breakfast:
   tips for improving, 276
   for working women, 283–85
breastfeeding, 76–88
   benefits of, 76–77
   diet and, 83–85
   folacin during, 49
   health concerns in, 79–85
   physical changes during, 77–78
   psychological changes during, 78–79
   sample meal plan for, 86
   supplements during, 279
   by working women, 85, 87, 88
breast tenderness, premenstrual, 38
brewer's yeast, 263
British Diabetic Association, 200, 205
brown fat theory, 129
Bruch, Hilde, 138, 170, 173
Buchwald, Art, 141
Bulimia, 145, 175, 177–81
Burkitt, Denis, 230
buying food, 165, 262–72
   estimating nutrient needs and, 267–68
   in health food stores, 262–67
   labels and, 268–72
   at supermarkets, 267
   time-saving tips for, 300–01
B vitamins, 327–30
   stress and, 298
   see also specific vitamins

caesarean section, 75
caffeine, 285–90
   birth defects and, 289–90
   breast tenderness and, 38
   breastfeeding and, 82
   cancer and, 288–89
   content of beverages and foods, 287
   fibrocystic breast disease and, 289
   heart disease and, 219, 288
   during pregnancy, 64
calcium, 333
   in adolescence, 29

Index

for athletes, 198
breastfeeding and, 85
for elderly, 114
food sources of, 358–59
inadequate, 51
osteoporosis and, 95–96
during pregnancy, 66–67
supplements, 98
Caldwell, Sarah, 123–24
calories, 133, 136–38
for adolescents, 20–22
in alcoholic beverages, 310
amount needed, resting and activity, 136–38
for athletes, 183
in reducing diet, 137–38
cancer, 15, 64, 223–33
caffeine and, 288–89
development of, 223–24
diet and, 225–33
in elderly, 105–06
in middle-age, 100
obesity and, 124
quack cures for, 231–32
saccharin and, 139
treatment of, diet during, 232–33
in young adulthood, 50–51
Cann, Christopher, 197
carbohydrate loading, 186–87
carbohydrates, 318–20
in athlete's diet, 182–84
craving for, 37–38
in diabetic diet, 238–39
digestion of, 242–43
during pregnancy, 56–58
in weight-loss diet, 136
carcinogens, 223
natural, in foods, 228–29
cardiovascular disease, *see* heart disease; high blood pressure
carotene, 24, 28
aging and, 112
amenorrhea and, 42
as cancer fighter, 229
megadoses of, 281
Carpenter, Karen, 171
Castelli, William, 213, 274
cavities, 25–26
cellulite, 143
cellulose, 244
Center for Disease Control, 65

Center for Science in the Public Interest, 257–59
Chanel, Gabrielle, 202
charting exercise, 163
charting three meals a day, 161
chelation therapy, 201–02
chemotherapy, 232
Cherry, Donna Grace, 122
Chesler, Phyllis, 54
chicken Korma, 348–49
Child, Julia, 253
chloride, 333
cholesterol, 216–217
blood levels of, 212–13
in breast milk, 76
caffeine and, 288
cancer and, 225–26
in foods, 360
Christie, Agatha, 103–04
chromium, 114, 335
cigarette smoking, 294
breastfeeding and, 82
caffeine and, 286
heart disease and, 215
during pregnancy, 65
supplements and, 279
climacterium, 89
cobalamin, *see* vitamin B$_{12}$
coffee, 290
cancer and, 226
decaffeinated, 289
see also caffeine
Colette, 119
collagen, 203
colonic irrigation, 252
colostrum, 78
competitive weight, determining, 195
complex carbohydrates, 319–20
conditioners, 206
constipation, 104–05, 246–47
during pregnancy, 59
copper, 50, 335
Coronary Primary Prevention Trial, 211, 213
corpus luteum, 36
cosmetics, natural and organic, 204
Cowley, Malcolm, 103
cramps:
leg and back, during pregnancy, 60
menstrual, 39
Crapo, Phyllis, 238

Index

crash diets, 16–20
cruciferous vegetables, 231
cytotoxic testing, 250

dancers, anorexia nervosa among, 172
decaffeinated coffee, 289
deoxyribonucleic acid (DNA), 321
depression:
  in adolescence, 21–22
  in elderly 114
  menstrual, 39
diabetes, 33, 234–41
  artificial sweeteners and, 139
  damage caused by, 235–36
  diet and, 238–39
  in elderly, 105
  exercise and, 239
  gestational, 62–63
  heart disease and, 215
  menstrual cycle and, 36
  obesity and, 124
  oral contraceptives and, 45
  risk factors for, 237–38
  symptoms of, 236
Dickinson, Emily, 209
diet:
  acne and, 24–26
  in adolescence, 30–33
  for athletes, 189–94
  breastfeeding and, 83–85
  cancer and, 225–33
  cavities and, 25–26
  diabetes and, 238–39
  for elderly, 113–16
  guidelines for improving, 272–78
  hair and, 199–201
  headaches and, 299
  iron in, 26–27, 47–48
  menopause and, 100–01
  oral contraceptives and, 43–45
  osteoporosis and, 51, 96–98
  during pregnancy, 67–68, 69
  premenstrual syndrome and, 40
  skin and, 202–06
  stress and, 297–99
  vegetarian, see vegetarianism
  weight-loss, see weight-loss diet
  Western diet, 219–22
  in young adulthood, 51–53
digestion, process of, 242–43
dinner, tips for improving, 277–78

disaccharides, 319
diuretics, 39
  bulimia and, 179
  for high blood pressure, 214
  for weight loss, 140–41
diverticulitis, 247
drugs:
  appetite controlling, 20, 140–41, 173
  breastfeeding and, 82
  elderly and, 108–09
  during pregnancy, 65
dysmenorrhea, 40–41

eating disorders, 19–20, 170–81
  amenorrhea and, 42
  among athletes, 196–97
  see also anorexia nervosa
eating habits:
  adolescent, 30–33
  of elderly, 114–15
  investigating, 157, 159–60
  in middle age, 100–01
  in young adulthood, 51–53
eating out, see restaurants
eclampsia, 61–62
edema, 61–62
eicosapentaenoic acid (EPA), 217
elastin, 203
elderly, 102–17
  eating strategy for, 113–16
  extending life of, 113
  health concerns of, 103–09
  living alone, 109
  physical and psychological changes in, 102–03
  on tight budget, 109–10
electrolytes, 323
Eliot, T. S., 116
emotions, obesity and, 130
endorphins, 147
enemas, 252
enriched products, 271
epidermis, 202
epinephrine, 309
ergogenic aids, 186
estrogen:
  appetite and, 37–38
  cancer and, 225
  heart disease and, 50–51
  hormone replacement therapy, 95–96

Index

menarche and, 15
menopause and, 89–90
menstrual cycle and, 35–36
in oral contraceptives, 43
estrone, 89–90
exercise:
in adolescence, 17
anorexia nervosa and, 172
calorie needs and, 137
on coffee breaks, 285
diabetes and, 239
for elderly, 102–03
lack of, heart disease and, 215
osteoporosis and, 98–99
pregnancy and, 71–72
skin and, 204, 206
weight-loss and, 145, 152–53
what to drink before, during, and after, 193
external cues, obesity and, 130

fad diets, 141–45
dry skin and, 203
side effects of, 144–45
Farnsworth, Alice, 244
fast foods, 31–32
fasting, 20, 143
supplemented, 143
fasting hypoglycemia, 239–40
fat-cell theory, 128
fatigue:
breastfeeding and, 79–80
nutritional factors in, 282
fats, 320–21
in athlete's diet, 184
blood levels of, 215–16
in breast milk, 76–77
cancer and, 225–26
comparison of, in diets, 220–21
in diabetic diet, 238–39
digestion of, 242–43
heart disease and, 216–18
fetal alcohol syndrome, 63–64
fiber, 105
as cancer fighter, 230–31
in diabetic diet, 238–39
food sources of, 360–62
gastrointestinal disorders and, 246–51
heart disease and, 219
in weight-loss diet, 139
fibrocystic breast disease, 289

fitness, see shape-up plan
fluoride, 336
osteoporosis and, 98
during pregnancy, 67
folacin, 49–50, 331
food sources of, 357–58
megadoses of, 281
oral contraceptives and, 43
during pregnancy, 60–61, 66, 68
food additives, see additives
food allergies, see allergies
food cravings:
during pregnancy, 59–60
premenstrual, 37–38
food exchange, 341–44
food and exercise diaries, 158
food groups, basic four, 257–58
fortified foods, 271–72
Framingham study, 211, 213
free radicals, 112
Frisch, Rose, 14
fructose, 307
fruitarian diet, 261

gallbladder disease, 124
gas, 248–49
gastrointestinal disorders, 242–52
and anatomy of gut (tract), 242–43
fiber and, 244–48
of elderly, 104–105
Gerovital H-3, 112
gestational diabetes, 62–63
gingerbread squares, 347
glucagon, 239
glycemic index, 238
glycogen, 182–83, 186
Godwin, Gail, 91
goiter, congenital, 64
Goodman, Ellen, 11, 123
Grace, Princess of Monaco, 88
growth spurt, 13–18, 29
gums, 244–45

hair, 199–202
headaches, 299
health foods, 262–64
heart disease, 15, 33, 209–22
alcohol and, 219, 310–11
caffeine and, 219, 288
diet and, 216–22
in elderly, 105–106
in middle age, 100

Index

obesity and, 215
research on, 211–12
risk factors for, 211–16
in young adulthood, 50–51
height-weight tablets, 125
hematocrit, 47
hemicellulose, 244–45
hemochromatosis, 49
hemoglobin, 45–47, 71
of athletes, 188
hemorrhoids, 247–48
herb blends, 349
herbal remedies, 265–66
high blood pressure, 33, 213–14
alcohol and, 311
in middle age, 100
obesity and, 102
high-density lipoproteins (HDLs), 212–13
Hippocrates, 58
hitting the wall, 183
hormonal imbalances:
among athletes, 197
obesity caused by, 129–30
hormone-replacement, therapy, 95–96
Hosmer, Trina, 68
hot flashes, 90
Howard Allen, 142
hypertension, *see* high blood pressure
hypoglycemia, 239–40
hypothermia, 104

identity crisis, adolescent, 15
indigestion, 104–05, 248
during pregnancy, 58–59
infections:
breast, 81
vitamin A and resistance to, 24
infertility, 42
among athletes, 197
ingredients, list of, 269–70
insulin, 234–35
intrauterine device (IUD), 42
breastfeeding and, 83
iodine, 336
acne and, 25
during pregnancy, 65
iron, 336
food sources of, 355–56
iron-deficiency anemia, 26–27
after abortion or miscarriage, 72

antacids and, 105
in athletes, 188
in IUD users, 45
during pregnancy, 60–61, 72
in young adulthood, 45–49
iron overload, 49
iron supplements, 48–49
for athletes, 188–89
breastfeeding and, 85
for elderly, 105
during pregnancy, 68
Irvin, Juno, 68

Jessop, Carol, 41

Kaye, Elizabeth, 173
Kerr, Jean, 57
keratin, 202
ketosis, 142

La Leche League of Great Britain, 88
labels, food, 268–72
lacto-ovovegetarian diet, 256
lactose, intolerance, 251
laetrile, 231
laxatives, 251–52
bulimia and, 179
lentil soup, 351
let-down reflex, 78, 81
poor, 80
life span, 111
Lifshitz, Fima, 19
lignin, 244, 245
Linn, Robert, 142
linoleic acid, 76, 184, 320
lipids, *see* fats
lipoproteins, 21
liquid protein diets, 142
Longworth, Alice Roosevelt, 34
low birth weight babies, 56, 57, 73
low-carbohydrate diets, 141–42
low-density lipoproteins (LDLs), 212
caffeine and, 288
lunch:
tips for improving, 272–78
for working women, 294–97

McCullers, Carson, 18
MacMahon, Dr, 288
macrobiotic diet, 74, 261
macrominerals, 323, 333–35
magnesium, 333

Index

premenstrual syndrome and, 39, 40
Maisner Centre, 181
manganese, 336
marijuana, breastfeeding and, 82–83
Marsh Annabel, 89
Marshall, Paule, 131
Mauriceau, 58
Mazel, Judy, 181
Meals on Wheels, 109
meconium, 78
megadosing:
   by alcoholics, 312
   by athletes, 187–88
   breastfeeding and, 85
   during pregnancy, 65
Memorial Sloan-Kettering Cancer Center, 231
menarche, 14–15, 19, 27
menopause, 89–101
   eating strategy for, 100–01
   health concerns in, 91–100
   physical changes in, 89–90
   psychological changes in, 91
   supplements after, 279
   surgical, 90
   weight control and, 99–100
menorrhagia, 46
menstrual cycle and menstruation, 35–36
   in adolescence, 14–15
   alcohol and, 311
   anemia and, 26–27, 45–49
   anorexia nervosa and, 173–74
   among athletes, 197–98
   bulimia and, 179
   disorders of, 37–42
Merrill, Caroline, 89
Metropolitan Life Insurance Company, 125
Mexican casserole, 352–53
middle adulthood, *see* menopause
minerals, 323–24, 333–37
   see also specific minerals
Minton, John, 289
miscarriage, 72
Moertel, C. G., 231
molybdenum, 337
monoamine oxidase inhibitors, 109
monosaccharides, 318
monosodium glutimate (MSG), 315
monounsaturated fats, 217

Morgagni, Giovanni, 209
morning sickness, 58
Morrison, Toni, 76
Moses, Grandma, 103
Muske, Carol, 199
mutagens, 223, 227, 228

Nachman, Gerald, 52
nails, 206
National Cancer Institute of America, 231
natural foods, 271–72
niacin, 328
   for athletes, 187
night blindness, 28
night-eating syndrome, 131
nitrosamines, 227–28
norepinephrine, 239
NutraSweet, *see* aspartame
nutrition information:
   on food labels, 270–71
   sources of, 338–40
nutritional therapies:
   for osteoporosis, 96–98
   for premenstrual syndrome, 40
Nyad, Diana, 182

obesity:
   in adolescence, 16–20, 30–31
   alcohol and, 311–12
   amenorrhea and, 42
   cancer and, 225
   causes of, 128–32
   cultural attitudes toward, 123–24
   diabetes and, 237–38
   determination of, 125–27
   heart disease and, 215
   medically supervised diets for, 153
   menopause and, 90, 99
   menstrual cycle and, 37–38
   osteoporosis and, 99–100
   physical and psychological problems of, 123–25
oligomenorrhea, 42
Oliver, Dean, 245–46
oral contraceptives, 43–45
   breastfeeding and, 83
   depression and, 39
   supplements and, 279
organic foods, 264–65
osteoarthritis, 106–07
   obesity and, 124

Index

osteopenia, 107
osteoporosis, 15, 29, 92–99
  athlete's risk of, 198
  beginnings of, 92–93
  risk factors for, 93–95
  treatment of, 95–99
  young adulthood and, 51
Overeaters Anonymous, 156
ovulation, 36
oxytocin, 77

pangamic acid, 188
pantothenic acid, 331
parties, eating at, 167
pastas, health-food, 264
Pearson, Durk, 111
pectins, 244–45
penicilamine, 107
periodontal disease, 107–108
pernicious anemia, 49
  during pregnancy, 60–61
pesticides, breastfeeding and, 83
phenylketonuria, 140
phenylpropanolamine (PPA), 141
phosphorous, 334
pica, 60
placebo effect, 340
placenta, 55, 66
plaque, 210
pollen, 263
polyunsaturated fats, 217, 320
  cancer and, 225–26
Porter, Katherine Anne, 282
postpartum period, 71
potassium, 334
precompetition liquid meal, 190, 350
preeclampsia, 61–62
pregnancy, 54–75
  after age thirty-five, 72–73
  checklist for, 72
  complications of, 75
  eating strategy in, 65–72
  folacin during, 49
  health concerns of, 56–65
  physical changes in, 54–55
  psychological changes in, 55–56
  sample meal plan for, 69
  supplements during, 279
  teenage, 73
  terminated, 72
  after use of oral contraceptives, 44
  vegetarianism and, 74
  vitamin A during, 24
  zinc during, 29
premenstrual syndrome (PMS), 37–40
preparation of food, 165, 271–72
  cancer and methods of, 226–27
  time-saving tips for, 300–01
Pritikin, Nathan, 218–19
product descriptions, 271–72
progesterone, 37
  appetite and, 37–38
  menopause and, 89
  in oral contraceptives, 43
  during pregnancy, 58–59
prolactin, 77, 79
prostaglandins, 41
proteins, 321–22
  in athlete's diet, 184–86
  in breast milk, 76
  cancer and, 226
  combinations of, 260–61
  digestion of, 242–43
  during pregnancy, 66, 74
  in vegetarian diet, 257–61
  in weight-loss diet, 136
Pym, Barbara, 114
pyramid guide, 275
pyridoxine, 39, 329
  breastfeeding and, 85
  morning sickness relieved by, 58
  oral contraceptives and, 43
  during pregnancy, 65, 67

reactive hypoglycemia, 240
reactive obesity, 21
Recommended Daily Amounts (ROA) 267–69
restaurants, 167, 313–17
  food additives used in, 315, 317
  terms used in, 314
  tips for ordering in, 316–17
Retin-A, 24
retinoic acid, 24
Retton, Mary Lou, 197
rheumatoid arthritis, 106–07
riboflavin, 328
  for athletes, 187
ribonucleic acid (RNA), 321

saccharin, 139, 228
  during pregnancy, 64
safrole, 228

Index

Saline, Carol, 89
saturated fats, 216–18
Sclafani, Anthony, 131
Scott-Maxwell, Florida, 103
Searle Pharmaceutical Company, 140
sebum, 23
selenium, 112, 337
    as cancer fighter, 230
senility, 109
serotonin, 38, 142
setpoint theory, 128–29
Shakespeare, William, 55, 59, 306
shampoos, 200
shape-up plan, 157–70
    balanced diet in, 164–65
    eating habits and, 157–60
    exercise in, 162–64
    reaching goals of, 165–69
    three meals a day in, 160–62
Shaw, Sandy, 111
Shultz, Susan, 181
sickle-cell anemia, 321
single-food diets, 143
skin, 202–06
    effects of nutrition on, 205
snacking, 160–61
    in adolescence, 30–32
    on health foods, 263
    at work, 293–94
sodium, 214, 218–19, 334
soft drinks, 290–92
    caffeine content of, 287
sorbitol, 307
spirulina, 263–64
    London Sports Medicine Institute, 198
Springer, Deleri, 131
Stacy, Hollis, 182
starch blockers, 141
Steinem, Gloria, 35
Stevenson, Alice, 111
stir-fry sauce, 350
storage of food, 165, 271–72
    time saving and, 300–05
Stowe, Harriet Beecher, 121
stress, 297–99
    acne and, 23
    adolescent obesity and, 21
    allergies and, 249
    bingeing and, 131
    body's response to, 297
    diet and, 297–99
    hair and, 200–01
    heart disease and, 216
    hypoglycemia and, 239
    skin and, 204, 206
    smoking and, 294
    supplements and, 279
stroke, 209
sucrose, 307
suction lipectomy, 143
sugar, 306–09
suicide, eating disorders and, 174, 179
sulfiting agents, 315, 317
sulfur, 335
supermarkets, 267
superoxide dismutase (SOD), 112
supplements, 278–81
    for athletes, 187–89
    breastfeeding and, 85
    choosing, 279–80
    during pregnancy, 68
    see also megadosing
Swanson, Gloria, 204
sweets, 306–09

Taylor, Elizabeth, 122
tea, 290
teenagers, *see* adolescence
Thayer, Robert, 285
thiamin, 327
Thomas, Fannie, 111
thyroid hormone, 129–30
tocopherol, *see* vitamin E
tofu, 262
toxemia of pregnancy, 61–62, 73
trace minerals, 323, 335–37
traveling, 305
tretinoin, 24
triglycerides, 215–16
tryptophan, 38
Tucker, Sophie, 102
Twain, Mark, 157, 242
twins, 57

underweight women, 155–56
uterus, pregnant, 54–55, 59

Van Horne, Harriet, 255
vegans, 256, 261
vegetarianism, 256, 261–62
    in adolescence, 29, 33

Index

breastfeeding and, 85
pregnancy and, 74
vitamin A, 323, 325
  acne and, 74
  in adolescence, 28–29
  breastfeeding and, 85
  for elderly, 114
  food sources of, 355
  megadoses of, 280–81
  during pregnancy, 65, 67
  premenstrual syndrome and, 42
  stress and, 298
vitamin B_1, 328
vitamin B_2 see riboflavin
vitamin B_3, see niacin
vitamin B_6, see pyridoxine
vitamin B_{12}, 330
  for athletes, 187
  breastfeeding and, 85
  deficiency of, 50
  for elderly, 105
  during pregnancy, 60, 61, 66
  vegetarian diet and, 256, 261
vitamin C, 332
  aging and, 112
  for athletes, 187
  as cancer fighter, 229–30
  for elderly, 112
  food sources of, 357
  megadoses of, 280–81
  nitrosamines and, 227–28
  during pregnancy, 65, 67, 70
  stress and 298
vitamins D, 323, 326
  osteoporosis and, 98
  during pregnancy, 66
vitamin E, 326
  acne and, 24
  aging and, 112
  for athletes, 187–88
  as cancer fighter, 230
  for elderly, 112, 114
  megadoses of, 280–81
  menopause and, 90
vitamin K, 327
vitamins, 322–23, 326–32
  food preparation and storage to protect, 271–72
  see also specific vitamins

vomiting in bulimia, 177–79

Walford, Roy, 111
water, 292–93, 322
  athlete's need for, 190–94
Weaver, Eula, 102
Webster, John, 59
Wernicke-Korsakoff syndrome, 312
weight control, treatment for, 134–35
weight gain during pregnancy, 56–58
weight-loss diet, 133–45
  in adolescence, 20–22
  aritificial sweeteners and, 139–40
  breastfeeding and, 83–84
  diuretics and diet pills and, 140–41
  exercise and, 151
  fad, 141–45
  guidelines for, 151–53
  medically supervised, 153
  planning of, 132–39
  during pregnancy, 57
Weight Watchers, 148, 156
wheat germ, 263
Woodhead, Cynthia, 182
working women, 282–05
  breakfast for, 282–85
  coffee breaks for, 285–88
  headaches of, 299
  lunch for, 294–97
  stress and, 297–99
  time-saving tips for, 300–05
  traveling by, 305
Wurtman, Judith, 38

yogurt-herb dressing, 347–48
young adulthood, 34–53
  eating strategy for, 51–53
  health concerns of, 35–51
  obesity in, 50
  physical changes in, 34–35
  psychological changes in, 35
  supplements in, 279
Yudkin, John, 308

Zen macrobiotic diet, 74, 261
zinc, 50, 337
  acne and, 25
  in adolescence, 19